Concise English–Chinese Vocabulary Handbook of Traditional Chinese Medicine

简明英汉
中医词汇手册

Chief Reviewers 主审

Chen Lixin　陈立新　　Song Ping　宋坪

Chief Editors 主编

Fang Jiliang　方继良　　Cui Yongqiang　崔永强

U0382967

SPM 南方出版传媒
广东科技出版社 | 全国优秀出版社
·广 州·

图书在版编目（CIP）数据

简明英汉中医词汇手册 / 方继良，崔永强主编. —广州：广东科技出版社，2022.1
ISBN 978-7-5359-7766-3

Ⅰ．①简…　Ⅱ．①方…　②崔…　Ⅲ．①中医学—词典—英、汉—手册　Ⅳ．①R2-62

中国版本图书馆CIP数据核字（2021）第216162号

简明英汉中医词汇手册
Jianming Yinghan Zhongyi Cihui Shouce

出　版　人：严奉强
责任编辑：李　芹
封面设计：林少娟
责任校对：陈　静　李云柯
责任印制：彭海波
出版发行：广东科技出版社
　　　　　（广州市环市东路水荫路11号　邮政编码：510075）
销售热线：020-37607413
http://www.gdstp.com.cn
E-mail: gdkjbw@nfcb.com.cn
经　　销：广东新华发行集团股份有限公司
印　　刷：佛山市浩文彩色印刷有限公司
　　　　　（佛山市南海狮山科技工业园A区　邮政编码：528225）
规　　格：889 mm×1 194mm　1/48　印张9.875　字数200千
版　　次：2022年1月第1版
　　　　　2022年1月第1次印刷
定　　价：48.00元

如发现因印装质量问题影响阅读，请与广东科技出版社印制室联系调换（电话：020-37607272）。

Acknowledgments

致　　谢

Our gratitude specially goes to Li Peilu for her contribution in parts of the compiling work.

感谢李沛璐参与部分编书工作。

Introduction of Chief Editors
主编简介

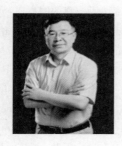

Fang Jiliang, Chief Physician, Professor, M.D., Ph.D.. Ph.D. supervisor and postdoctoral co-supervisor, Chief Researcher of China Academy of Chinese Medical Sciences (CACMS) and Deputy Director of Department of Radiology/Director of the Functional Imaging Research Lab at Guang An Men Hospital . Prof. Fang was a visiting scholar at Universität zu Köln, Germany from 2001–2002. In 2009, he finished his 4 years' postdoctor and research fellow training program (2005–2009) in the Athinoula A. Martinos Center for Biomedical Imaging at Massachusetts General Hospital in Harvard University, USA.

方继良，主任医师，教授，医学博士，博士生导师和博士后联合导师，担任中国中医科学院首席研究员和广安门医院放射科副主任/功能影像研究室主任。2001-2002年，方教授曾在德国科隆大学做访问学者。2009年，他在美国哈佛大学马萨诸塞州总医院Athinoula A. Martinos生物医学成像中心完成了为期四年的博士后和研究员培训项目（2005-2009）。

Prof. Fang has compiled several professional books, such as *Concise Chinese-English Vocabulary Handbook of Traditional Chinese Medicine* (chief editor), *Medical Imaging for Acupuncture* (chief editor), and was co-editor in 8 professional books on medical imaging, auricular needle and systematic acupuncture.

方教授编著了多部专业书籍，如《简明中医汉英词汇手册》（主编）、《针灸医学影像学》（主编），并参与了医学影像学、耳针和系统针灸等8部专业书籍的编写。

Prof. Fang, as a part-time medical English teacher at the Graduate School of CACMS, has been responsible for teaching medical English course for post-graduate students since 2010, which makes him rich in teaching English experience. In many years of teaching, clinical practice and scientific research, he deeply feel the necessity of publishing an English-Chinese glossary of Traditional Chinese medicine in line with international standards and in a modern style.

方教授是中国中医科学院研究生院的兼职医学英语教师，自2010年起负责研究生医学英语课程的教学，具有丰富的英语教学经验。在多年的教学、临床实践和科研工作中，他深深感受到出版一本与国际接轨、具有现代风格的中医药英汉词汇的必要性。

Prof. Fang is an expert in the integrated medicine, and as a pioneer has been engaged in the study of neuromechanism of acupuncture by using brain functional magnetic resonance imaging (fMRI) for 20 years. As a Project Investigator, he has completed 12 projects funded by the Ministry of Science and Technology, the National Natural Foundation of China, the United States National Institutes of Health and others. He published over 45 articles in peer-reviewed international SCI journals and more than 50 articles in domestic journals. He has been honored with

11 provincial-level awards for his scientific work, such as the first prize in science and technology from Chinese Association of Traditional Chinese Medicine, the second prize from Beijing Municipal Science & Technology Award.

方教授是中西医结合领域的专家，20多年来利用脑功能磁共振成像（fMRI）研究针刺神经机制。作为项目研究者，他完成了科技部、国家自然科学基金及美国国立卫生研究院等资助的12个项目。在国际SCI期刊上发表论文45余篇，在国内期刊上发表论文50余篇。他的科研成果获得了中华中医药学会科学技术一等奖、北京市科学技术二等奖等11项省部级奖项。

Prof. Fang is academically appointed as: Chairman of the Expert's Committee of Medical Imaging, China Association of Acupuncture-Moxibustion, Vice Chairman of Medical Imaging Branch, China Society of Integrated Traditional Chinese and Western Medicine. He is also the corresponding reviewer on the grant of National Natural Science Foundation, Beijing Municipal Natural Science Foundation, the Health and Medical Research Fund under the Government of the Hong Kong Special Administrative Region (HKSAR) and international and national professional journals.

方教授现为中国针灸学会针灸医学影像专业委员会主任委员、中国中西医结合学会影像专委会副主任委员。他也是国家自然科学基金、北京市自然科学基金及香港特别行政区政府卫生与医学研究基金项目及多本国际、国内期刊的通讯评委。

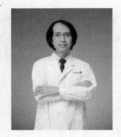

Cui Yongqiang, served as a World Health Organization (WHO) consultant on traditional medicine programs, is a medical professor and practicing acupuncturist at Guang An Men Hospital of China Academy of Chinese Medical Sciences. He is the director of Beijing Guidance and Evaluation Center for International Services of TCM and Beijing Research Center for International Traditional Chinese Medicine (TCM) Tourism, as well as the deputy editor-in-chief of Journal of Integrative Nursing.

崔永强，世界卫生组织（WHO）传统医学项目顾问，医学教授，中国中医科学院广安门医院针灸师。他现任北京市中医药国际服务指导评价中心主任、北京市中医药国际旅游研究中心主任，《中西医结合护理》杂志副主编。

Prof. Cui has more than 20 years of front-line experience in international exchange of TCM and integrated TCM and Western medicine, and has had direct dialogues with a number of foreign heads of state, including 130 foreign health ministers on the development of TCM, integrated TCM and Western medicine, public health, and internationalization of TCM. More than 10 years ago, he took the lead in achieving the accreditations of TCM by two fortune 500 insurance companies in the United States and Britain.

崔教授拥有超过20年的一线中医药国际交流和中西医结合经验，直接对话一些外国元首，包括130名外国卫生部长，对中医的发展、中西医结合、公共卫生、中医药国际化的见解。十多年前，他率先获得了美国和英国两家财富500强保险公司对中医的认证。

He has special interest in running short-term courses on TCM for American doctors and nurses, medical students from Harvard, John Hopkins, Cornell, Ohio State University, Bristol Medical School, etc and nurse students from the U.S, Germany and Sweden through continuing medical education (CME) and continuing nursing education (CNE). Over the past decade, Dr. Cui has been focusing on sharing China's experience in integrating TCM into its national health system with its neighboring ASEAN countries, League of Arab States (LAS) and African nations through a series of well-designed seminars and field study programs for senior health officials under the auspices of National Health Commission of PRC and regional organizations.

他对为美国的医生和护士、哈佛大学、约翰霍普金斯大学、康奈尔大学、俄亥俄州立大学、布里斯托尔医学院等医学院的学生，以及美国、德国和瑞典的护士学生开设中医短期课程特别感兴趣，这些学生通过继续医学教育（CME）和继续护理教育（CNE）来学习中医。在过去的十年里，他一直致力于与东盟邻国分享中国将中医药融入国家卫生体系的经验，在中华人民共和国国家卫生健康委员会和区域组织的主持下，通过一系列为高级卫生官员设计的研讨会和实地考察项目，向阿拉伯国家联盟和非洲国家提供培训。

Prof. Cui is the founder for TCM LED Talk, a weekly talk program onsite and online-Let's Explore and Discover

（LED）TCM which has been run for 8 years for the International community in Beijing in an attempt to raise public awareness of TCM. He is in charge of China's first TCM package program for international medical tourists, Beijing Annual International TCM Nursing Seminar and Field Study to share "culturally appropriate, scientifically sound, technically safe practice" of TCM nursing, and the world's first TCM English-Speaking Helpline which is the only free government-approved service of its kind, providing quality, authentic TCM and health information for the general public.

崔教授是"中医LED讲座"的创始人，"让我们探索和发现中医"是一个每周线上和线下的谈话节目，已经在北京国际社区运营了8年，旨在提高公众对中医的认识。他负责中国首个面向国际医疗游客的中医服务包项目，北京年度国际中医护理研讨会和实地考察，分享"文化兼容、科学合理、技术安全"的中医护理实践，以及世界上第一条也是唯一经政府批准的为公众提供优质、真实的中医药和健康信息的中医药英语咨询免费服务热线。

He is the founder for TCM Mind-Body Qi Meditation theory based on stress as a trigger. With a decade of study of TCM for stress reduction, he literally coined the terms Qi meditation for stress reduction or Qi focus for stress relief, which means "qi nian jian ya" in Chinese, and stress as a trigger of diseases or "ya li shi fa wu". He convincingly interprets the concepts and value of Qi and meridians appearing in the latest compendium of WHO, ICD-11. His English-Chinese bilingual courses for stress reduction are widely recognized among local medical workers.

他是中医"心身气冥想"理论的创始人，该理论认为压力是发物。 在对中医减压研究了十年之后，他创造了"气冥想"这个词来减压，或者"气关注"来减压，中文意思是"气念减压"，压力是疾病的诱因，或者"压力是发物"。 他令人信服地解释了世界卫生组织最新汇编ICD-11中出现的气和经络的概念和价值。 他的中英双语减压课程得到当地医务工作者的广泛认可。

Prof. Cui is the co-author of two bestselling medical monographs in English for almost three decades, which are *TESTS Chinese Acupuncture and Moxibustion*（ISBN 7-119-01587-7）and *Handbook to Chinese Auricular Therapy*（ISBN 7-119-01224-X）.

崔教授是畅销国外近30年的两部英文医学专著的合著者，分别是《中国针灸试验》（ISBN 7- 119-01587-7）和《中国耳穴治疗手册》（ISBN 7- 119-01224-X）。

Preface
前　　言

In 2019, the World Health Organization (WHO) released *the 11th revision of the International Classification of Diseases* (ICD-11) with a supplementary chapter on traditional medicine originated from Traditional Chinese Medicine (TCM) for the first time. It has laid a foundation for countries around the world to know, understand and use TCM. TCM has shown its unique value worldwide, and has been widely recognized and concerned by the international community. In the global fight against COVID-19 in 2020, TCM also has played a great role in the prevention, treatment and rehabilitation, and has won wide acclaim at home and abroad.

2019年，世界卫生组织（WHO）首次将中医药传统医学纳入新制定的《国际疾病分类第十一次修订本（ICD-11）》，为世界各国认识中医药、了解中医药、使用中医药奠定了基础。中医药显示了其在世界范围内的独特价值，越来越受到国际社会的广泛认可和关注。2020年，在抗击新型冠状病毒肺炎的全球性战役中，中医药在预防、治疗和康复方面更是发挥了巨大的作用，获得国内外的广泛赞誉。

To make TCM go global and promote TCM in countries and regions along the "Belt and Road", improve TCM international service and promote the exchange among medical staffs and patients at home and abroad, based on the work of Concise *Chinese-English Vocabulary Handbook of Traditional Chinese Medicine* in 2019, this year, a team of experts with rich experience in TCM international exchange and cooperation has been gathered for compiling its companion book—*Concise English—Chinese Vocabulary Handbook of Traditional Chinese Medicine* by careful study on the TCM terms' translation and international standardization system. The handbook introduces the most common TCM terms and expressions in international language and discourse system, and facilitates readers to learn TCM with much convenience.

为推进中医药国际化进程，推动中医药在"一带一路"沿线国家和地区的发展，更好地服务于国内外医生和患者交流，提升中医药国际化服务水平，继2019年《简明汉英中医词汇手册》出版后，今年我们又组建了具有丰富的中医药对外交流和合作经验的编写专家团队，认真研究和总结中医药术语英译和国际标准化体系，编写了姊妹篇《简明英汉中医词汇手册》，用国际通用的语言以及话语体系向读者介绍最常见的中医药知识和词汇，具有较强的实用性，利于广大读者学习掌握。

The handbook is co-edited by two teams of chief editors, Prof. Fang Jiliang and Prof. Cui Yongqiang. Prof. Fang Jiliang is the lead researcher for the integrated medicine in China Academy of Chinese Medical Sciences (CACMS) and chairman of Medical Imaging for Acupuncture Committee of China Association of Acupuncture-

Moxibustion, and Prof. Cui Yongqiang is the director of the International Cooperation Office of Guang An Men Hospital of the CACMS. It contains about 5,000 terms of TCM basic theories and clinical disciplines. Besides the common TCM terms, it also includes appendixes on the supplementary traditional medicine chapter of WHO ICD-11. All terms are originated from the standard TCM terms reviewed and published by the China National Committee for Terms in Sciences and Technologies and other authoritative TCM dictionaries, each term attached with standard Chinese translation and Pinyin spelling. The handbook is not only an essential tool for medical staffs, scientific researchers, college students, graduates and translators in the field of TCM and integrative medicine at home and abroad, but also a reference for a large number of Chinese and foreigners who love and learn TCM and Chinese culture, or seek TCM medical help.

《简明英汉中医词汇手册》由中国中医科学院首席研究员、中国针灸学会针灸医学影像专业委员会主任委员方继良教授和中国中医科学院广安门医院国际合作办公室主任崔永强教授共同主编。本书收录中医基本理论及临床各科词目约5000条，除收录中医药常见的名词术语外，还兼收录ICD-11传统医学补充章节中的病证诊断术语，方便读者对照查阅。本书区别于其他同类书籍的是所有词条均来源于全国科学技术名词审定委员会审定公布的中医药学类名词以及权威词典，为读者提供了科学、规范的中译文及拼音参考。本书不仅是一本可供国内外广大中医药、中西医结合医务人员及科研人员、大学生、研究生和中医学翻译人员参阅的工具书,还是一本可供大批热爱中医药和中华文化的海外人士在求医问药时学习参考的工具书。

ICD-11 includes TCM and sets a standard for TCM globally, which is of great practical and far-reaching historical significance. Echoing to the world's recognition of TCM, the handbook elaborates the profound TCM culture between the lines, the unique appeal of Chinese culture, and in a global perspective, tells TCM story of "Chinese characteristics, Chinese style", thus to promote the wide spread of TCM culture around the world. In the future, the digital network and intelligent technology will be applied for the handbook, and the TCM knowledge and information would attract more readers all over the world to dive into the TCM treasure house and truly enjoy the essence of TCM.

ICD-11纳入中医药,具有非常重要的现实意义和极为深远的历史意义,也为中医药树立了国际通用名词术语标准。本书作为世界对中医药认可的回礼,力争在翻译的字里行间展示中医药文化的博大精深、中华文化的独特魅力,推动中医药文化在世界范围内更广泛地传播和产生影响,助推在全球视角下讲好"中国特色、中国风格"的中医故事。未来,数字化、智能化技术还会被应用于本书,真正为国内外读者在中医药宝库里畅享漫游、发掘精华提供便利。

Instructions
说　　明

1. Each term lists in a sequence of English expression, phonetic transcription, and Chinese expression, Chinese Pinyin spelling. ";" is used to separate two or more Chinese expressions.

一、每个词汇按英文、音标、中文、拼音排列。有两个及两个以上释义时，用"；"隔开。

2. All terms are originated from TCM terms reviewed and published by the China National Committee for Terms in Sciences and Technologies and some authoritative dictionaries.

二、所有词条均来源于全国科学技术名词审定委员会审定公布的中医药学类名词及权威词典。

3. All English entries and phonetic transcriptions come from the Collins dictionary's official website, https://www.collinsdictionary.com/zh/. American phonetic transcriptions are used in this book. Example: Water in Chinese Pinyin spelling is shuǐ, according to the China National Committee for Terms in Sciences and Technologies. And water in American phonetic transcription is / wɔtər / with reference to the Collins dictionary's official website.When it is not

possible to find the entire English entry based on Chinese Pinyin spelling, the initials and finals of Chinese Pinyin spelling need to be transformed respectively. The standards for transformation confirms with *the Comparison table of Chinese Pinyin spelling and International Phonetic Symbols* (IPS) and *the Comparison of the latest IPS and British as well as Phonetic transcriptions*. When the phonetic transcriptions cannot be founded in the Collins dictionary's official website, it need to take any further actions as follows: Chinses expression "术", zhú / dʒu /, ch in IPS is t͡ʂʰ, which is not included in American phonetic transcriptions. eng/ rŋ/ in IPS is another typical example, it is needed to replace its American phonetic transcription with eng in surname Deng.

三、所有英文词条、音标均来自科林斯词典官网，网址https://www.collinsdictionary.com/zh/。音标统一为美音音标。来源示例如下：①根据中国规范术语网的拼音shuǐ，可在科林斯词典查询到美音音标结果/ wɔtər/。②当无法根据拼音查找整个英文词条的音标时，需要对拼音的声母或者韵母进行各自音标的分别替换，替换规则来源于《汉语拼音与国际音标对照表》，而后进行美式音标的转换，规则根据《最新国际音标与英式美式音标对比》。③当情况②中需要把声母、韵母分别对照转换，但无法在英汉词典中找到相对应的音标的时候，则用含有相同的拼音的词查找确定，例如，ch对应的音标为ts^h（根据《汉语拼音与国际音标对照表》），但美音音标体系中无ts^h，则通过科林斯词典官网查找词条，进一步确定ch的音标为ʧ。④其他较为典型的例子包括：eng的音标对应/ɤŋ/（根据《汉语拼音与国际音标对照表》），但在美音词典无法找到对应音标，则根据邓姓的姓氏拼音deng中的eng来替换。

Regarding the issue of long vowel and short vowel i, because there are no vowel i in the American phonetic transcription, we unified the long vowel i as i and the short vowel i as ɪ after spending long time studying.

关于长元音、短元音的i的问题，由于美音的音标无长元音i，根据最后资料查阅，将长元音i统一为i，将短元音i统一为ɪ。

4. The Pinyin writing rules of this book are based on the basic rules of Chinese Pinyin Orthography（GB），"in terms of Chinese information processing, the polysyllabic structure representing an overall concept can be written all together". Considering the particularity of traditional Chinese medicine, its vocabulary is a polysyllabic word with the overall concept, so pinyin is all connected.

四、本书的拼音书写规则根据《汉语拼音正词法基本规则（GB）》中的"在中文信息处理方面，表示一个整体概念的多音节结构，可全部连写"。由于中医学的特殊性，其词汇作为具有整体概念的多音节词，将其拼音全部连写。

5．All terms are arranged and indexed in alphabetical order.

五、本词汇按首英文字母的次序进行排列及索引。

6．"*" in the appendix of ICD-11 terms marks different expression in the book.

六、ICD-11内的词汇与正文有差异的标注了星号"*"。

7．"#" represents no phonetic symbol for the word.

七、"#"代表此词没有音标。

8．Standard terms and expressions of TCM based on the lastest ICD-11 of WHO can be used directly in electronic health records and electronic medical records for effective communication and better interoperability.

八、基于世界卫生组织（WHO）《国际疾病分类第十一次修订本（ICD-11）》收录的标准中医术语可直接用于电子保健及电子医学记录，促进有效交流及操作互动性。

Introduction to the 11th revision of the International Classification of Diseases（ICD–11）

国际疾病分类第十一次修订本 （ICD–11）介绍

The International Classification of Diseases（ICD）is the basis for identifying global health trends and statistics. It contains about 55，000 unique codes related to injuries，diseases and causes of death，enabling health practitioners to exchange health information around the world through a common language.

《国际疾病分类》是确定全球卫生趋势和统计数据的基础，其中含有约5.5万个与损伤、疾病以及死因有关的独特代码，使卫生从业人员能够通过一种通用语言来交换世界各地的卫生信息。

The 11th revision of the latest released ICD by the World Health Organization（WHO）includes traditional medicine in the classification system for the first time. The inclusion of traditional medicine in ICD–11 has far–reaching implications and will accelerate the further expansion of the currently thriving traditional medicine to become a necessary part of global health care. The WHO's decision on TCM can be understood as a mainstream endorsement that will have a major global impact. In the appendix of this book, ICD-11 traditional medicine chapters are compiled by the National Health Commission both in English and Chinese for your reference.

世界卫生组织（WHO）最新发布的《国际疾病分类》第十一次修订本（ICD-11）首次将传统医学纳入分类系统。将传统医学写入ICD-11影响深远，将进一步扩大目前正蓬勃发展的传统医学的影响力，使其最终成为全球医疗保健不可或缺的一部分。WHO关于中医药的决策可以理解成是一种主流认可，将在全球范围内产生重大影响。本书附录中收录的是ICD-11传统医学章节并经国家卫生健康委员会官方组织编译形成的英汉版。

Contents
目　　录

Chapter 1　History of Traditional Chinese Medicine and Classics

第一章　医史文献

A Supplement to Recipes Worth a Thousand Gold / əˈsʌplɪmənt tə ˈrɛsəpiz wɜrθ ə ˈθaʊznd ɡoʊld / 千金翼方 qiānjīnyìfāng

acupuncture and moxibustion chart / ˈækjupʌŋktʃə ənd mɑksɪˈbʌstʃən tʃɑrt / 明堂图 míngtángtú

adaptation array / ˌædæpˈteɪʃn əˈreɪ / 因阵 yīnzhèn

alchemy / ˈælkəmi / 炼丹术 liàndānshù

astringent formula / əˈstrɪndʒənt ˈfɔrmjələ / 涩剂 sèjì

Beiji Qianjin Yao Fang / peɪdʒi ˈtʃɪˈændʒɪn jɑʊ fæŋ / 备急千金要方 bèijíqiānjīnyàofāng

Bencao Gangmu / pentsɑʊ ɡæŋmu / 本草纲目 běncǎogāngmù

Bencao Gangmu Shiyi / pentsɑʊ ɡæŋmu ʃiji / 本草纲目拾遗 běncǎogāngmùshíyí

Bianque / pjæntʃue / 扁鹊 biǎnquè

Bureau for Compounding / ˈbjʊroʊ fər kəmˈpaʊndɪŋ / 和剂局 héjìjú

Bureau of Administration of Royal Medicinal Affairs / ˈbjʊroʊ əv ədmɪnɪˈstreɪʃn əv ˈrɔɪəl məˈdɪsɪnl əˈferz / 尚药局 shàngyàojú

case record / keɪs ˈrekərd / 诊籍 zhěnjí

Chao Yuanfang / tʃɑʊ jwanfæŋ / 巢元方 cháoyuánfāng

Chen Cangqi / tʃen tsɑŋtʃi / 陈藏器 chéncángqì

Chen Ziming / tʃen tsimɪŋ / 陈自明 chénzìmíng

chi / tsi / 尺 chǐ

Classified Case Records of Celebrated Physicians / ˈklæsɪfaɪd keɪs ˈrɛkədz əv ˈselɪbreɪtɪd fəˈzɪʃənz / 名医类案 míngyīlèiàn

clearing method / ˈklɪrɪŋ ˈmeθəd / 清法 qīngfǎ

cold array / koʊld əˈreɪ / 寒阵 hánzhèn

Collected Exegesis of Recipes / kəˈlektɪd ˌeksɪˈdʒɪsɪs əv ˈrɛsəpiz / 医方集解 yīfāngjíjiě

Compendium of Acupuncture and Moxibustion / kəmˈpendiəm əv ˈækjupʌŋktʃər ənd ˌmɑksɪˈbʌstʃən / 针灸大成 zhēnjiǔdàchéng

Compendium of Materia Medica / kəmˈpendiəm əv məˈtiəriə ˈmedikə / 本草纲目 běncǎogāngmù

Compendium of Medicine / kəmˈpendiəm əv ˈmedɪsn / 医学纲目 yīxuégāngmù

compound recipe / ˈkɑmpaʊnd ˈresəp / 重方 zhòngfāng

Correction on Errors in Medical Classics / kəˈrekʃn ɑn ˈɛrəz ɪn ˈmedɪkl ˈklæsɪks / 医林改错 yīlíngǎicuò

cun / tswən / 寸 cùn

diaphoresis / daɪəfəˈrisɪs / 汗法 hànfǎ

dietetician / ˈdaɪətetɪʃn / 食医 shíyī

diffusing formula / dɪˈfjʊzɪŋ ˈfɔrmjələ / 宣剂 xuānjì

dissipating array / ˈdɪsɪpeɪtɪŋ əˈreɪ / 散阵 sànzhèn

drastic prescriptions / ˈdræstɪk prɪˈskrɪpʃəns / 急方 jífāng

dry formula / draɪ ˈfɔrmjələ / 燥剂 zàojì

Effective Formulae Handed Down for Generations / ɪˈfektɪv ˈfɔrmjəli ˈhændɪd daʊn fər ˌdʒenəˈreɪʃnz / 世医得效方 shìyīdéxiàofāng

eight methods / eɪt ˈmeθədz / 八法 bāfǎ

eight tactical arrays / eɪt ˈtæktɪkl əˈreɪs / 八阵 bāzhèn

emesis method / ˈɛməsɪs ˈmeθəd / 吐法 tǔfǎ

Essence of External Diseases / ˈesns əv ɪkˈstɜrnl dɪˈzizɪs / 外科精要 wàikējīngyào

Essential Recipes for Emergent Use Worth a Thousand Gold / ɪˈsenʃl ˈrɛsəpiz fər ɪˈmɜrdʒənt juz wɜrθ ə ˈθaʊznd goʊld / 备急千金要方 bèijíqiānjīnyàofāng

even-ingredient prescriptions / ˈivn ɪnˈgridiənt prɪˈskrɪpʃəns / 偶方 ǒufāng

fen / fen / 分 fēn

four scholastic sects of Jin-Yuan dynasties / fɔr skə ˈlæstɪk sekts əv dʒɪn jwan ˈdɪnəstɪs / 金元四家 jīnyuánsìjiā

ge / kɛ / 合 gě

Ge Hong / kɛ hʊŋ / 葛洪 gěhóng

general medicine / ˈdʒenrəl ˈmedɪsn / 疾医 jíyī

General Treatise on Causes and Manifestations of All Diseases / ˈdʒenrəl ˈtritɪs ɑn kɔziz ənd ˌmænəfɛsˈteʃəns əv ɔl dɪˈzizɪs / 诸病源候论 zhūbìngyuánhòulùn

gentle prescriptions / ˈdʒentl prɪˈskrɪpʃəns / 缓方 huǎnfāng

Gong Tingxian / gʊŋ tɪŋʃjæn / 龚廷贤 gōngtíngxián

Handbook of Prescriptions for Emergency / ˈhændbʊk əv prɪˈskrɪpʃən fər ɪˈmɜrdʒənsi / 肘后备急方

zhǒuhòubèijífāng

harmonizing array / ˈhɑrmənaɪzɪŋ əˈreɪ / 和阵 hézhèn

harmonizing method / ˈhɑrmənaɪzɪŋ ˈmeθəd / 和法 héfǎ

heat array / hit əˈreɪ / 热阵 rèzhèn

heavy formula / ˈhevi ˈfɔrmjələ / 重剂 zhòngjì

Hua Tuo / huɑ tuo / 华佗 huàtuó

Huangdi / hwɑŋdi / 黄帝 huángdì

Huangdi Neijing / hwɑŋdɪ neɪdʒɪŋ / 黄帝内经 huáng dìnèijīng

Huangfu Mi / hwɑŋfu mi / 皇甫谧 huángfǔmì

Imperial Academy of Medicine / ɪmˈpɪriəl əˈkædəmi əv ˈmedɪsn / 太医院 tàiyīyuàn

Imperial Medical Academy / ɪmˈpɪriəl ˈmedɪkl əˈkædə mi / 太医署 tàiyīshǔ

Imperial Medical Service / ɪmˈpɪriəl ˈmedɪkl ˈsɜrvɪs / 太医局 tàiyījú

Inner Canon of Huangdi / ˈɪnər ˈkænən əv hwɑŋdɪ / 黄帝内经 huángdìnèijīng

Inner Canon of Yellow Emperor / ˈɪnər ˈkænən əv ˈjɛlo ˈempərər / 黄帝内经 huángdìnèijīng

jin / dʒɪn / 斤 jīn

Jingui Yaolüe / dʒɪngweɪ jɑuluə / 金匮要略 jīnguì yàolüè

Jingyue Quanshu / dʒɪŋjue tʃwɑnʃu / 景岳全书 jǐng yuèquánshū

Jing-yue's Complete Works / dʒɪŋjue kəmˈplit wɜrks / 景岳全书 jǐngyuèquánshū

Jiuhuang Bencao / ˈdʒjuhwɑŋ pentsɑu / 救荒本草 jiù

huāngběncǎo

Jiyin Gangmu / ˈdʒijɪn gæŋmu / 济阴纲目 jìyīngāngmù

Key to Therapeutics of Children's Diseases / ki tə ˌθer əˈpjutɪks əv ˈtʃɪldrən dɪˈzizɪs / 小儿药证直诀 xiǎoʼéryàozhèngzhíjué

king of medicine / kɪŋ əv ˈmedɪsn / 药王 yàowáng

Lei Xiao / leɪ ʃaʊ / 雷斅 léixiào

Leigong Paozhi Lun / leɪgʊŋ pɑʊdʒi lwən / 雷公炮炙论 léigōngpáozhìlùn

li / li / 厘 lí

Li Gao / li kɑʊ / 李杲 lǐgǎo

Li Shizhen / li ʃidʒen / 李时珍 lǐshízhēn

liang / ljɑŋ / 两 liǎng

light formula / laɪt ˈfɔrmjələ / 轻剂 qīngjì

Lingshu Jing / lɪŋ ʃu dʒɪŋ / 灵枢经 língshūjīng

lubricating formula / ˈlʊbrɪketɪŋ ˈfɔrmjələ / 滑剂 huájì

Mai Jing / mai dʒɪŋ / 脉经 màijīng

major prescriptions / ˈmeɪdʒər prɪˈskrɪpʃəns / 大方 dàfāng

Master Lei's Discourse on Drug Processing / ˈmæstər leɪz ˈdɪskɔrs ɑn drʌg ˈprɑsesɪŋ / 雷公炮炙论 léigōngpáozhìlùn

materia medica / məˈtiəriə ˈmedikə / 本草 běncǎo

Materia Medica for Famines / məˈtiəriə ˈmedikə fər ˈfæmənz / 救荒本草 jiùhuāngběncǎo

medical classic / ˈmedɪkl ˈklæsɪk / 医经 yījīng

Medical Institute of Benevolence / ˈmedɪkl ˈɪnstɪtut əv bəˈnevələns / 惠民局 huìmínjú

medical sage / ˈmedɪkl seɪdʒ / 医圣 yīshèng

Mingyi Leian / mɪŋji leɪɑn / 名医类案 míngyīlèi'àn

minor prescriptions / ˈmaɪnər prɪˈskrɪpʃəns / 小方 xiǎofāng

Miraculous Pivot / mɪrækjələs pɪvət / 灵枢经 língshū jīng

moist formula / mɔɪst ˈfɔrmjələ / 湿剂 shījì

New Compilation of Effective Recipes / nu ˌkɑmpɪˈleɪʃn əv ɪˈfektɪv ˈresəpɪz / 验方新编 yànfāngxīnbiān

Newly Revised Materia Medica / ˈnuli rɪˈvaɪzd məˈtiəriə ˈmedikə / 新修本草 xīnxiūběncǎo

obstruction-removing formula / əbˈstrʌkʃn riˈmuvɪŋ ˈfɔrmjələ / 通剂 tōngjì

odd-ingredient prescriptions / ɑd ɪnˈgridiənt prɪˈskrɪpʃəns / 奇方 jīfāng

offensive array / əˈfensɪv əˈreɪ / 攻阵 gōngzhèn

On Blood Syndromes / ɑn blʌd ˈsɪndrəʊmz / 血证论 xuèzhènglùn

On Plague Diseases / ɑn pleɪg dɪˈzizɪs / 温疫论 wēnyìlùn

Orthodox Manual of External Diseases / ˈɔrθədɑks ˈmænjuəl əv ɪkˈstɜrnl dɪˈzizɪs / 外科正宗 wàikē zhèngzōng

Outline for Women's Diseases / ˈaʊtlaɪn fər ˈwɪmɪn dɪˈzizɪs / 济阴纲目 jìyīngāngmù

palace physician / ˈpæləs fɪˈzɪʃn / 太医 tàiyī

Pang Anshi / pæŋ anʃi / 庞安时 páng'ānshí

Piwei Lun / pɪweɪ lwən / 脾胃论 píwèilùn

Plain Questions / pleɪn ˈkwestʃənz / 素问 sùwèn

powder for anesthesia / ˈpaʊdər fər ænəsˈθiʒə / 麻沸散 máfèisǎn

powder for boiling / ˈpaʊdər fər ˈbɔɪlɪŋ / 煮散 zhǔsǎn

powder of five minerals / ˈpaʊdər əv faɪv ˈmɪnərəls / 五石散 wǔshísǎn

powder taken cold / ˈpaʊdər ˈtekən koʊld / 寒食散 hánshísǎn

Prescriptions for Universal Relief / prɪˈskrɪpʃənz fər ˌjunɪˈvɜrsl rɪˈlif / 普济方 pǔjìfāng

Prescriptions of the Bureau of Taiping People's Welfare Pharmacy / prɪˈskrɪpʃənz əv ðə ˈbjʊroʊ əv taɪˈpɪŋ ˈpipls ˈwelfer ˈfɑrməsi / 太平惠民和剂局方 tàipíng huìmínhéjìjúfāng

processing / ˈprɑsesɪŋ / 炮炙 páozhì

Puji Fang / puʤi fæŋ / 普济方 pǔjìfāng

Pulse Classic / pʌls ˈklæsɪk / 脉经 màijīng

purgative formula / ˈpɜrgətɪv ˈfɔrmjələ / 泄剂 xièjì

purgative method / ˈpɜrgətɪv ˈmeθəd / 下法 xiàfǎ

Qi Dezhi / tʃi dəʤi / 齐德之 qídézhī

Qian Yi / tʃɪˈænd ji / 钱乙 qiányǐ

Qianjin Yi Fang / tʃɪˈændʒɪn jifæŋ / 千金翼方 qiānjīnyìfāng

Qibo / tʃipo / 岐伯 qíbó

Recipes in Rhymes / ˈrɛsəpɪz ɪn raɪmz / 汤头歌诀

tāngtóugējué

Records for Washing Away of Wrong Cases / ˈrɛkɚdz fər ˈwɑʃɪŋ əˈweɪ əv rɔŋ kesɪz / 洗冤录 xǐyuānlù

resolving method / rɪˈzɑlvɪŋ ˈmɛθəd / 消法 xiāofǎ

Royal Drug Museum / ˈrɔɪəl drʌg mjuˈziəm / 御药院 yùyàoyuàn

royal surgeon / ˈrɔɪəl ˈsɜrdʒən / 疡医 yángyī

* **school of warm diseases** / skul əv wɔrm dɪˈzizɪs / 温病学派 wēnbìngxuépài

securing array / sɪˈkjʊrɪŋ əˈreɪ / 固阵 gùzhèn

seven kinds of prescriptions / ˈsevn kaɪndz əv prɪˈskrɪpʃəns / 七方 qīfāng

Shanghan Lun / ʃæŋhan lwən / 伤寒论 shānghánlùn

Shanghan Zabing Lun / ʃæŋhan zaˈpɪŋ lwən / 伤寒杂病论 shānghánzábìnglùn

sheng / ʃeŋ / 升 shēng

Shennong / ʃennʊŋ / 神农 shénnóng

Shennong Bencao Jing / ʃennʊŋ pentsɑʊ dʒɪŋ / 神农本草经 shénnóngběncǎojīng

Shennong's Classic of Materia Medica / ʃennʊŋsˈklæsɪk əv məˈtiəriə ˈmedikə / 神农本草经 shénnóngběncǎojīng

Shiyi Dexiao Fang / ʃiji dəʃɑʊ fæŋ / 世医得效方 shìyīdéxiàofāng

Song Ci / sʊŋ tsi / 宋慈 sòngcí

Sun Simiao / swən simjɑʊ / 孙思邈 sūnsīmiǎo

Supplement to Compendium of Materia Medica / ˈsʌplɪmənt tə kəmˈpendiəm əv məˈtiəriə ˈmedikə /

本草纲目拾遗 běncǎogāngmùshíyí

supplementing array / ˈsʌplɪməntɪŋ əˈreɪ / 补阵 bǔ zhèn

Suwen / su wən / 素问 sùwèn

Synopsis of Golden Chamber / sɪˈnɑpsɪs əv ˈɡouldən ˈtʃeɪmbər / 金匮要略 jīnguìyàolüè

Taiping Holy Prescriptions for Universal Relief / taɪˈpɪŋ ˈhouli prɪˈskrɪpʃənz fər ˌjunɪˈvɜrsl rɪˈlif / 太平圣惠方 tàipíngshènghuìfāng

Taiping Huimin Heji Ju Fang / taɪˈpɪŋ huɪmɪn hɜdʒi dʒu fæŋ / 太平惠民和剂局方 tàipínghuìmínhéjìjúfāng

Taiping Shenghui Fang / taɪˈpɪŋ ʃʌŋhuɪ fæŋ / 太平圣惠方 tàipíngshènghuìfāng

take at dawn / teɪk ət dɔn / 平旦服 píngdànfú

Tangtou Gejue / tɑŋtou kɛʤuə / 汤头歌诀 tāngtóugējué

Tao Hongjing / tɑu huŋdʒɪŋ / 陶弘景 táohóngjǐng

ten functional types of formularies / ten ˈfʌŋkʃənl taɪps əv ˈfɔrmjələrɪs / 十剂 shíjì

Textual Research on Reality and Titles of Plants / ˈtekstʃuəl ˈrisɜrtʃ ɑn riˈælətɪ ənd ˈtaɪtlz əv plænts / 植物名实图考 zhíwùmíngshítúkǎo

tonifying formula / ˈtoʊnɪfaɪŋ ˈfɔrmjələ / 补剂 bǔjì

tonifying method / ˈtoʊnɪfaɪŋ ˈmeθəd / 补法 bǔfǎ

Treatise on Cold Pathogenic and Miscellaneous Diseases / ˈtritɪs ɑn kould ˌpæθəˈdʒenɪk ənd ˌmɪsəˈleɪnɪəs dɪˈzizɪs / 伤寒杂病论 shānghánzábìnglùn

Treatise on Cold Pathogenic Diseases / ˈtritɪs ɑn koʊld ˌpæθəˈdʒenɪk dɪˈzizɪs / 伤寒论 shānghánlùn

Treatise on Spleen and Stomach / ˈtritɪs ɑn splin ənd ˈstʌmək / 脾胃论 píwèilùn

variolation / vɛəriəˈleiʃən / 人痘接种术 réndòujiē zhòngshù

Waike Jingyao / waɪke dʒɪŋjɑʊ / 外科精要 wàikē jīngyào

Waike Zhengzong / waɪkɛ dʒɛŋtsɒŋ / 外科正宗 wàikēzhèngzōng

Wang Ang / wæŋ æŋ / 汪昂 wāng'áng

Wang Bing / wɑŋ bɪŋ / 王冰 wángbīng

Wang Hongxu / wæŋ hʊŋsu / 王洪绪 wánghóngxù

Wang Qingren / wæŋ qɪŋrən / 王清任 wángqīngrèn

Wang Shuhe / wæŋ ʃuhɛsu / 王叔和 wángshūhé

warming method / ˈwɔrmɪŋ ˈmeθəd / 温法 wēnfǎ

Wenyi Lun / wənji lwən / 温疫论 wēnyìlùn

Wu Kun / wu kwən / 吴昆 wúkūn

Wu Youxing / wu joʊʃɪŋ / 吴有性 wúyǒuxìng

Xiao'er Yao Zheng Zhi Jue / ˈʃɑʊɑr jɑʊ ʤɛŋ ʤi ʤue / 小儿药证直诀 xiǎo'éryàozhèngzhíjué

Xinxiu Bencao / ʃɪnʃju pentsɑʊ / 新修本草 xīnxiū běncǎo

Xiyuan Lu / ʃi juˈɑn lu / 洗冤录 xǐyuānlù

Xue Ji / ʃuə dʒi / 薛己 xuējǐ

Xue Xue / ʃuə ʃuə / 薛雪 xuēxuě

Xuezheng Lun / ʃuə ʤɛŋ lwən / 血证论 xuèzhènglùn

Yanfang Xinbian / jənfæŋ ʃɪnbjɑn / 验方新编 yàn

fāngxīnbiān

Yang Jizhou / jæŋ dʒidʒoʊ / 杨继洲 yángjìzhōu

Yang Shangshan / jæŋ ʃæŋʃan / 杨上善 yángshàng shàn

Yao Wang / jɑʊ wæŋ / 药王 yàowáng

Ye Gui / jɛ gweɪ / 叶桂 yèguì

Yellow Emperor / ˈjeloʊ ˈempərə(r) / 黄帝 huángdì

Yifang Jijie / jifæŋ ʤiʤæ / 医方集解 yīfāngjíjiě

Yilin Gaicuo / jilɪn gaɪtswəʊ / 医林改错 yīlíngǎicuò

Yixue Gangmu / jɪʃuə gæŋmu / 医学纲目 yīxuégāng mù

Zhang Jingyue / ʤæŋ dʒɪŋjue / 张景岳 zhāngjǐngyuè

Zhang Zhongjing / dʒæŋ dʒʊŋdʒɪŋ / 张仲景 zhāng zhòngjǐng

Zhao Xuemin / ʤɑʊ ʃuəmɪn / 赵学敏 zhàoxuémǐn

Zhenjiu Dacheng / dʒɛndʒju dɑtʃʌŋ / 针灸大成 zhēn jiǔdàchéng

Zhiwu Mingshi Tukao / dʒiwu mɪŋʃi tukɑʊ / 植物名 实图考 zhíwùmíngshítúkǎo

Zhouhou Beiji Fang / dʒoʊhoʊ peɪdʒi fæŋ / 肘后备急 方 zhǒuhòubèijífāng

Zhu Bing Yuan Hou Lun / dʒu pɪŋ jwan hoʊ lwən / 诸病源候论 zhūbìngyuánhòulùn

Chapter 2　Basic Theories of Traditional Chinese Medicine

第二章　中医基础理论

Section 1　General Introduction

第一节　概　　论

child qi / tʃaɪld tʃi / 子气 zǐqì

correspondence between human body and natural environment / ˌkɔrəˈspɑndəns bɪˈtwin ˈhjumən ˈbɑdi ənd ˈnætʃrəl ɪnˈvaɪrənmənt / 天人相应 tiānrén xiāngyìng

counter-restriction of five phases / ˈkauntər ɪˈstrɪkʃn əv faɪvˈfesiz / 五行相侮 wǔxíngxiāngwǔ

earth / ɜrθ / 土 tǔ

earth generating metal / ɜrθ ˈdʒɛnəretɪŋ ˈmetl / 土生金 tǔshēngjīn

earth restricting water / ɜrθ rɪˈstrɪktɪŋ ˈwɔtər / 土克水 tǔkèshuǐ

extreme yang changing into yin / ɪkˈstrim jæŋ tʃendʒ ˈɪntə jɪn / 重阳必阴 chóngyángbìyīn

extreme yin changing into yang / ɪkˈstrim jɪn tʃendʒ ˈɪntə jæŋ / 重阴必阳 chóngyīnbìyáng

fire / ˈfaɪər / 火 huǒ

fire generating earth / ˈfaɪər ˈdʒɛnəretɪŋ ɜrθ / 火生土 huǒshēngtǔ

fire restricting metal / ˈfaɪə rɪˈstrɪktɪŋ ˈmetl / 火克金 huǒkèjīn

five evolutive phases / faɪv ˈevəˌlutɪv ˈfesiz / 五运 wǔyùn

five evolutive phases and six climatic factors / faɪv ˈevəlutɪv ˈfesiz ənd sɪks klaɪˈmætɪk ˈfæktəz / 运气 yùnqì

five orientations / faɪv ˌɔriənˈteɪʃnz / 五方 wǔfāng

five phases / faɪv ˈfesiz / 五行 wǔxíng

five seasons / faɪv siznz / 五时 wǔshí

five-phase theory / faɪv ˈfesiz ˈθiəri / 五行学说 wǔxíng xuéshuō

heavenly stems and earthly branches / ˈhevnli stemz ənd ˈɜrθli bræntʃɪz / 干支 gānzhī

holism / ˈhoʊlɪzəm / 整体观念 zhěngtǐguānniàn

illness of child viscera affecting mother one / ˌɪlnəs əv tʃaɪld ˈvɪsərə əˈfektɪŋ ˈmʌðər wʌn / 子病及母 zǐbìngjímǔ

illness of mother viscera affecting the child one / ˌɪlnəs əv ˈmʌðər ˈvɪsərə əˈfektɪŋ ðə tʃaɪld wʌn / 母病及子 mǔbìngjízǐ

manifestation and root cause / mænɪfeˈsteɪʃn ənd rut kɔz / 标本 biāoběn

metal / ˈmetl / 金 jīn

metal generating water / ˈmetl ˈdʒɛnəretɪŋ ˈwɔtər / 金生水 jīnshēngshuǐ

metal restricting wood / ˈmetl rɪˈstrɪktɪŋ wʊd / 金克木 jīnkèmù

mother qi / ˈmʌðər tʃi / 母气 mǔqì

mutual convertibility of yin-yang / ˈmjutʃuəl kənvɜrtəˈbɪləti əv jɪn jæŋ / 阴阳转化 yīnyángzhuǎnhuà

mutual generation of five phases / ˈmjutʃuəl ˌdʒenəˈreɪʃn əv faɪv ˈfesiz / 五行相生 wǔxíngxiāngshēng

mutual restriction of five phases / ˈmjutʃuəl rɪˈstrɪkʃn əv faɪv ˈfesiz / 五行相克 wǔxíngxiāngkè

mutual rooting of yin-yang / ˈmjutʃuəl ˈrutɪŋ əv jɪn jæŋ / 阴阳互根 yīnyánghùgēn

natural harmony of yin-yang / ˈnætʃrəl ˈhɑrməni əv jɪn jæŋ / 阴阳自和 yīnyángzìhé

over-restriction of five phases / ˈəuvə-rɪˈstrɪkʃn əv faɪv ˈfesiz / 五行相乘 wǔxíngxiāngchéng

principle-method-recipe-medicines / ˈprɪnsəpl ˈmeθəd ˈresəpi ˈmedɪsnz / 理法方药 lǐfǎfāngyào

relative equilibrium of yin-yang / ˈrelətɪv ˌikwɪˈlɪbriəm əv jɪn jæŋ / 阴平阳秘 yīnpíngyángmì

six climatic factors / sɪks klaɪˈmætɪk ˈfæktəz / 六气 liùqì

sixty-year cycle / sɪks jɪrˈ saɪkl / 甲子 jiǎzǐ

steady yin and vexed yang / ˈstedi jɪn ənd veksd jæŋ / 阴阳对立 yīnyángduìlì

treatment based on syndrome differentiation / ˈtritmənt beɪst ɑn ˈsɪndroʊm ˌdɪfəˌrenʃiˈeɪʃn / 辨证论治 biànzhènglùnzhì

water / ˈwɔtər / 水 shuǐ

water generating wood / ˈwɔtər ˈdʒɜnəretɪŋ wʊd / 水

生木 shuǐshēngmù

water restricting fire / ˈwɔtər rɪˈstrɪktɪŋ ˈfaɪər / 水克火 shuǐkèhuǒ

waxing and waning of yin-yang / ˈwæksɪŋ ənd ˈweɪnɪŋ əv jɪn jæŋ / 阴阳消长 yīnyángxiāozhǎng

wood / wʊd / 木 mù

wood generating fire / wʊd ˈdʒɛnəretɪŋ ˈfaɪər / 木生火 mùshēnghuǒ

wood restricting earth / wʊd rɪˈstrɪktɪŋ ɝθ / 木克土 mùkètǔ

yang qi / jæŋ tʃi / 阳气 yángqì

yin qi / jɪn tʃi / 阴气 yīnqì

yin-yang / jɪn jæŋ / 阴阳 yīnyáng

yin-yang theory / jɪn jæŋ ˈθiəri / 阴阳学说 yīnyáng xuéshuō

Section 2　Visceral Manifestations

第二节　脏　　象

bile / baɪl / 胆汁 dǎnzhī

bladder / ˈblædər / 膀胱 pángguāng

bone / boʊn / 骨 gǔ

bone-length measurement / boʊn lɛŋθ ˈmɛʒərmənt / 骨度 gǔdù

brain / breɪn / 脑 nǎo

brain marrow / breɪn ˈmæroʊ / 脑髓 nǎosuǐ

door of brain / dɔr əv breɪn / 脑户 nǎohù

essence chamber / ˈɛsns ˈtʃeɪmbər / 精室 jīngshì

extraordinary Fu-viscera / ɪkˈstrɔrdəneri fuˈvɪsərə /

奇恒之腑 qíhéngzhīfǔ

five body constituents / faɪv ˈbɑdi kənˈstɪtʃʊənts / 五体 wǔtǐ

five emotions / faɪv ɪˈmoʃənz / 五神 wǔshén

five humors / faɪv ˈhjʊməz / 五液 wǔyè

five lustre / faɪv lystr / 五华 wǔhuá

five minds / faɪv maɪndz / 五志 wǔzhì

five Zang viscera / faɪv zæŋ ˈvɪsərə / 五脏 wǔzàng

fontanel / ˌfɒntəˈnel / 囟门 xìnmén

functioning of bladder / ˈfʌŋkʃənɪŋ əv ˈblædər / 膀胱气化 pángguāngqìhuà

Fu-viscera of marrow / fuˈvɪsərə əv ˈmærou / 髓之府 suǐzhīfǔ

Fu-viscera of mental activity / fuˈvɪsərə əv ˈmentl ækˈtɪvəti / 元神之府 yuánshénzhīfǔ

gallbladder / ˈgɔlˌblædə / 胆 dǎn

gallbladder qi / ˈgɔlˌblædə tʃi / 胆气 dǎnqì

heart / hɑrt / 心 xīn

heart being connected with small intestine / hɑrt ˈbiɪŋ kəˈnektɪd wɪθ smɔl ɪnˈtestɪn / 心合小肠 xīnhéxiǎocháng

heart governing blood and vessels / hɑrt ˈgəvərnɪŋ blʌd ənd ˈvɛslz / 心主血脉 xīnzhǔxuèmài

heart opening at tongue / hɑrt ˈoupənɪŋ ət tʌŋ / 心开窍于舌 xīnkāiqiàoyúshé

heart storing spirit / hɑrt storɪŋ ˈspɪrɪt / 心藏神 xīncángshén

heart yang / hɑrt jæŋ / 心阳 xīnyáng

heart yin / hɑrt jɪn / 心阴 xīnyīn

homogeny of liver and kidney / hoˈmɑdʒəni əv ˈlɪvər ənd ˈkɪdni / 肝肾同源 gānshèntóngyuán

house of blood / haʊs əv blʌd / 血之府 xuèzhīfǔ

ileum / ˈɪliəm / 回肠 huícháng

interconnection of Zang-Fu viscera / ˌɪntərkəˈnekʃn əv zæŋ fu ˈvɪsərə / 脏腑相合 zàngfǔxiānghé

intercourse between heart and kidney / ˈɪntərkɔrs bɪˈtwin hɑrt ənd ˈkɪdni / 心肾相交 xīnshèn xiāngjiāo

kidney / ˈkɪdni / 肾 shèn

kidney being averse to dryness / ˈkɪdni ˈbiɪŋ əˈvɜrs tə ˈdraɪnəs / 肾恶燥 shènwùzào

kidney being congenital origin / ˈkɪdni ˈbiɪŋ kənˈdʒenɪtl ˈɔrɪdʒɪn / 肾为先天之本 shènwéi xiāntiānzhīběn

kidney being connected with bladder / ˈkɪdni ˈbiɪŋ kəˈnektɪd wɪθ ˈblædər / 肾合膀胱 shènhépáng guāng

kidney essence / ˈkɪdni ˈesns / 肾精 shènjīng

kidney governing bones / ˈkɪdni ˈgəvərnɪŋ bonz / 肾主骨 shènzhǔgǔ

kidney governing inspiration / ˈkɪdni ˈgəvərnɪŋ ˌɪnspəˈreɪʃn / 肾主纳气 shènzhǔnàqì

kidney governing reproduction / ˈkɪdni ˈgəvərnɪŋ ˌrɪprəˈdʌkʃn / 肾主生殖 shènzhǔshēngzhí

kidney governing storage / ˈkɪdni ˈgəvərnɪŋ ˈstɔrɪdʒ / 肾主封藏 shènzhǔfēngcáng

kidney governing water metabolism / ˈkɪdni ˈɡəvərnɪŋ ˈwɔtər məˈtæbəlɪzəm / 肾主水液 shènzhǔshuǐyè

kidney opening at ear / ˈkɪdni ˈoʊpənɪŋ ət ɪr / 肾开窍于耳 shènkāiqiàoyúěr

kidney qi / ˈkɪdni tʃi / 肾气 shènqì

kidney storing essence / ˈkɪdni storɪŋ ˈesns / 肾藏精 shèncángjīng

kidney storing will / ˈkɪdni storɪŋ wɪl / 肾藏志 shèncángzhì

kidney yang / ˈkɪdni jæŋ / 肾阳 shènyáng

kidney yin / ˈkɪdni jɪn / 肾阴 shèn yīn

large intestine / lɑrdʒ ɪnˈtestɪn / 大肠 dàcháng

liver / ˈlɪvər / 肝 gān

liver being averse to wind / ˈlɪvər ˈbiɪŋ əˈvɜrs tə wɪnd / 肝恶风 gānwùfēng

liver being connected with gallbladder / ˈlɪvər ˈbiɪŋ kəˈnektɪd wɪθ ˈɡɔlˌblædə / 肝合胆 gānhédǎn

liver controlling conveyance and dispersion / ˈlɪvər kənˈtrolɪŋ kənˈveɪəns ənd dɪˈspɜrʒn / 肝主疏泄 gānzhǔshūxiè

liver governing ascending and dredging / ˈlɪvər ˈɡəvərnɪŋ əˈsɛndɪŋ ənd ˈdrɛdʒɪŋ / 肝主升发 gānzhǔshēngfā

liver governing tendons / ˈlɪvər ˈɡəvərnɪŋ ˈtendənz / 肝主筋 gānzhǔjīn

liver opening at eye / ˈlɪvər ˈoʊpənɪŋ ət aɪ / 肝开窍于目 gānkāiqiàoyúmù

liver storing blood / ˈlɪvər storɪŋ blʌd / 肝藏血 gān

cángxuè

liver storing soul / ˈlɪvər stɔrɪŋ soʊl / 肝藏魂 gān cánghún

liver yang / ˈlɪvər jæŋ / 肝阳 gānyáng

liver yin / ˈlɪvər jɪn / 肝阴 gānyīn

lower jiao / ˈloə dʒjɑʊ / 下焦 xiàjiāo

lung / lʌŋ / 肺 fèi

lung being connected with large intestine / lʌŋ ˈbiɪŋ kəˈnektɪd wɪθ lɑrdʒ ɪnˈtestɪn / 肺合大肠 fèihé dàcháng

lung governing diffusion / lʌŋ ˈgəvərnɪŋ dɪˈfjuʒən / 肺主宣发 fèizhǔxuānfā

lung governing management and regulation / lʌŋ ˈgəvərnɪŋ ˈmænɪdʒmənt ənd ˌregjuˈleɪʃn / 肺主治节 fèizhǔzhìjié

lung governing purification and descending / lʌŋ ˈgəvərnɪŋ ˌpjʊrɪfɪˈkeɪʃn ənd dɪˈsendɪŋ / 肺主肃降 fèizhǔsùjiàng

lung governing skin and hair / lʌŋ ˈgəvərnɪŋ skɪn ənd her / 肺主皮毛 fèizhǔpímáo

lung opening at nose / lʌŋ ˈoʊpənɪŋ ət noʊz / 肺开窍于鼻 fèikāiqiàoyúbí

lung qi / lʌŋ tʃi / 肺气 fèiqì

lung storing inferior spirit / lʌŋ stɔrɪŋ ɪnˈfɪriər ˈspɪrɪt / 肺藏魄 fèicángpò

lung yang / lʌŋ jæŋ / 肺阳 fèiyáng

lung yin / lʌŋ jɪn / 肺阴 fèiyīn

marrow / ˈmæroʊ / 髓 suǐ

menstruation / ˌmenstruˈeɪʃn / 月经 yuèjīng

middle jiao / ˈmɪdl dʒɑʊ / 中焦 zhōngjiāo

mutually promotion of lung and kidney / ˈmjutʃuəli prəˈmoʊʃn əv lʌŋ ənd ˈkɪdni / 肺肾相生 fèishèn xiāngshēng

official of transportation / əˈfɪʃl əv ˌtrænspɔrˈteɪʃn / 传导之官 chuándǎozhīguān

pancreas / ˈpæŋkriəs / 胰 yí

reservoir of food and drink / ˈrezərvwɑr əv fud ənd drɪŋk / 水谷之海 shuǐgǔzhīhǎi

sanjiao / sandʒɑʊ / 三焦 sānjiāo

separating clear and excreting turbid / ˈsepəreitiŋ klɪr ənd ɪkˈskritiŋ ˈtɜrbɪd / 分清泌浊 fēnqīngmìzhuó

seven emotions / ˈsevn ɪˈmoʃənz / 七情 qīqíng

six Fu viscera / sɪks fu ˈvɪsərə / 六腑 liùfǔ

small intestine / smɔl ɪnˈtestɪn / 小肠 xiǎocháng

spleen / splin / 脾 pí

spleen being acquired foundation / splin ˈbiɪŋ əˈkwaɪrd faʊnˈdeɪʃn / 脾为后天之本 píwéihòutiānzhīběn

spleen being connected with stomach / splin ˈbiɪŋ kəˈnektɪd wɪθ stomach / 脾合胃 píhéwèi

spleen governing ascending clear / splin ˈgəvərniŋ əˈsendiŋ klɪr / 脾主升清 pízhǔshēngqīng

spleen governing transportation and transformation / splin ˈgəvərniŋ ˌtrænspɔrˈteɪʃn ənd ˌtrænsfərˈmeɪʃn / 脾主运化 pízhǔyùnhuà

spleen liking dryness and disliking dampness / splin ˈlaɪkɪŋ ˈdraɪnəs ənd dɪsˈlaɪkɪŋ ˈdæmpnəs / 脾喜燥

恶湿 píxǐzàowùshī

spleen opening at mouth / splin ˈoʊpənɪŋ ət maʊθ / 脾开窍于口 píkāiqiàoyúkǒu

spleen storing idea / splin ˈstɔːrɪŋ ˈdiə / 脾藏意 pícángyì

spleen storing nutrients / splin ˈstɔːrɪŋ ˈnjutrɪənts / 脾藏营 pícángyíng

spleen yang / splin jæŋ / 脾阳 píyáng

spleen yin / splin jɪn / 脾阴 píyīn

stomach / ˈstʌmək / 胃 wèi

stomach fluid / ˈstʌmək ˈfluɪd / 胃津 wèijīn

stomach liking moistness and disliking dryness / ˈstʌmək ˈlaɪkɪŋ ˈmɔɪstnəs ənd dɪsˈlaɪkɪŋ ˈdraɪnəs / 胃喜润恶燥 wèixǐrùnwùzào

stomach qi / ˈstʌmək tʃi / 胃气 wèiqì

stomach receiving food and drink / ˈstʌmək rɪˈsivɪŋ fud ənd drɪŋk / 胃主受纳 wèizhǔshòunà

stomach yang / ˈstʌmək jæŋ / 胃阳 wèiyáng

stomach yin / ˈstʌmək jɪn / 胃阴 wèiyīn

theory of visceral manifestations / ˈθɪəri əv ˈvɪsərəl ˌmænəfesˈteʃənz / 脏象学说 zàngxiàngxuéshuō

upper jia / ˈʌpər dʒjɑʊ / 上焦 shàngjiāo

uterine vessels / ˈjutəraɪn ˈvɛslz / 胞脉 bāomài

uterus / ˈjutərəs / 胞宫 bāogōng

vagina / vəˈdʒaɪnə / 阴道 yīndào

vessel / ˈvesl / 脉 mài

visceral manifestations / ˈvɪsərəl ˌmænəfesˈteʃənz/ 脏象 zàngxiàng

vital gate / ˈvaɪtl ɡeɪt / 命门 mìngmén

vital gate fire / ˈvaɪtl ɡeɪt ˈfaɪər / 命门之火 mìngmén zhīhuǒ

womb / wum / 胞宫 bāogōng

Zang-Fu viscera / zæŋfu ˈvɪsərə / 脏腑 zàngfǔ

Section 3　Meridians
第三节　经　　络

aponeurotic system / ˌæpənjuˈrɔtik ˈsɪstəm / 经筋 jīngjīn

Belt Channel / belt ˈtʃænl / 带脉 dàimài

Belt Vessel / belt ˈvesl / 带脉 dàimài

branched channel / brɑntʃt ˈtʃænl / 经别 jīngbié

channel / ˈtʃænl / 经络 jīngluò

channel / ˈtʃænl / 经脉 jīngmài

channel qi / ˈtʃænl tʃi / 经气 jīngqì

channel theory / ˈtʃænl ˈθiəriˌ / 经络学说 jīngluòxuéshuō

Chong Channel / ˈtʃʊŋ ˈtʃænl / 冲脉 chōngmài

Chong Vessel / ˈtʃʊŋ ˈvesl / 冲脉 chōngmài

collaterals / kəˈlætərəlz / 络脉 luòmài

Conception Channel / kənˈsepʃn ˈtʃænl / 任脉 rènmài

Conception Vessel / kənˈsepʃn ˈvesl / 任脉 rènmài

connecting collaterals / kəˈnektiŋ kəˈlætərəlz / 别络 biéluò

dermal parts / ˈdɚməl pɑrts / 皮部 píbù

Eight Extraordinary Channels / eɪt ɪkˈstrɔrdəneri ˈtʃænlz / 奇经八脉 qíjīngbāmài

Eight Extraordinary Meridians / eɪt ɪkˈstrɔrdəneri məˈrɪdɪənz / 奇经八脉 qíjīngbāmài

four seas / fɔr siz / 四海 sìhǎi

fourteen channels / ˌfɔrˈtin ˈtʃænlz / 十四经 shísìjīng

Governor Channel / ˈgʌvərnər ˈtʃænl / 督脉 dūmài

Governor Vessel / ˈgʌvərnər ˈvesl / 督脉 dūmài

Jueyin Liver Channel of Foot / dʒuəjɪn ˈlɪvər ˈtʃænl əv fʊt / 足厥阴肝经 zújuéyīngānjīng

Jueyin Liver Meridian of Foot / dʒuəjɪn ˈlɪvər məˈ rɪdɪən əv fʊt / 足厥阴肝经 zújuéyīngānjīng

Jueyin Pericardium Channel of Hand / dʒuəjɪn ˌpɛrɪˈkɑrdɪəm ˈtʃænl əv hænd / 手厥阴心包经 shǒu juéyīnxīnbāojīng

Jueyin Pericardium Meridian of Hand / dʒuəjɪn ˌpɛrɪˈkɑrdɪəm məˈrɪdɪən əv hænd / 手厥阴心包经 shǒujuéyīnxīnbāojīng

meridian / məˈrɪdɪən / 经络 jīngluò

pathway of qi / ˈpæθweɪ əv tʃi / 气街 qìjiē

root and knot / rut ənd nɑt / 根结 gēnjié

Shaoyang Gallbladder Channel of Foot / ʃaʊjæŋ ˈgɔlˌblædə ˈtʃænl əv fʊt / 足少阳胆经 zúshàoyáng dǎnjīng

Shaoyang Gallbladder Meridian of Foot / ʃaʊjæŋ ˈgɔlˌblædə məˈrɪdɪən əv fʊt / 足少阳胆经 zúshào yángdǎnjīng

Shaoyang Sanjiao Channel of Hand / ʃaʊjæŋ sandʒjɑʊ ˈtʃænl əv hænd / 手少阳三焦经 shǒushào yángsānjiāojīng

Shaoyang Sanjiao Meridian of Hand / ʃaʊjæŋ sandʒjaʊ məˈrɪdɪən əv hænd / 手少阳三焦经 shǒushàoyángsānjiāojīng

Shaoyin Heart Channel of Hand / ʃaʊjɪn hɑrt ˈtʃænl əv hænd / 手少阴心经 shǒushàoyīnxīnjīng

Shaoyin Heart Meridian of Hand / ʃaʊjɪn hɑrt məˈrɪdɪən əv hænd / 手少阴心经 shǒushàoyīnxīnjīng

Shaoyin Kidney Channel of Foot / ʃaʊjɪn ˈkɪdni ˈtʃænl əv fʊt / 足少阴肾经 zúshàoyīnshènjīng

Shaoyin Kidney Meridian of Foot / ʃaʊjɪn ˈkɪdni məˈrɪdɪən əv fʊt / 足少阴肾经 zúshàoyīnshènjīng

superficial collaterals / ˌsupərˈfɪʃl kəˈlætərəlz / 浮络 fúluò

Taiyang Bladder Channel of Foot / taɪˈjæŋ ˈblædə ˈtʃænl əv fʊt / 足太阳膀胱经 zútàiyángpángguāngjīng

Taiyang Bladder Meridian of Foot / taɪˈjæŋ ˈblædə məˈrɪdɪən əv fʊt / 足太阳膀胱经 zútàiyángpángguāngjīng

Taiyang Small Intestine Channel of Hand / taɪˈjæŋ smɔl ɪnˈtestɪn ˈtʃænl əv hænd / 手太阳小肠经 shǒutàiyángxiǎochángjīng

Taiyang Small Intestine Meridian of Hand / taɪˈjæŋ smɔl ɪnˈtestɪn məˈrɪdɪən əv hænd / 手太阳小肠经 shǒutàiyángxiǎochángjīng

Taiyin Lung Channel of Hand / taɪˌjɪn lʌŋ ˈtʃænl əv hænd / 手太阴肺经 shǒutàiyīnfèijīng

Taiyin Lung Meridian of Hand / taɪˌjɪn lʌŋ məˈrɪdɪən

əv hænd / 手太阴肺经 shǒutàiyīnfèijīng

Taiyin Spleen Channel of Foot / taɪˌjɪn splin ˈtʃænl əv fʊt / 足太阴脾经 zútàiyīnpíjīng

Taiyin Spleen Meridian of Foot / taɪˌjɪn splin məˈrɪdɪən əv fʊt / 足太阴脾经 zútàiyīnpíjīng

tertiary collaterals / ˈtɜrʃieri kəˈlætərəlz / 孙络 sūn luò

three yang channels of foot / θri jæŋ ˈtʃænlz əv fʊt / 足三阳经 zúsānyángjīng

three yang channels of hand / θri jæŋ ˈtʃænlz əv hænd / 手三阳经 shǒusānyángjīng

three yang meridians of foot / θri jæŋ məˈrɪdɪənz əv fʊt / 足三阳经 zúsānyángjīng

three yang meridians of hand / θri jæŋ məˈrɪdɪənz əv hænd / 手三阳经 shǒusānyángjīng

three yin channels of foot / θri jɪn ˈtʃænlz əv fʊt / 足三阴经 zúsānyīnjīng

three yin channels of hand / θri jɪn ˈtʃænlz əv hænd / 手三阴经 shǒusānyīnjīng

three yin meridians of foot / θri jɪn məˈrɪdɪənz əv fʊt / 足三阴经 zúsānyīnjīng

three yin meridians of hand / θri jɪn məˈrɪdɪənz əv hænd / 手三阴经 shǒusānyīnjīng

twelve regular channels / twelv ˈregjələr ˈtʃænlz / 十二经脉 shíèrjīngmài

twelve regular meridians / twelv ˈregjələr məˈrɪdɪənz / 十二经脉 shíèrjīngmài

Yang Link Channel / jæŋ lɪŋk ˈtʃænl / 阳维脉 yáng

wéimài

Yang Link Vessel / jæŋ lɪŋk ˈvesl / 阳维脉 yángwéi mài

Yangming Large Intestine Channel of Hand / jæŋmɪŋ lɑrdʒ ɪnˈtestɪn ˈtʃænl əv hænd / 手阳明大肠经 shǒuyángmíngdàchángjīng

Yangming Large Intestine Meridian of Hand / jæŋmɪŋ lɑrdʒ ɪnˈtestɪn məˈrɪdɪən əv hænd / 手阳明大肠经 shǒuyángmíngdàchángjīng

Yangming Stomach Channel of Foot / jæŋmɪŋ ˈstʌmək ˈtʃænl əv fʊt / 足阳明胃经 zúyángmíng wèijīng

Yangming Stomach Meridian of Foot / jæŋmɪŋ ˈstʌmək məˈrɪdɪən əv fʊt / 足阳明胃经 zúyángmíng wèijīng

Yin Heel Channel / jɪn hil ˈtʃænl / 阴跷脉 yīnqiāo mài

Yin Heel Vessel / jɪn hil ˈvesl / 阴跷脉 yīnqiāomài

Yin Link Channel / jɪn lɪŋk ˈtʃænl / 阴维脉 yīnwéi mài

Yin Link Vessel / jɪn lɪŋk ˈvesl / 阴维脉 yīnwéimài

Section 4　Body and Orifices

第四节　形体官窍

abdomen / ˈæbdəmən / 腹 fù

acupoint chart / ˈækjuˈpɔint tʃɑrt / 明堂 míngtáng

anus / ˈeɪnəs / 魄门 pòmén

anus / ˈeɪnəs / 后阴 hòuyīn

auricle / ˈɔrɪkl / 耳郭 ěrguō

back / bæk / 背 bèi

black eye / blæk aɪ / 黑睛 hēijīng

bones / boʊnz / 百骸 bǎihái

bottom of throat / ˈbɑtəm əv θroʊt / 喉底 hóudǐ

bulbar conjunctiva and sclera / ˈbʌlbə ˌkɑndʒʌŋkˈtaɪvə ənd ˈsklɪrə / 白睛 báijīng

canthus / ˈkænθəs / 眦 zì

cervical vertebra / ˈsɜrvɪkl ˈvɜrtɪbrə / 颈骨 jǐnggǔ

coccyx / ˈkɑksɪks / 尾闾骨 wěilǘgǔ

convergent tendon / kənˈvɜrdʒənt ˈtendən / 宗筋 zōngjīn

cornea and iris / ˈkɔrniə ənd ˈaɪrɪs / 黑睛 hēijīng

crystal pearl / ˈkrɪstl pɜl / 晶珠 jīngzhū

diaphragm / ˈdaɪəfræm / 膈 gé

ear / ɪr / 耳 ěr

external genitalia / ekˈstɜrnəl dʒɛnəˈteljə / 前阴 qiányīn

external orifice of male urethra / ekˈstɜrnəl ˈɔrɪfɪs əv meɪl jʊˈriθrə / 精窍 jīngqiào

eye / aɪ / 目 mù

eye connector / aɪ kəˈnektər / 目系 mùxì

eye socket / aɪ ˈsɑkɪt / 目窠 mùkē

eyelash / ˈaɪlæʃ / 睫毛 jiémáo

eyelid / ˈaɪˌlɪd / 眼睑 yǎnjiǎn

five sense apertures / faɪv sens ˈæpərtʃʊrz / 五官 wǔguān

five wheels and eight regions / faɪv hwilz ənd eɪt ˈridʒənz / 五轮八廓 wǔlúnbākuò

four limbs / fɔr lɪmz / 四极 sìjí

four poles / fɔr polz / 四极 sìjí

genuine tooth / ˈdʒenjuɪn tuθ / 真牙 zhēnyá

gum / gʌm / 龈 yín

hand bone / hænd boʊn / 手骨 shǒugǔ

hard palate / hɑrd ˈpælət / 硬腭 yìng'è

head / hed / 头 tóu

hip / hɪp / 髋 kuān

hip bone / hɪp boʊn / 髋骨 kuāngǔ

house of intelligence / haʊs əv ɪnˈtelɪdʒəns / 精明之府 jīngmíngzhīfǔ

house of kidney / haʊs əv ˈkɪdni / 肾之府 shènzhīfǔ

house of tendons / haʊs əv ˈtendənz / 筋之府 jīnzhīfǔ

inner canthus / ˈɪnər ˈkænθəs / 目内眦 mùnèizì

interpleuro-diaphragmatic space / ɪnˈtɜrˈpluərə ˌdaɪəfræɡˈmætik speɪs / 膜原 móyuán

joint / dʒɔɪnt / 关节 guānjié

knee / ni / 膝 xī

lachrymal punctum / ˈlækrəml ˈpʌŋktəm / 泪窍 lèiqiào

lachrymal spring / ˈlækrəml sprɪŋ / 泪泉 lèiquán

lateral lower abdomen / ˈlætərəl ˈloə ˈæbdəmən / 少腹 shàofù

lateral thorax / ˈlætərəl ˈθɔræks / 胁肋 xiélèi

lens / lenz / 晶珠 jīngzhū

lip / lɪp / 唇 chún

lower abdomen / ˈloə ˈæbdəmən / 小腹 xiǎofù

lumbar bone / ˈlʌmbər boʊn / 腰骨 yāogǔ

mandibular angle / mænˈdɪbjələ ˈæŋgl / 曲牙 qǔyá

mastoid process / ˈmæstɔɪd proˈsɛs / 完骨 wángǔ

medial malleolus / ˈmidiəl məˈliələs / 合骨 hégǔ

membrane / ˈmembreɪn / 膜 mó

mo yuan / moʊ juɑn / 膜原 móyuán

mouth / maʊθ / 口 kǒu

muscle / ˈmʌsl / 肌肉 jīròu

nasal apex / ˈneɪzl ˈeɪpeks / 鼻准 bízhǔn

nasopharynx / ˌnezoˈfærɪŋks / 颃颡 hángsǎng

nine orifices / naɪn ˈɔrəfɪsɪz / 九窍 jiǔqiào

node of throat / noʊd əv θroʊt / 喉核 hóuhé

nose / noʊz / 鼻 bí

nose / noʊz / 明堂 míngtáng

occipital bone / ɑkˈsɪpətl boʊn / 枕骨 zhěngǔ

ocular band / ˈɑkjələr bænd / 眼带 yǎndài

ocular orbit / ˈɑkjələr ˈɔrbɪt / 目眶 mùkuàng

outer canthus / ˈaʊtər ˈkænθəs / 目外眦 mùwàizì

palate / ˈpælət / 腭 è

penis / ˈpinɪs / 茎 jīng

penis and testes / ˈpinɪs ənd ˈtestiz / 宗筋 zōngjīn

peri-navel region / ˈperiˈneɪvl ˈridʒən / 脐腹 qífù

pharynx / ˈfærɪŋks / 咽 yān

physique / fɪˈzik / 形 xíng

plantar / ˈplæntər / 跖 zhí

posterior pharyngeal wall / pɑˈstɪriər fəˈrɪndʒiəl wɔl / 喉底 hóudǐ

protruding bones / prəˈtrudɪŋ boʊnz / 高骨 gāogǔ

pubis bone / ˈpjubɪs boʊn / 交骨 jiāogǔ

seminal orifice / ˈsemɪnl ˈɔrɪfɪs / 精窍 jīngqiào

seven orifices / ˈsevn ˈɔrəfɪsɪz / 七窍 qīqiào

skin and hair / skɪn ənd her / 皮毛 pímáo

skull / skʌl / 头颅骨 tóulúgǔ

soft palate / sɔft ˈpælət / 软腭 ruǎn'è

soft tissue / sɔft ˈtɪʃu / 筋 jīn

spine / spaɪn / 脊 jǐ

striae and interstitial space / ˈstraɪɪ ənd ˌɪntərˈstɪʃl speɪs / 腠理 còulǐ

sublingual vessels and ligament / sʌbˈlɪŋgwəl ˈvɛsəlz ənd ˈlɪgəmənt / 舌系 shéxì

sweat pore / swet pɔr / 玄府 xuánfǔ

tear / ˈter / 泪 lèi

tendon / ˈtendən / 筋 jīn

testicle / ˈtestɪkl / 睾 gāo

throat / θroʊt / 喉 hóu

throat bar / θroʊt bɑr / 喉关 hóuguān

tongue / tʌŋ / 舌 shé

tongue connector / tʌŋ kəˈnektər / 舌系 shéxì

tonsil / ˈtɑnsl / 喉核 hóuhé

tooth / tuθ / 齿 chǐ

vaginal door / vəˈdʒaɪnl dɔr / 阴户 yīnhù

vaginal orifice / vəˈdʒaɪnl ˈɔrɪfɪs / 阴门 yīnmén

waist / weɪst / 腰 yāo

white eye / hwaɪt aɪ / 白睛 báijīng

wisdom tooth / ˈwɪzdəm tuθ / 真牙 zhēnyá

Section 5 Qi Blood and Body Fluid

第五节　气　血　津　液

acquired essence / əˈkwaɪrd ˈesns / 后天之精 hòutiān

zhījīng

anxiety / æŋ'zaɪəti / 虑 lǜ

ascending, descending, exiting and entering / ə'sɛndɪŋ dɪ'sɛndɪŋ 'eksɪtɪŋ ənd 'entərɪŋ / 升降出入 shēng jiàngchūrù

blood / blʌd / 血 xuè

blood being mother of qi / blʌd 'biɪŋ 'mʌðər 'əv tʃi / 血为气母 xuèwéiqìmǔ

blood being responsible for nurturing body / blʌd 'biɪŋ rɪ'spɑnsəbl fər 'nɜrtʃərɪŋ 'bɑdi / 血主濡之 xuè zhǔrúzhī

changing steaming in infant / 'tʃeɪndʒɪŋ 'stimɪŋ ɪn 'ɪnfənt / 变蒸 biànzhēng

clear fluid / klɪr 'fluɪd / 津 jīn

congenital essence / kən'dʒenɪtl 'esns / 先天之精 xiāntiānzhījīng

defensive qi / dɪ'fensɪv tʃi / 卫气 wèiqì

essence / 'esns / 精 jīng

essential qi / ɪ'senʃl tʃi / 精气 jīngqì

fluid / 'fluɪd / 津液 jīnyè

genuine qi / 'dʒenjuɪn tʃi / 真气 zhēnqì

growing fever and perspiration / 'groʊɪŋ 'fivər ənd ˌpəspə'reɪʃn / 变蒸

homogeny of clear fluid and blood / hɔ'mɔdʒəni əv klɪr 'fluɪd ənd blʌd / 津血同源 jīnxuètóngyuán

homogeny of essence and blood / hɔ'mɔdʒəni əv 'esns ənd blʌd / 精血同源 jīngxuètóngyuán

idea / aɪ'diə / 意 yì

inferior spirit / ɪnˈfɪriər ˈspɪrɪt / 魄 pò

mental activity / ˈmentl ækˈtɪvətɪ / 神 shén

middle qi / ˈmɪdl tʃi / 中气 zhōngqì

natural endowment / ˈnætʃrəl ɪnˈdaʊmənt / 禀赋 bǐngfù

nutrient qi / ˈnutriənt tʃi / 营气 yíngqì

nutrient-blood / ˈnutriənt blʌd / 营血 yíngxuè

pectoral qi / ˈpektərəl tʃi / 宗气 zōngqì

primordial qi / praɪˈmɔrdiəl tʃi / 元气 yuánqì

primordial spirit / praɪˈmɔrdiəl ˈspɪrɪt / 元神 yuánshén

qi / tʃi / 气 qì

qi being commander of blood / tʃi ˈbiɪŋ kəˈmændər əv blʌd / 气为血帅 qìwéixuèshuài

qi movement / tʃi ˈmuvmənt / 气机 qìjī

qi of Zang-Fu viscera / tʃi əv zæŋ fu ˈvɪsərə / 脏腑之气 zàngfǔzhīqì

qi transformation / tʃi ˌtrænsfərˈmeɪʃn / 气化 qìhuà

qi warming body / tʃi ˈwɔrmɪŋ ˈbɑdi / 气主煦之 qì zhǔxùzhī

root of body / rut əv ˈbɑdi / 身之本 shēnzhīběn

semen / ˈsimən / 精 jīng

soul / soʊl / 魂 hún

spirit / ˈspɪrɪt / 神 shén

spiritual mechanism / ˈspɪrɪtʃuəl ˈmekənɪzəm / 神机 shénjī

tender yang / ˈtendər jæŋ / 稚阳 zhìyáng

tender yin / ˈtendər jɪn / 稚阴 zhìyīn

thought / θɔt / 思 sī

turbid fluid / ˈtɜrbɪd ˈfluɪd / 液 yè

vitality / vaɪˈtæləti / 神 shén

will / wɪl / 志 zhì

wisdom / ˈwɪzdəm / 智 zhì

Section 6　Etiology

第六节　病　因

bitten by animal and insect / ˈbɪtn baɪ ˈænɪml ənd ˈɪnsekt / 虫兽伤 chóngshòushāng

cause of disease / kɔz əv dɪˈziz / 病因 bìngyīn

characteristic of dampness being descending / ˌkærəktəˈrɪstɪk əv ˈdæmpnəs ˈbiɪŋ dɪˈsɛndɪŋ / 湿性趋下 shīxìngqūxià

characteristic of dampness being heavy and turbid / ˌkærəktəˈrɪstɪk əv ˈdæmpnəs ˈbiɪŋ ˈhevi ənd ˈtɜrbɪd / 湿性重浊 shīxìngzhòngzhuó

characteristic of dampness being sticky and stagnant / ˌkærəktəˈrɪstɪk əv ˈdæmpnəs ˈbiɪŋ ˈstɪki ənd ˈstægnənt / 湿性黏滞 shīxìngniánzhì

characteristic of dryness being dry and puckery / ˌkærəktəˈrɪstɪk əv ˈdraɪnəs ˈbiɪŋ draɪ ənd ˈpʌkəri / 燥性干涩 zàoxìnggānsè

characteristic of fire being flaring up / ˌkærəktəˈrɪstɪk əv ˈfaɪər ˈbiɪŋ ˈflɛrɪŋ ʌp / 火性炎上 huǒxìngyán shàng

characteristic of summer-heat being ascending and dispersive / ˌkærəktəˈrɪstɪk əv ˈsʌmər hit ˈbiɪŋ əˈsɛndɪŋ ənd dɪˈspɝˑsɪv / 暑性升散 shǔxìngshēng sàn

characteristic of summer-heat being scorching-hot / ˌkærəktəˈrɪstɪk əv ˈsʌmər hit ˈbiɪŋ ˈskɔrtʃɪŋ hɑt / 暑性炎热 shǔxìngyánrè

characteristic of wind being mobile / ˌkærəktəˈrɪstɪk əv wɪnd ˈbiɪŋˈmoʊbl / 风性主动 fēngxìngzhǔdòng

cold having property of coagulation and stagnation / koʊld ˈhævɪŋ ˈprɑpərti əv koʊægjuˈleɪʃn ənd stægˈneɪʃn / 寒性凝滞 hánxìngníngzhì

cold having property of contraction / koʊld ˈhævɪŋ ˈprɑpərti əv kənˈtrækʃn / 寒性收引 hánxìngshōu yǐn

cold pathogen / koʊld ˈpæθədʒən / 寒邪 hánxié

cold pathogen being apt to attack yang / koʊld ˈpæθədʒən ˈbiɪŋ æpt tə əˈtæk jæŋ / 寒易伤阳 hán yìshāngyáng

cool dryness / kul ˈdraɪnəs / 凉燥 liángzào

damaged by excess of seven emotions / ˈdæmɪdʒd baɪ ɪkˈses əv ˈsevn ɪˈmoʃəns / 七情所伤 qīqíng suǒshāng

dampness hampering qi movement / ˈdæmpnəs ˈhæmpərɪŋ tʃi ˈmuvmənt / 湿阻气机 shīzǔqìjī

dampness pathogen / ˈdæmpnəs ˈpæθədʒən / 湿邪 shīxié

deficient pathogen / dɪˈfɪʃnt ˈpæθədʒən / 虚邪 xūxié

drinker / ˈdrɪŋkər / 酒客 jiǔkè

dryness likely to injure lung / ˈdraɪnəs ˈlaɪkli tə

'ɪndʒər lʌŋ / 燥易伤肺 zàoyìshāngfèi

dryness pathogen / 'draɪnəs 'pæθədʒən / 燥邪 zàoxié

etiology / ˌiti'ɑlədʒi / 病因学说 bìngyīnxuéshuō

excessive joy and anger impairing qi / ɪk'sesɪv dʒɔɪ ənd 'æŋgər ɪm'perɪŋ tʃi / 喜怒伤气 xǐnùshāngqì

excessive pathogen / ɪk'sesɪv 'pæθədʒən / 实邪 shíxié

excessive sexual intercourse / ɪk'sesɪv 'sekʃuəl 'ɪntərkɔrs / 房劳 fángláo

exogenous disease / ek'sɑdʒənəs dɪ'ziz / 外感 wàigǎn

external cause / ɪk'stɜrnl kɔz / 外因 wàiyīn

external injury / ɪk'stɜrnl 'ɪndʒəri / 外伤 wàishāng

fear impairing kidney / fɪr ɪm'perɪŋ 'kɪdni / 惊恐伤肾 jīngkǒngshāngshèn

fetal toxicity / 'fitl tɑk'sɪsəti / 胎毒 tāidú

fire being likely to cause convulsion and bleeding / 'faɪər 'biɪŋ 'laɪkli tə kɔz kən'vʌlʃn ənd 'blidɪŋ / 火易生风动血 huǒyìshēngfēngdòngxuè

fire being likely to disturb heart / 'faɪər 'biɪŋ 'laɪkli tə dɪ'stɜrb hɑrt / 火易扰心 huǒyìrǎoxīn

fire consuming qi and injuring yin / 'faɪər kən'sumɪŋ tʃi ənd 'ɪndʒərɪŋ jɪn / 火耗气伤阴 huǒhàoqìshāngyīn

fire pathogen / 'faɪər 'pæθədʒən / 火邪 huǒxié

five consumptions / faɪv kən'sʌmpʃns / 五劳 wǔláo

five pathogens / faɪv 'pæθədʒəns / 五邪 wǔxié

flavor predilection / 'flevə ˌpredl'ekʃn / 五味偏嗜 wǔwèipiānshì

fluid retention / 'fluɪd rɪ'tenʃn / 饮 yǐn

greasy and surfeit flavour / ˈgrisi ənd ˈsɜrfɪt ˈfleɪvər / 膏粱厚味 gāoliánghòuwèi

heat pathogen / hit ˈpæθədʒən / 热邪 rèxié

heat-toxicity / hit tɑkˈsɪsəti / 热毒 rèdú

injury due to diet / ˈɪndʒəri du tə ˈdaɪət / 饮食所伤 yǐnshísuǒshāng

insufficiency of natural endowment / ˌɪnsəˈfɪʃənsi əv ˈnætʃrəl ɪnˈdaʊmənt / 禀赋不足 bǐngfùbùzú

internal cause / ɪnˈtɜrnl kɔz / 内因 nèiyīn

internal damage / ɪnˈtɜrnl ˈdæmɪdʒ / 内伤 nèishāng

malarial pathogen / məˈleriəl ˈpæθədʒən / 疟邪 nüèxié

melancholy impairing lung / ˈmelənkɑli ɪmˈperɪŋ lʌŋ / 悲忧伤肺 bēiyōushāngfèi

miasma / miˈæzmə / 瘴气 zhàngqì

non-acclimatization / nɔn əklaɪmətəˈzeɪʃn / 水土不服 shuǐtǔbùfú

non-endo-non-exogenous cause / nɔn ˈendəu nɔn ekˈsɑdʒənəs kɔz / 不内外因 bùnèiwàiyīn

overstrain / ˈovəstren / 劳倦 láojuàn

overuse / ˌouvərˈjus / 过用 guòyòng

overuse causing disease / ˌouvərˈjus ˈkɔzɪŋ dɪˈziz / 病起过用 bìngqǐguòyòng

overwhelming joy impairing heart / ˌouvərˈwelmɪŋ dʒɔɪ ɪmˈperɪŋ hɑrt / 暴喜伤心 bàoxǐshāngxīn

pathogenic qi / ˌpæθəˈdʒenɪk tʃi / 邪气 xiéqì

person suffering from dampness / ˈpɜrsn ˈsʌfərɪŋ frəm ˈdæmpnəs / 湿家 shījiā

person suffering from jaundice / ˈpɝrsn ˈsʌfərɪŋ frəm ˈdʒɔndɪs / 黄家 huángjiā

person suffering from seminal loss / ˈpɝrsn ˈsʌfərɪŋ frəm ˈsemɪnl lɔs / 失精家 shījīngjiā

pestilent toxicity / ˈpestɪlənt tɑkˈsɪsəti / 瘟毒 wēndú

pestilential qi / ˌpestɪˈlenʃl tʃi / 疠气 lìqì

phlegm / flem / 痰 tán

phlegm and fluid retention / flem ənd ˈfluɪd rɪˈtenʃn / 痰饮 tányǐn

rage impairing liver / reɪdʒ ɪmˈperɪŋ ˈlɪvər / 大怒伤肝 dànùshānggān

seasonal pathogen / ˈsizənl ˈpæθədʒən / 时邪 shíxié

seven damages / ˈsevn ˈdæmɪdʒɪz / 七伤 qīshāng

six climatic exopathogens / sɪks klaɪˈmætɪk ˈeksəuˈpæθədʒəns / 六淫 liùyín

static blood / ˈstætɪk blʌd / 瘀血 yūxuè

summer-heat being likely to be mixed with dampness / ˈsʌmər hit ˈbiɪŋ ˈlaɪkli tə bi mɪkst wɪð ˈdæmpnəs / 暑易夹湿 shǔyìjiāshī

summer-heat being likely to disturb heart / ˈsʌmər hit ˈbiɪŋ ˈlaɪkli tə dɪˈstɝrb hɑrt / 暑易扰心 shǔyìrǎoxīn

summer-heat pathogen / ˈsʌmər hit ˈpæθədʒən / 暑邪 shǔxié

theory of three types of disease causes / ˈθiəri əv θri taɪps əv dɪˈziz kɔziz / 三因学说 sānyīnxuéshuō

three types of disease causes / θri taɪps əv dɪˈziz kɔziz / 三因 sānyīn

toxic pathogen causing measles / ˈtɑksɪk ˈpæθədʒən ˈkɔzɪŋ ˈmizlz / 麻毒 mádú

visiting pathogen / ˈvɪzɪtɪŋ ˈpæθədʒən / 客邪 kèxié

warm dryness / wɔrm ˈdraɪnəs / 温燥 wēnzào

wind being apt to attack yang portion of body / wɪnd ˈbiɪŋ æpt tə əˈtæk jæŋ ˈpɔrʃn əv ˈbɑdi / 风易伤阳位 fēngyìshāngyángwèi

wind being mobile and changeable / wɪnd ˈbiɪŋ ˈmoʊbl ənd ˈtʃeɪndʒəbl / 风善行数变 fēngshànxíngshuòbiàn

wind being primary pathogen / wɪnd ˈbiɪŋ ˈpraɪmeri ˈpæθədʒən / 风为百病之长 fēngwéibǎibìngzhīzhǎng

wind dryness / wɪnd ˈdraɪnəs / 风燥 fēngzào

wind pathogen / wɪnd ˈpæθədʒən / 风邪 fēngxié

wind pathogen being characterized by opening-dispersing / wɪnd ˈpæθədʒən ˈbiɪŋ ˈkærɪktəˈraɪzd baɪ ˈoʊpənɪŋ dɪˈspɝsɪŋ / 风性开泄 fēngxìngkāixiè

worry impairing spleen / ˈwɜri ɪmˈperɪŋ splin / 思虑伤脾 sīlǜshāngpí

wrong treatment / rɔŋ ˈtritmənt / 误治 wùzhì

yang pathogen / jæŋ ˈpæθədʒən / 阳邪 yángxié

yin pathogen / jɪn ˈpæθədʒən / 阴邪 yīnxié

Section 7　Pathogenesis
第七节　病　机

* **dampness stagnancy due to spleen deficiency** / ˈdæmpnəs ˈstægnənsi du tə splin dɪˈfɪʃnsi / 脾虚

脾虚湿困 píxūshīkùn

* **deficiency of both heart and spleen** / dɪˈfɪʃnsi əv bouθ hɑrt ənd splin / 心脾两虚 xīnpíliǎngxū

* **deficiency of lung qi** / dɪˈfɪʃnsi əv lʌŋ tʃi / 肺气虚 fèiqìxū

* **deficiency of spleen qi** / dɪˈfɪʃnsi əv splin tʃi / 脾气虚 píqìxū

* **disharmony between heart and kidney** / dɪsˈhɑrməni bɪˈtwin hɑrt ənd ˈkɪdni / 心肾不交 xīnshènbùjiāo

* **disharmony between nutrient qi and defensive qi** / dɪsˈhɑrməni bɪˈtwin ˈnutriənt tʃi ənd dɪˈfensɪv tʃi / 营卫不和 yíngwèibùhé

* **flaring up of heart fire** / ˈflɛrɪŋ ʌp əv hɑrt ˈfaɪər / 心火上炎 xīnhuǒshàngyán

* **qi deficiency of heart and lung** / tʃi dɪˈfɪʃnsi əv hɑrt ənd lʌŋ / 心肺气虚 xīnfèiqìxū

* **wind-heat invading lung** / wɪnd hit ɪnˈvedɪŋ lʌŋ / 风热犯肺 fēngrèfànfèi

* **yang deficiency of spleen and kidney** / jæŋ dɪˈfɪʃnsi əv splin ənd ˈkɪdni / 脾肾阳虚 píshènyángxū

accumulation of dry feces / əˌkjumjəˈleɪʃn əv draɪ ˈfisiz / 燥结 zàojié

adverse rising of stomach qi / ədˈvɜrs ˈraɪzɪŋ əv ˈstʌmək tʃi / 胃气上逆 wèiqìshàngnì

alternate cold and heat / ˈɔltərnət kould ənd hit / 厥热胜复 juérèshèngfù

anorexia / ˌænəˈreksiə / 胃纳呆滞 wèinàdāizhì

bleeding due to qi reversed flow / ˈblidɪŋ du tə tʃi

rɪˈvɜst floʊ / 血随气逆 xuèsuíqìnì

blocked heat / blɑkt hit / 热遏 rè'è

blood deficiency / blʌd dɪˈfɪʃnsi / 血虚 xuèxū

blood deficiency causing wind / blʌd dɪˈfɪʃnsi ˈkɔzɪŋ wɪnd / 血虚生风 xuèxūshēngfēng

blood deficiency of heart and liver / blʌd dɪˈfɪʃnsi əv hɑrt ənd ˈlɪvər / 心肝血虚 xīngānxuèxū

blood depletion / blʌd dɪˈpliʃn / xuètuō 血脱

blood disease involving qi / blʌd dɪˈziz ɪnˈvɑlvɪŋ tʃi / 血病及气 xuèbìngjíqì

blood dryness causing wind / blʌd ˈdraɪnəs ˈkɔzɪŋ wɪnd / 血燥生风 xuèzàoshēngfēng

blood stasis / blʌd ˈsteɪsɪs / 血瘀 xuèyū

blood stasis due to qi deficiency / blʌd ˈsteɪsɪs du tə tʃi dɪˈfɪʃnsi / 气虚血瘀 qìxūxuèyū

blood tier / blʌd tɪr / 血分 xuèfēn

clear fluid depletion / klɪr ˈfluɪd dɪˈpliʃn / 津脱 jīntuō

cold accumulation of large intestine / koʊld əˌkjumjəˈleɪʃn əv lɑrdʒ ɪnˈtestɪn / 大肠寒结 dàchánghánjié

cold attack on paired channels / koʊld əˈtæk ɑn pɛrd ˈtʃænlz / 两感 liǎnggǎn

cold in blood / koʊld ɪn blʌd / 血寒 xuèhán

cold manifestation due to yang deficiency / koʊld mænɪfeˈsteɪʃn də tə jæŋ dɪˈfɪʃnsi / 阳虚生寒 yángxūshēnghán

cold transformation of Shaoyin disease / koʊld ˌtrænsfərˈmeɪʃn əv ʃaʊjɪn dɪˈziz / 少阴寒化 shàoyīn hánhuà

cold transformed from yin / koʊld trænsˈfɔrmd frəm jɪn / 从阴化寒 cóngyīnhuàhán

cold-dampness disturbing spleen / koʊld ˈdæmpnəs dɪˈstɜrbɪŋ splin / 寒湿困脾 hánshīkùnpí

consumption of vital essence / kənˈsʌmpʃn əv ˈvaɪtl ˈesns / 精气夺 jīngqìduó

damage of collaterals in lung / ˈdæmɪdʒ əv kəˈlætərəlz ɪn lʌŋ / 肺络损伤 fèiluòsǔnshāng

damaged lung not functioning normally / ˈdæmɪdʒd lʌŋ nɑt ˈfʌŋkʃənɪŋ ˈnɔrməli / 金破不鸣 jīnpòbùmíng

dampness-heat in lower jiao / ˈdæmpnəs hit ɪn ˈloə dʒjɑʊ / 下焦湿热 xiàjiāoshīrè

dampness-heat in middle jiao / ˈdæmpnəs hit ɪn ˈmɪdl dʒjɑʊ / 中焦湿热 zhōngjiāoshīrè

dampness-heat in upper jiao / ˈdæmpnəs hit ɪn ˈʌpər dʒjɑʊ / 上焦湿热 shàngjiāoshīrè

dampness-heat of bladder / ˈdæmpnəs hit əv ˈblædər / 膀胱湿热 pángguāngshīrè

dampness-heat of large intestine / ˈdæmpnəs hit əv lɑrdʒ ɪnˈtestɪn / 大肠湿热 dàchángshīrè

dampness-heat of liver and gallbladder / ˈdæmpnəs hit əv ˈlɪvər ənd ˈgɔlˌblædə / 肝胆湿热 gāndǎnshīrè

dampness-heat of liver channel / ˈdæmpnəs hit əv ˈlɪvər ˈtʃænl / 肝经湿热 gānjīngshīrè

dampness-heat of spleen and stomach / ˈdæmpnəs hit əv splin ənd ˈstʌmək / 脾胃湿热 píwèishīrè

dampness-heat stagnating in spleen / ˈdæmpnəs hit ˈstægneɪtɪŋ ɪn splin / 湿热蕴脾 shīrèyùnpí

decline of vital gate fire / dɪˈklaɪn əv ˈvaɪtl geɪt ˈfaɪər / 命门火衰 mìngménhuǒshuāi

defense tier / dɪˈfɛns tɪr / 卫分 wèifēn

defensive yang being obstructed / dɪˈfensɪv jæŋ ˈbiɪŋ əbˈstrʌktɪd / 卫阳被遏 wèiyángbèi'è

deficiency / dɪˈfɪʃnsi / 虚 xū

deficiency complicated with excess / dɪˈfɪʃnsi ˈkɑmplɪkeɪtɪd wɪð ɪkˈses / 虚中夹实 xūzhōngjiáshí

deficiency of both lung and spleen / dɪˈfɪʃnsi əv boʊθ lʌŋ ənd splin / 肺脾两虚 fèipíliǎngxū

deficiency of both qi and yin / dɪˈfɪʃnsi əv boʊθ tʃi ənd jɪn / 气阴两虚 qìyīnliǎngxū

deficiency of both yin and yang / dɪˈfɪʃnsi əv boʊθ jɪn ən jæŋ / 阴阳两虚 yīnyángliǎngxū

deficiency of defensive qi / dɪˈfɪʃnsi əv dɪˈfensɪv tʃi / 卫气虚 wèiqìxū

deficiency of either yin or yang / dɪˈfɪʃnsi əv ˈiðər jɪn ɔr jæŋ / 阴阳偏衰 yīnyángpiānshuāi

deficiency of heart qi / dɪˈfɪʃnsi əv hɑrt tʃi / 心气虚 xīnqìxū

deficiency of kidney qi / dɪˈfɪʃnsi əv ˈkɪdni tʃi / 肾气虚 shènqìxū

deficiency of kidney qi failing to control respiring qi / dɪˈfɪʃnsi əv ˈkɪdni tʃi ˈfeɪlɪŋ tə kənˈtroʊl rɪˈspaɪərɪŋ tʃi / 肾不纳气 shènbùnàqì

deficiency of kidney yang / dɪˈfɪʃnsi əv ˈkɪdni jæŋ

肾阳虚 shènyángxū

deficiency of kidney yin / dɪ'fɪʃnsi əv 'kɪdni jɪn / 肾阴虚 shènyīnxū

deficiency of liver blood / dɪ'fɪʃnsi əv 'lɪvər blʌd / 肝血虚 gānxuèxū

deficiency of liver qi / dɪ'fɪʃnsi əv 'lɪvər tʃi / 肝气虚 gānqìxū

deficiency of liver yang / dɪ'fɪʃnsi əv 'lɪvər jæŋ / 肝阳虚 gānyángxū

deficiency of liver yin / dɪ'fɪʃnsi əv 'lɪvər jɪn / 肝阴虚 gānyīnxū

deficiency of lung yin / dɪ'fɪʃnsi əv lʌŋ jɪn / 肺阴虚 fèiyīnxū

deficiency of spleen and stomach / dɪ'fɪʃnsi əv splin ənd 'stʌmək / 脾胃虚弱 píwèixūruò

deficiency of spleen yang / dɪ'fɪʃnsi əv splin jæŋ / 脾阳虚 píyángxū

deficiency of spleen yin / dɪ'fɪʃnsi əv splin jɪn / 脾阴虚 píyīnxū

deficiency of stomach qi / dɪ'fɪʃnsi əv 'stʌmək tʃi / 胃气虚 wèiqìxū

deficiency of stomach yin / dɪ'fɪʃnsi əv 'stʌmək jɪn / 胃阴虚 wèiyīnxū

deficiency transformed from excess / dɪ'fɪʃnsi træns 'fɔrmd frəm ɪk'ses / 由实转虚 yóushízhuǎnxū

deficiency transmitted from lower body to upper body / dɪ'fɪʃnsi trænz'mɪtɪd frəm 'loə 'bɑdi tə 'ʌpər 'bɑdi / 下损及上 xiàsǔnjíshàng

deficiency transmitted from upper body to lower body / dɪˈfɪʃnsi trænzˈmɪtɪd frəm ˈʌpər ˈbɑdi tə ˈloʊ ˈbɑdi / 上损及下 shàngsǔnjíxià

deficient cold of bladder / dɪˈfɪʃnt koʊld əv ˈblædər / 膀胱虚寒 pángguāngxūhán

deficient cold of large intestine / dɪˈfɪʃnt koʊld əv lɑrdʒ ɪnˈtestɪn / 大肠虚寒 dàchángxūhán

deficient cold of small intestine / dɪˈfɪʃnt koʊld əv smɔl ɪnˈtestɪn / 小肠虚寒 xiǎochángxūhán

deficient cold of spleen and stomach / dɪˈfɪʃnt koʊld əv splin ənd ˈstʌmək / 脾胃虚寒 píwèixūhán

deficient disease located in Taiyin / dɪˈfɪʃnt dɪˈziz ˈloʊkeɪtɪd ɪn taɪˌjɪn / 虚则太阴 xūzétàiyīn

deficient yang with upper manifestation / dɪˈfɪʃnt jæŋ wɪð ˈʌpər ˌmænɪfeˈsteɪʃn / 虚阳上浮 xūyángshàngfú

depletion of essence / dɪˈpliʃn əv ˈesns / 精脱 jīngtuō

depletion of fluid causing blood dryness / dɪˈpliʃn əv ˈfluɪd ˈkɔzɪŋ blʌd ˈdraɪnəs / 津枯血燥 jīnkūxuèzào

depletion of fluid involving qi desertion / dɪˈpliʃn əv ˈfluɪd ɪnˈvɑlvɪŋ tʃi dɪˈzɜrʃn / 气随液脱 qìsuíyètuō

depletion of yin causing yang collapse / dɪˈpliʃn əv jɪn ˈkɔzɪŋ jæŋ kəˈlæps / 阴竭阳脱 yīnjiéyángtuō

devitalization of heart yang / diˌvaɪtəlɪˈzeʃən əv hɑrt jæŋ / 心阳不振 xīnyángbùzhèn

direct attack / dəˈrekt əˈtæk / 直中 zhízhòng

discomfort in stomach / dɪsˈkʌmfərt ɪn ˈstʌmək / 胃不和 wèibùhé

disease arising from yang / dɪˈziz əˈraɪzɪŋ frəm jæŋ / 病发于阳 bìngfāyúyáng

disease arising from yin / dɪˈziz əˈraɪzɪŋ frəm jɪn / 病发于阴 bìngfāyúyīn

disease caused by disorder of this channel / dɪˈziz kɔzd baɪ dɪsˈɔrdər əv ðɪs ˈtʃænl / 是动病 shìdòngbìng

disease involving other channel / dɪˈziz ɪnˈvɑlvɪŋ ˈʌð ˈtʃænl / 再经 zàijīng

disease involving two or more channels / dɪˈziz ɪnˈvɑlvɪŋ tu ɔr mɔr ˈtʃænlz / 合病 hébìng

disease involving weifen and qifen / dɪˈziz ɪnˈvɑlvɪŋ weɪfen ənd tʃifen / 卫气同病 wèiqìtóngbìng

disease involving weifen and yingfen / dɪˈziz ɪnˈvɑlvɪŋ weɪfen ənd jɪŋfen / 卫营同病 wèiyíngtóngbìng

disease of one channel involving another channel / dɪˈziz əv wʌn tʃænl ɪnˈvɑlvɪŋ əˈnʌðər tʃænl / 并病 bìngbìng

disease of one channel without transmission / dɪˈziz əv wʌn ˈtʃænl wɪˈðaʊt trænzˈmɪʃn / 经尽 jīngjìn

disease of viscera connecting with this channel / dɪˈziz əv ˈvɪsərə kəˈnektɪŋ wɪð ðɪs ˈtʃænl / 所生病 suǒshēngbìng

disease transmitting from one channel to another / dɪˈziz trænzˈmɪtɪŋ frəm wʌn ˈtʃænl tə əˈnʌðər / 过经 guòjīng

disharmony of Chong and Conception Channels / dɪsˈhɑrməni əv tʃʊŋ ənd kənˈsepʃn ˈtʃænlz / 冲任不调 chōngrènbùtiáo

disorder of qi and blood / dɪsˈɔrdər əv tʃi ənd blʌd / 气血失调 qìxuèshītiáo

disorder of qi movement / dɪsˈɔrdər əv tʃi ˈmuvmənt / 气机不利 qìjībùlì

divorce of yin-yang / dɪˈvɔrs əv jɪn jæŋ / 阴阳离决 yīnyánglíjué

dry qi impairing lung / draɪ tʃi ɪmˈperɪŋ lʌŋ / 燥气伤肺 zàoqìshāngfèi

dry-heat impairing lung / draɪ hit ɪmˈperɪŋ lʌŋ / 燥热伤肺 zàorèshāngfèi

dryness affecting clear orifices / ˈdraɪnəs əˈfektɪŋ klɪr ˈɔrəfɪsɪz / 燥干清窍 zàogānqīngqiào

dryness-heat / ˈdraɪnəs hit / 燥热 zàorè

dysfunction of spleen in transportation / dɪsˈfʌŋkʃn əv splin ɪn ˌtrænspɔrˈteɪʃn / 脾失健运 píshījiànyùn

endogenous cold / enˈdɑdʒənəs koʊld / 内寒 nèihán

endogenous dampness / enˈdɑdʒənəs ˈdæmpnəs / 内湿 nèishī

endogenous dryness / enˈdɑdʒənəs ˈdraɪnəs / 内燥 nèizào

endogenous heat / enˈdɑdʒənəs hit / 内热 nèirè

endogenous wind / enˈdɑdʒənəs wɪnd / 内风 nèifēng

excess / ɪkˈses / 实 shí

excess complicated with deficiency / ɪkˈses ˈkɑmplɪkeɪtɪd wɪð dɪˈfɪʃnsi / 实中夹虚 shízhōngjiáxū

excess of either yin or yang / ɪkˈses əv ˈiðər jɪn ɔr jæŋ / 阴阳偏盛 yīnyángpiānshèng

excess of pathogenic qi / ɪkˈses əv ˌpæθəˈdʒenɪk tʃi / 邪气盛 xiéqìshèng

excess of stomach and intestine / ɪkˈses əv ˈstʌmək ənd ɪnˈtestɪn / 胃家实 wèijiāshí

excess resulted from deficiency / ɪkˈses rɪˈzʌltɪd frəm dɪˈfɪʃnsi / 因虚致实 yīnxūzhìshí

excessive disease located in yangming / ɪkˈsesɪv dɪˈziz ˈloʊkeɪtɪd ɪn jæŋmɪŋ / 实则阳明 shízéyángmíng

excessive heat of liver and gallbladder / ɪkˈsesɪv hit əv ˈlɪvər ənd ˈgɔlˌblædə / 肝胆实热 gāndǎnshírè

excessive heat of small intestine / ɪkˈsesɪv hit əv smɔl ɪnˈtestɪn / 小肠实热 xiǎochángshírè

excessive joy leading to qi loose / ɪkˈsesɪv dʒɔɪ ˈlidɪŋ tə tʃi lus / 喜则气缓 xǐzéqìhuǎn

excessive sorrow leading to qi consumption / ɪkˈsesɪv ˈsɑroʊ ˈlidɪŋ tə tʃi kənˈsʌmpʃn / 悲则气消 bēizéqìxiāo

expulsion of yin-yang / ɪkˈspʌlʃn əv jɪn jæŋ / 阴阳格拒 yīnyánggéjù

extreme heat causing wind / ɪkˈstrim hit ˈkɔzɪŋ wɪnd / 热极生风 rèjíshēngfēng

extreme yang with yin manifestation / ɪkˈstrim jæŋ wɪð jɪn ˌmænɪfeˈsteɪʃn / 阳极似阴 yángjísìyīn

extreme yin with yang manifestation / ɪkˈstrim jɪn wɪð jæŋ ˌmænɪfeˈsteɪʃn / 阴极似阳 yīnjísìyáng

exuberance of heart fire / ɪgˈzubərəns əv hɑrt ˈfaɪər /

心火亢盛 xīnhuǒkàngshèng

exuberance of stomach fire / ɪgˈzubərəns əv ˈstʌmək ˈfaɪər / 胃火炽盛 wèihuǒchìshèng

exuberant fire of heart and stomach / ɪgˈzubərənt ˈfaɪər əv hɑrt ənd ˈstʌmək / 心胃火燔 xīnwèihuǒfán

failure in qi transformation / ˈfeɪljər ɪn tʃi ˌtrænsfərˈmeɪʃn / 气化无权 qìhuàwúquán

failure of keeping fluid due to qi deficiency / ˈfeɪljər əv ˈkipɪŋ ˈfluɪd du tə tʃi dɪˈfɪʃnsi / 气虚不摄 qìxūbùshè

failure of lung qi in dispersion / ˈfeɪljər əv lʌŋ tʃi ɪn dɪˈspɜrʒn / 肺气不宣 fèiqìbùxuān

failure of qi transforming fluid / ˈfeɪljər əv tʃi trænsˈfɔrmɪŋ ˈfluɪd / 气不化津 qìbùhuàjīn

failure of stomach qi to descend / ˈfeɪljər əv ˈstʌmək tʃi tə dɪˈsend / 胃气不降 wèiqìbùjiàng

fear leading to qi sinking / fɪr ˈlidɪŋ tə tʃi ˈsɪŋkɪŋ / 恐则气下 kǒngzéqìxià

fetal infection / ˈfitl ɪnˈfekʃn / 胎传 tāichuán

fever due to yin deficiency / ˈfivər du tə jɪn dɪˈfɪʃnsi / 阴虚发热 yīnxūfārè

fire stagnation / ˈfaɪər stægˈneɪʃn / 火郁 huǒyù

five exhaustions / faɪv ɪgˈzɔstʃəns / 五夺 wǔduó

five minds transforming into fire / faɪv maɪndz trænsˈfɔrmɪŋ ˈɪntə ˈfaɪər / 五志化火 wǔzhìhuàhuǒ

flaring heat in qifen and xuefen / ˈflɛrɪŋ hit ɪn tʃifen ənd ʃuɛfen / 气血两燔 qìxuèliǎngfán

flaring heat in qifen and yingfen / ˈflɛrɪŋ hit ɪn tʃifen ənd jɪŋfen / 气营两燔 qìyíngliǎngfán

flaring up of deficient fire / ˈflɛrɪŋ ʌp əv dɪˈfɪʃnt ˈfaɪər / 虚火上炎 xūhuǒshàngyán

flatulence caused by qi deficiency / ˈflætʃələns kɔzd baɪ tʃi dɪˈfɪʃnsi / 气虚中满 qìxūzhōngmǎn

fluid insufficiency of large intestine / ˈfluɪd ˌɪnsəˈfɪʃənsi əv lɑrdʒ ɪnˈtestɪn / 大肠液亏 dàchángyèkuī

fright leading to qi turbulence / fraɪt ˈlidɪŋ tə tʃi ˈtɜrbjələns / 惊则气乱 jīngzéqìluàn

Fu-viscera disease involving Zang-viscera / fu ˈvɪsərə dɪˈziz ɪnˈvɑlvɪŋ zæŋ ˈvɪsərə / 腑病及脏 fǔbìng jízàng

half-superficies and half-interior / hæf ˌsʊpəˈfɪʃˌiz ənd hæf ɪnˈtɪriər / 半表半里 bànbiǎobànlǐ

heart spirit confused by phlegm / hɑrt ˈspɪrɪt kənˈfjuzd baɪ flem / 痰蒙心窍 tánméngxīnqiào

heat accumulation / hit əˌkjumjəˈleɪʃn / 热结 rèjié

heat accumulation of bladder / hit əkjumjəˈleɪʃn əv ˈblædər / 热结膀胱 rèjiépángguāng

heat accumulation of large intestine / hit əˌkjumjəˈleɪʃn əv lɑrdʒ ɪnˈtestɪn / 大肠热结 dàchángrèjié

heat affecting spirit / hit əˈfektɪŋ ˈspɪrɪt / 热伤神明 rèshāngshénmíng

heat blockade / hit blɑˈkeɪd / 热闭 rèbì

heat in blood / hit ɪn blʌd / 血热 xuèrè

heat invading blood chamber / hit ɪnˈvedɪŋ blʌd ˈtʃeɪmber / 热入血室 rèrùxuèshì

heat invading large intestine / hit ɪnˈvedɪŋ lɑrdʒ

ɪnˈtestɪn / 热迫大肠 rèpòdàcháng

heat invading xuefen / hit ɪnˈvedɪŋ ʃuɛfen / 热入血分 rèrùxuèfēn

heat lodging in Chong and Conception Channels / hit ˈlɑdʒɪŋ ɪn tʃʊŋ ənd kənˈsepʃn ˈtʃænlz / 热伏冲任 rèfúchōngrèn

heat stagnation / hit stægˈneɪʃn / 热郁 rèyù

heat transformation of Shaoyin disease / hit trænsfərˈmeɪʃn əv ʃɑʊjɪn dɪˈziz / 少阴热化 shàoyīnrèhuà

heat transformed from yang / hit trænsˈfɔrmd frəm jæŋ / 从阳化热 cóngyánghuàrè

heat-toxicity in xuefen / hit tɑkˈsɪsəti ɪn ʃuɛfen / 血分热毒 xuèfēnrèdú

hidden pathogen / ˈhɪdn ˈpæθədʒən / 伏邪 fúxié

hyperactive liver yang causing wind / ˌhaɪpərˈæktɪv ˈlɪvər jæŋ ˈkɔzɪŋ wɪnd / 肝阳化风 gānyánghuàfēng

hyperactivity of fire due to yin deficiency / ˌhaɪpəræktˈɪvəti əv ˈfaɪər du tə jɪn dɪˈfɪʃnsi / 阴虚火旺 yīnxūhuǒwàng

hyperactivity of heart-liver fire / ˌhaɪpəræktˈɪvəti əv hɑrt ˈlɪvər ˈfaɪər / 心肝火旺 xīngānhuǒwàng

hyperactivity of ministerial fire / ˌhaɪpəræktˈɪvəti əv ˌmɪnɪˈstɪriəl ˈfaɪər / 相火妄动 xiànghuǒwàngdòng

hyperactivity of yang due to yin deficiency / ˌhaɪpəræktˈɪvəti əv jæŋ du tə jɪn dɪˈfɪʃnsi / 阴虚阳亢 yīn xūyángkàng

impaired depurative descending of lung qi / ɪmˈperd dɪˈpjʊərətɪv dɪˈsɛndɪŋ əv lʌŋ tʃi / 肺失清肃 fèishīqīngsù

impairment of fluid / ɪmˈpermənt əv ˈfluɪd / 伤津 shāngjīn

infection / ɪnˈfekʃn / 传染 chuánrǎn

injury of fluid due to exuberant heat / ˈɪndʒəri əv ˈfluɪd du tə ɪgˈzubərənt hit / 热炽津伤 rèchìjīnshāng

inner blocking causing collapse / ˈɪnər ˈblɑkɪŋ ˈkɔzɪŋ kəˈlæps / 内闭外脱 nèibìwàituō

insidious onset / ɪnˈsɪdiəs ˈɑnset / 徐发 xúfā

insufficiency of gallbladder qi causing timidity / ˌɪnsəˈfɪʃənsi əv ˈgɔlˌblædə tʃi ˈkɔzɪŋ tɪˈmɪdəti / 胆虚气怯 dǎnxūqìqiè

insufficiency of heart yin / ˌɪnsəˈfɪʃənsi əv hɑrt jɪn / 心阴不足 xīnyīnbùzú

insufficiency of kidney essence / ˌɪnsəˈfɪʃənsi əv ˈkɪdni ˈesns / 肾精不足 shènjīngbùzú

interior cold / ɪnˈtɪriər koʊld / 里寒 lǐhán

interior deficiency / ɪnˈtɪriər dɪˈfɪʃnsi / 里虚 lǐxū

interior disease involving superficies / ɪnˈtɪriər dɪˈziz ɪnˈvɑlvɪŋ ˌsupəˈfɪʃɪˌiz / 里病出表 lǐbìngchūbiǎo

interior excess / ɪnˈtɪriər ɪkˈses / 里实 lǐshí

interior heat / ɪnˈtɪriər hit / 里热 lǐrè

intermingled cold and heat / ˌɪntərˈmɪŋgld koʊld ənd hit / 寒热错杂 hánrècuòzá

intermingled deficiency and excess / ˌɪntərˈmɪŋgld dɪˈfɪʃnsi ənd ɪkˈses / 虚实夹杂 xūshíjiāzá

invasion of pericardium by heat / ɪnˈveɪʒn əv ˌpɛrɪˈkɑrdɪəm baɪ hit / 热入心包 rèrùxīnbāo

kidney failing to nourish liver / ˈkɪdni ˈfeɪlɪŋ tə ˈnɜrɪʃ ˈlɪvər / 水不涵木 shuǐbùhánmù

liver fire flaring up / ˈlɪvər ˈfaɪər ˈflɛrɪŋ ʌp / 肝火上炎 gānhuǒshàngyán

liver fire invading lung / ˈlɪvər ˈfaɪər ɪnˈvedɪŋ lʌŋ / 肝火犯肺 gānhuǒfànfèi

liver qi invading spleen / ˈlɪvər tʃi ɪnˈvedɪŋ splin / 肝气犯脾 gānqìfànpí

liver qi invading stomach / ˈlɪvər tʃi ɪnˈvedɪŋ ˈstʌmək / 肝气犯胃 gānqìfànwèi

lung being reservoir of phlegm / lʌŋ ˈbiɪŋ ˈrezərvwɑr əv flem / 肺为贮痰之器 fèiwéizhùtánzhīqì

malnutrition of heart blood / ˌmælnuˈtrɪʃn əv hɑrt blʌd / 心血失养 xīnxuèshīyǎng

mistreatment by warming therapy / ˌmɪsˈtritmənt baɪ ˈwɔrmɪŋ ˈθerəpi / 火逆 huǒnì

new affection / nu əˈfekʃn / 新感 xīngǎn

non-consolidation of kidney qi / nɔn kənˌsɑlɪˈdeɪʃn əv ˈkɪdni tʃi / 肾气不固 shènqìbùgù

nutrient qi and yin fluid being damaged / ˈnutriənt tʃi ənd jɪn ˈfluɪd ˈbiɪŋ ˈdæmɪdʒd / 气阴两伤 qìyīn liǎngshāng

nutrient tier / ˈnutriənt tɪr / 营分 yíngfēn

obstructed lung not functioning normally / əbˈstrʌktɪd lʌŋ nɑt ˈfʌŋkʃənɪŋ ˈnɔrməli / 金实不鸣 jīnshíbùmíng

over consumption of heart nutrient / ˈouvər kənˈsʌmpʃn əv hɑrt ˈnutriənt / 心营过耗 xīnyíngguòhào

overexertion leading to qi consumption / ˌouvərigˈzəʃən ˈlidɪŋ tə tʃi kənˈsʌmpʃn / 劳则气耗 láozéqìhào

overheat causing qi leakage / ˌouvərˈhit ˈkɔzɪŋ tʃi ˈlikɪdʒ / 炅则气泄 jiǒngzéqìxiè

pathogenesis / ˌpæθəˈdʒenɪsɪs / 病机 bìngjī

pensiveness leading to qi knotting / ˈpensɪvnɪs ˈlidɪŋ tə tʃi nɒtɪŋ / 思则气结 sīzéqìjié

phlegm stasis causing wind / flem ˈsteɪsɪs ˈkɔzɪŋ wɪnd / 痰瘀生风 tányūshēngfēng

phlegm-fire disturbing heart / flem ˈfaɪər dɪˈstɜrbɪŋ hɑrt / 痰火扰心 tánhuǒrǎoxīn

predominant dampness causing diarrhea / prɪˈdɑmɪnənt ˈdæmpnəs ˈkɔzɪŋ ˌdaɪəˈriə / 湿胜[则]濡泻 shīshèng[zé]rúxiè

predominant dampness causing weak yang / prɪˈdɑmɪnənt ˈdæmpnəs ˈkɔzɪŋ wik jæŋ / 湿胜阳微 shīshèngyángwēi

predominant dryness causing withering / prɪˈdɑmɪnənt ˈdraɪnəs ˈkɔzɪŋ ˈwɪðərɪŋ / 燥胜则干 zàoshèngzégān

predominant heat causing swelling / prɪˈdɑmɪnənt hit ˈkɔzɪŋ ˈswelɪŋ / 热胜则肿 rèshèngzézhǒng

predominate wind causing motion / prɪˈdɑmɪneɪt wɪnd ˈkɔzɪŋ ˈmouʃn / 风胜则动 fēngshèngzédòng

qi blockage / tʃi ˈblɑkɪdʒ / 气闭 qìbì

qi deficiency / tʃi dɪˈfɪʃnsi / 气虚 qìxū

qi deficiency of lung and kidney / tʃi dɪˈfɪʃnsi əv lʌŋ ənd ˈkɪdni / 肺肾气虚 fèishènqìxū

qi depression transforming into fire / tʃi dɪˈpreʃn trænsˈfɔrmɪŋ ˈɪntə ˈfaɪər / 气郁化火 qìyùhuàhuǒ

qi depression / tʃi dɪˈpreʃn / 气郁 qìyù

qi desertion / tʃi dɪˈzɜrʃn / 气脱 qìtuō

qi desertion due to blood depletion / tʃi dɪˈzɜrʃn du tə blʌd dɪˈpliʃn / 气随血脱 qìsuíxuètuō

qi disease involving blood / tʃi dɪˈziz ɪnˈvɑlvɪŋ blʌd / 气病及血 qìbìngjíxuè

qi failing to control blood / tʃi ˈfeɪlɪŋ tə kənˈtroʊl blʌd / 气不摄血 qìbùshèxuè

qi stagnation / tʃi stægˈneɪʃn / 气滞 qìzhì

qi tier / tʃi tɪr / 气分 qìfēn

qifen / tʃifən / 气分 qìfén

rage leading to qi ascending / reɪdʒ ˈlidɪŋ tə tʃi əˈsɛndɪŋ / 怒则气上 nùzéqìshàng

recurrence caused by dietary irregularity / rɪˈkɜrəns kɔzd baɪ ˈdaɪəteri ɪˌregjəˈlærəti / 食复 shífù

recurrence caused by overexertion / rɪˈkɜrəns kɔzd baɪ ˌoʊvərigˈzɜʃən / 劳复 láofù

rehabilitation / ˌriəbɪlɪˈteɪʃn / 康复 kāngfù

reverse transmission / rɪˈvɜrs trænzˈmɪʃn / 逆传 nìchuán

reversed flow of qi / rɪˈvɜrst floʊ əv tʃi / 气逆 qìnì

reversed transmission to pericardium / rɪˈvɜrst trænzˈmɪʃn tə ˌperɪˈkɑrdiəm / 逆传心包 nìchuánxīnbāo

rising and falling of vital qi and pathogen / ˈraɪzɪŋ ənd ˈfɔlɪŋ əv ˈvaɪtl tʃi ənd ˈpæθədʒən / 邪正盛衰 xié zhèngshèngshuāi

sequelae / sɪ'kwili / 转归 zhuǎnguī

sequential transmission / sɪ'kwenʃl trænz'mɪʃn / 顺传 shùnchuán

sequential transmission along channel / sɪ'kwenʃl trænz'mɪʃn ə'lɔŋ 'tʃænl / 循经传 xúnjīngchuán

simultaneous superficies and interior syndromes / ˌsaɪml'teɪniəs ˌsʊpə'fɪʃɪiz ənd ɪn'tɪriər 'sɪndroʊmz / 表里同病 biǎolǐtóngbìng

sinking of spleen qi / 'sɪŋkɪŋ əv splin tʃi / 脾气下陷 píqìxiàxiàn

spleen being source of phlegm / splin 'biɪŋ sɔrs əv flem / 脾为生痰之源 píwéishēngtánzhīyuán

spleen deficiency causing wind / splin dɪ'fɪʃnsi 'kɔzɪŋ wɪnd / 脾虚生风 píxūshēngfēng

spleen deficiency generating phlegm / splin dɪ'fɪʃnsi 'dʒɛnəˌretŋ flem / 脾虚生痰 píxūshēngtán

spleen failing to manage blood / splin 'feɪlɪŋ tə 'mænɪdʒ blʌd / 脾不统血 píbùtǒngxuè

stagnant blockade of heart blood / 'stægnənt blɑ'keɪd əv hɑrt blʌd / 心血瘀阻 xīnxuèyūzǔ

stagnant pathogen of Shaoyang / 'stægnənt 'pæθədʒən əv ʃaʊjæŋ / 邪郁少阳 xiéyùshàoyáng

stagnated gallbladder qi with disturbing phlegm / 'stægneɪtɪd 'gɔlˌblædə tʃi wɪð dɪ'stɜrbɪŋ flem / 胆郁痰扰 dǎnyùtánrǎo

stagnated heat in xuefen / 'stægneɪtɪd hit ɪn ʃuɛfen / 血分瘀热 xuèfēnyūrè

stagnated heat of gallbladder channel / ˈstægneɪtɪd hit əv ˈgɔlˌblædə ˈtʃænl / 胆经郁热 dǎnjīngyùrè

stagnated heat of liver channel / ˈstægneɪtɪd hit əv ˈlɪvər ˈtʃænl / 肝经郁热 gānjīngyùrè

stagnation of liver qi / stægˈneɪʃn əv ˈlɪvər tʃi / 肝气郁结 gānqìyùjié

stagnation of liver qi and spleen deficiency / stægˈneɪʃn əv ˈlɪvər tʃi ənd splin dɪˈfɪʃnsi / 肝郁脾虚 gānyùpíxū

stagnation of qi and blood stasis / stægˈneɪʃn əv tʃi ənd blʌd ˈsteɪsɪs / 气滞血瘀 qìzhìxuèyū

stirring wind due to yin deficiency / ˈstɜrɪŋ wɪnd du tə jɪn dɪˈfɪʃnsi / 阴虚风动 yīnxūfēngdòng

stomach cold / ˈstʌmək koʊld / 胃寒 wèihán

stomach heat / ˈstʌmək hit / 胃热 wèirè

stomach heat accelerating digestion / ˈstʌmək hit ækˈsɛləˌretɪŋ daɪˈdʒestʃən / 胃热消谷 wèirèxiāogǔ

struggle between vital qi and pathogen / ˈstrʌgl bɪˈtwin ˈvaɪtl tʃi ənd ˈpæθədʒən / 正邪相争 zhèngxié xiāngzhēng

sudden onset / ˈsʌdn ˈɑnset / 卒发 zúfā

superficies cold / ˌsʊpəˈfɪʃɪˌiz koʊld / 表寒 biǎohán

superficies cold with interior heat / ˌsʊpəˈfɪʃɪˌiz koʊld wɪð ɪnˈtɪriər hit / 表寒里热 biǎohánlǐrè

superficies deficiency / ˌsʊpəˈfɪʃɪˌiz dɪˈfɪʃnsi / 表虚 biǎoxū

superficies excess / ˌsʊpəˈfɪʃɪˌiz ɪkˈses / 表实 biǎoshí

superficies heat / ˌsʊpəˈfɪʃɪˌiz hit / 表热 biǎorè

superficies heat with interior cold / ˌsʊpəˈfɪʃɪˌiz hit wɪð ɪnˈtɪriər koʊld / 表热里寒 biǎorèlǐhán

superficies pathogens involving interior / ˌsʊpəˈfɪʃɪˌiz ˈpæθədʒəns ɪnˈvɑlvɪŋɪn ˈtɪriər / 表邪入里 biǎo xiérùlǐ

Taiyin cold-dampness / taɪˌjɪn koʊld ˈdæmpnəs / 太阴寒湿 tàiyīnhánshī

Taiyin deficient cold / taɪˌjɪn dɪˈfɪʃnt koʊld / 太阴虚寒 tàiyīnxūhán

theory of pathogenesis / ˈθiəri əv pæθəˈdʒenɪsɪs / 病机学说 bìngjīxuéshuō

timidity due to deficiency of heart qi / tɪˈmɪdəti du tə dɪˈfɪʃnsi əv hɑrt tʃi / 心虚胆怯 xīnxūdǎnqiè

transformation in accord with constitution / ˌtræns fərˈmeɪʃn ɪn əˈkɔrd wɪð ˌkɑnstɪˈtuʃn / 从化 cóng huà

transmission / trænzˈmɪʃn / 传变 chuánbiàn

transmission of skipping to other channel / trænzˈmɪʃn əv skɪpɪŋ tə ˈʌðər ˈtʃænl / 越经传 yuèjīngchuán

transverse dysfunction of liver qi / ˈtrænzvɜrs dɪsˈfʌŋkʃn əv ˈlɪvər tʃi / 肝气横逆 gānqìhèngnì

true cold disease with false heat manifestation / tru koʊld dɪˈziz wɪð fɔls hit ˌmænɪfeˈsteɪʃn / 真寒假热 zhēnhánjiǎrè

true deficiency disease with false excessive manifestation / tru dɪˈfɪʃnsi dɪˈziz wɪð fɔls ɪkˈsesɪv ˌmænɪfeˈsteɪʃn / 真虚假实 zhēnxūjiǎshí

true excess disease with false deficient manifestation

/ tru ɪkˈses dɪˈziz wɪð fɔls dɪˈfɪʃnt ˌmænɪfeˈsteɪʃn / 真实假虚 zhēnshíjiǎxū

true heat disease with false cold manifestation / tru hit dɪˈziz wɪð fɔls koʊld ˌmænɪfeˈsteɪʃn / 真热假寒 zhēnrèjiǎhán

true-false of cold and heat / tru fɔls əv koʊld ənd hit / 寒热真假 hánrèzhēnjiǎ

true-false of excess-deficiency / tru fɔls əv ɪkˈses dɪˈfɪʃnsi / 虚实真假 xūshízhēnjiǎ

turbid fluid depletion / ˈtɜrbɪd ˈfluɪd dɪˈpliʃn / 液脱 yètuō

turbid phlegm obstructing lung / ˈtɜrbɪd flem əbˈstrʌktɪŋ lʌŋ / 痰浊阻肺 tánzhuózǔfèi

unconsolidation of Chong and Conception Channels / ʌnkənsɑlɪˈdeɪʃn əv tʃʊŋ ənd kənˈsepʃn ˈtʃænlz / 冲任不固 chōngrènbùgù

upper deficiency and lower excess / ˈʌpər dɪˈfɪʃnsi ənd ˈloə ɪkˈses / 上虚下实 shàngxūxiàshí

upper excess and lower deficiency / ˈʌpər ɪkˈses ənd ˈloə dɪˈfɪʃnsi / 上盛下虚 shàngshèngxiàxū

upper hyperactivity of liver yang / ˈʌpər ˌhaɪpərækˈtɪvəti əv ˈlɪvər jæŋ / 肝阳上亢 gānyángshàngkàng

vital qi / ˈvaɪtl tʃi / 正气 zhèngqì

water diffusion due to kidney deficiency / ˈwɔtər dɪˈfjuʒn du tə ˈkɪdni dɪˈfɪʃnsi / 肾虚水泛 shènxū shuǐfàn

water failing to nourish wood / ˈwɔtər ˈfeɪlɪŋ tə ˈnɜrɪʃ wud / 水不涵木 shuǐbùhánmù

water pathogen attacking heart / ˈwɔtər ˈpæθədʒən əˈtækɪŋ hɑrt / 水气凌心 shuǐqìlíngxīn

water-cold attacking lung / ˈwɔtər koʊld əˈtækɪŋ lʌŋ / 水寒射肺 shuǐhánshèfèi

weifen / weɪfen / 卫分 wèifēn

wind-cold attacking lung / wɪnd koʊld əˈtækɪŋ lʌŋ / 风寒袭肺 fēnghánxífèi

wind-heat of liver channel / wɪnd hit əv ˈlɪvər ˈtʃænl / 肝经风热 gānjīngfēngrè

xuefen / ʃuɛfen / 血分 xuèfēn

yang deficiency / jæŋ dɪˈfɪʃnsi / 阳虚 yángxū

yang deficiency involving yin / jæŋ dɪˈfɪʃnsi ɪnˈvɑlvɪŋ jɪn / 阳损及阴 yángsǔnjíyīn

yang depletion / jæŋ dɪˈpliʃn / 亡阳 wángyáng

yang disease involving yin / jæŋ dɪˈziz ɪnˈvɑlvɪŋ jɪn / 阳病入阴 yángbìngrùyīn

yang excessiveness / jæŋ ikˈsesivnis / 阳盛 yáng shèng

Yangming deficient cold / jæŋmɪŋ dɪˈfɪʃnt koʊld / 阳明虚寒 yángmíngxūhán

Yangming dryness-heat / jæŋmɪŋ ˈdraɪnəs hit / 阳明燥热 yángmíngzàorè

Yangming Fu-viscera excess / jæŋmɪŋ fu ˈvɪsərə ikˈses / 阳明腑实 yángmíngfǔshí

yin deficiency / jɪn dɪˈfɪʃnsi / 阴虚 yīnxū

yin deficiency involving yang / jɪn dɪˈfɪʃnsi ɪnˈvɑlvɪŋ jæŋ / 阴损及阳 yīnsǔnjíyáng

yin deficiency of liver and kidney / jɪn dɪˈfɪʃnsi əv ˈlɪvər ənd ˈkɪdni / 肝肾阴虚 gānshènyīnxū

yin deficiency of lung and kidney / jɪn dɪˈfɪʃnsi əv lʌŋ ənd ˈkɪdni / 肺肾阴虚 fèishènyīnxū

yin deficiency of spleen and stomach / jɪn dɪˈfɪʃnsi əv splin ənd ˈstʌmək / 脾胃阴虚 píwèiyīnxū

yin depletion / jɪn dɪˈpliʃn / 亡阴 wángyīn

yin disease involving yang / jɪn dɪˈziz ɪnˈvɑlvɪŋ jæŋ / 阴病出阳 yīnbìngchūyáng

yin excessiveness / jɪn ikˈsesivnis / 阴盛 yīnshèng

yingfen / jɪŋfen / 营分 yíngfēn

yin-yang disharmony / jɪn jæŋ dɪsˈhɑrməni / 阴阳失调 yīnyángshītiáo

Zang-viscera disease involving Fu-viscera / zæŋ ˈvɪsərə dɪˈziz ɪnˈvɑlvɪŋ fu ˈvɪsərə / 脏病及腑 zàngbìng jífǔ

61

Chapter 3 Diagnostics of Traditional Chinese Medicine

第三章 中医诊断学

Section 1 Diagnostic Methods

第一节 诊 法

* **abdominal pain** / æb'dɑmɪnl peɪn / 腹痛 fùtòng

abdominal examination / æb'dɑmɪnl ɪɡˌzæmɪ'neɪʃn / 腹诊 fùzhěn

abdominal pain / æb'dɑmɪnl peɪn / 里急 lǐjí

abdominal pain refusing to pressure / æb'dɑmɪnl peɪn ri'fjʊz tə 'preʃər / 腹痛拒按 fùtòngjù`àn

abnormal frequency pulse / æb'nɔrml 'frikwənsi pʌls / 离经脉 líjīngmài

abnormal pulse / æb'nɔrml pʌls / 病脉 bìngmài

acid regurgitation / 'æsɪd rɪˌɡɜrdʒɪ'teɪʃn / 泛酸，吞酸，吐酸 fànsuān, tūnsuān, tǔsuān

addiction to eating foreign bodies / ə'dɪkʃn tə 'itɪŋ 'fɔrən 'bɑdɪz / 喜食异物 xǐshíyìwù

afternoon tidal fever / ˌæftər'nun 'taɪdl 'fivər / 日晡潮热 rìbūcháorè

alternate attacks of chill and fever / 'ɔltərnət ə'tæks əv tʃɪl ənd 'fivər / 寒热往来 hánrèwǎnglái

alternative chill and fever / ɔl'tɜrnətɪv tʃɪl ənd 'fivər / 寒热起伏 hánrèqǐfú

analeptic / ˌænə'leptɪk / 但欲寐 dànyùmèi

anhidrosis / ˌænhaɪ'drəʊsɪs / 无汗 wúhàn

ankyloglossia / ˌæŋkələuˈglɔsiə / 绊舌 bànshé

anorexia / ˌænəˈreksiə / 纳呆 nàdāi

anorexia / ˌænəˈreksiə / 厌食 yànshí

aphtha / ˈæfθə / 口糜 kǒumí

arm pain / ɑrm peɪn / 臂痛 bìtòng

armpit sweating / ˈɑrmpɪt ˈswetɪŋ / 腋汗 yèhàn

arranging fingers in pulse taking / əˈreɪndʒɪŋ ˈfɪŋgərs ɪn pʌls ˈtekɪŋ / 布指 bùzhǐ

arthralgia / ɑrˈθrældʒə / 关节疼痛 guānjiéténgtòng

asexuality / æˌsɛkʃʊˈæləti / 房事淡漠 fángshìdànmò

aversion to cold / əˈvɜrʒn tə koʊld / 恶寒 wùhán

aversion to cold with fever / əˈvɜrʒn tə koʊld wɪθ ˈfivər / 恶寒发热 wùhánfārè

aversion to heat / əˈvɜrʒn tə hit / 恶热 wùrè

aversion to wind / əˈvɜrʒn tə wɪnd / 恶风 wùfēng

∗ **buzzing in brain** / ˈbʌzɪŋ ɪn breɪn / 脑鸣 nǎomíng

backache / ˈbækeɪk / 背痛 bèitòng

belching / beltʃɪŋ / 嗳气 ǎiqì

benign complexion / bɪˈnaɪn kəmˈplekʃn / 善色 shànsè

berry-sauce fur / ˈberi sɔs fɜr / 霉酱苔 méijiàngtāi

bitter taste in mouth / ˈbɪtər teɪst ɪn maʊθ / 口苦 kǒukǔ

black fur / blæk fɜr / 黑苔 hēitāi

blackening of teeth / ˈblækənɪŋ əv tiθ / 牙齿焦黑 yáchǐjiāohēi

bleeding from five aperture or subcutaneous tissue / ˈblidɪŋ frəm faɪv ˈæpərtʃʊr ɔr ˌsʌbkjuˈteɪniəs ˈtɪʃu / 衄血 nǜxuè

blockage in deglutition / ˈblɑkɪdʒ ɪn ˌdiglʊˈtɪʃən / 吞

食梗塞 tūnshígěngsè

blood stasis and pain of eyelid / blʌd ˈsteɪsɪs ənd peɪn əv ˈaɪlɪd / 眼胞瘀痛 yǎnbāoyūtòng

blue tongue / blu tʌŋ / 青舌 qīngshé

body palpation / ˈbɑdi pælˈpeɪʃn / 按诊 ànzhěn

body shaking / ˈbɑdi ˈʃeɪkɪŋ / 身振摇 shēnzhènyáo

bone steaming / boʊn ˈstimɪŋ / 骨蒸 gǔzhēng

borborygmus / ˌbɔrbəˈrɪgməs / 肠鸣 chángmíng

breast pain / brest peɪn / 乳房疼痛 rǔfángténgtòng

bromhidrosis / ˌbroʊmɪˈdroʊsɪs / 汗臭 hànchòu

bulging fontanel in infant / ˈbʌldʒɪŋ ˌfɑntəˈnel ɪn ˈɪnfənt / 囟门高突 xìnméngāotū

burning pain / ˈbɜrnɪŋ peɪn / 灼痛 zhuótòng

* **constipation** / ˌkɑnstɪˈpeɪʃn / 大便秘结 dàbiànmìjié

* **cough** / kɔf / 咳嗽 késou

* **coughing and dyspnea in semireclining position** / ˈkɔfɪŋ ənd dɪspˈniə ɪn ˈsemɪriˈklaɪnɪŋ pəˈzɪʃn / 咳逆倚息 kénìyǐxī

carphology / kɑˈfɒlədʒɪ / 循衣摸床 xúnyīmōchuáng

cheilectropion / kilɛktroʊpɪɒn / 唇反 chúnfǎn

chest pain / tʃest peɪn / 胸痛 xiōngtòng

chest sweating / tʃest ˈswetɪŋ / 胸汗 xiōnghàn

chill and fever similar to malaria / tʃɪl ənd ˈfivər ˈsɪmələr tə məˈleriə / 寒热如疟 hánrèrúnüè

chill without fever / tʃɪl wɪˈðaʊt ˈfivər / 但寒不热 dànhánbùrè

choke when drinking / tʃoʊk wen ˈdrɪŋkɪŋ / 饮水则呛 yǐnshuǐzéqiàng

ciliary hyperemia / ˈsɪlɪəri ˌhaipəˈrimiə / 抱轮红赤 bàolúnhóngchì

cinnabar palm / ˈsɪnəbɑr pɑm / 朱砂掌 zhūshāzhǎng

clear urine in large amounts / klɪr ˈjʊrɪn ɪn lɑrdʒ əˈmaʊnts / 小便清长 xiǎobiànqīngcháng

cloudy vision / ˈklaʊdi ˈvɪʒn / 目昏 mùhūn

coccygeal pain / kɑkˈsɪdʒɪəl peɪn / 尾闾痛 wěilútòng

cold pain / koʊld peɪn / 冷痛 lěngtòng

cold sweating / koʊld ˈswetɪŋ / 冷汗 lěnghàn

coldness in back / ˈkoʊldnəs ɪn bæk / 背冷 bèilěng

coldness in waist / ˈkoʊldnəs ɪn weɪst / 腰冷 yāolěng

coldness of external genitals / ˈkoʊldnəs əv ɪkˈstɜrnl ˈdʒenɪtlz / 阴冷 yīnlěng

colic / ˈkɑlɪk / 绞痛 jiǎotòng

collapsed eye / kəˈlæpst aɪ / 目下陷 mùxiàxiàn

complexion / kəmˈplekʃn / 面色 miànsè

comprehensive analysis of data gained by four diagnostic methods / ˌkɑmprɪˈhensɪv əˈnæləsɪs əv ˈdeɪtə geind baɪ fɔr daɪəgˈnɑstɪk ˈmeθədz / 四诊合参 sìzhěnhécān

comprehensive analysis to both pulse manifestation and symptoms / ˌkɑmprɪˈhensɪv əˈnæləsɪs tə boʊθ pʌls ˌmænɪfeˈsteɪʃn ənd ˈsɪmptəms / 脉症合参 màizhènghécān

comprehensive consideration of both complexion and pulse manifestation / ˌkɑmprɪˈhensɪv kənˌsɪdəˈreɪʃn əv boʊθ kəmˈplekʃn ənd pʌls ˌmænɪfeˈsteɪʃn / 色脉合参 sèmàihécān

concurrent pulse / kənˈkɜrənt pʌls / 相兼脉 xiāngjiān

mài

congruence of pulse with four seasons / ˈkɑŋgruəns əv pʌls wɪð fɔr siznz / 脉应四时 màiyìngsìshí

convulsion / kənˈvʌlʃn / 抽搐 chōuchù

coughing of phlegm / ˈkɔfɪŋ əv flem / 咳痰 kétán

critical pulse manifestation / ˈkrɪtɪkl pʌls ˌmænɪfeˈsteɪʃn / 真脏脉 zhēnzàngmài

cun-guan-chi / tsun gwɑn tʃi / 寸关尺 cùnguānchǐ

cunkou / tsunˌkɔʊ / 寸口 cùnkǒu

curdy fur / ˈkɜrdi fɜr / 腐苔 fǔtāi

curly tongue / ˈkɜrli tʌŋ / 舌卷 shéjuǎn

cyanotic lips / ˌsaɪəˈnɔtik lɪps / 口唇青紫 kǒuchún qīngzǐ

* **deafness** / ˈdefnəs / 耳聋 ěrlóng

darkish complexion / ˈdɑkɪʃ kəmˈplekʃn / 面色黧黑 miànsèlíhēi

deadly cold hand and foot / ˈdedli koʊld hænd ənd fʊt / 手足厥逆 shǒuzújuénì

deep and harsh voice / dip ənd hɑrʃ vɔɪs / 语声重浊 yǔshēngzhòngzhuó

deep blind fistula / dip blaɪnd ˈfɪstʃələ / 窦道 dòudào

deep pulse / dip pʌls / 沉脉 chénmài

deep red tongue / dip red tʌŋ / 绛舌 jiàngshé

deep-colored urine / dip ˈkʌlərd ˈjʊrɪn / 小便黄赤 xiǎobiànhuángchì

deep-sited pulse / dip saɪted pʌls / 伏脉 fúmài

deformed joints / dɪˈfɔrmd dʒɔɪnts / 关节变形 guānjiébiànxíng

delirium / dɪˈlɪriəm / 谵语 zhānyǔ

diagnostic method / ˌdaɪəgˈnɑstɪk ˈmeθəd / 诊法 zhěnfǎ

diagnostic significance of five colors / ˌdaɪəgˈnɑstɪk sɪgˈnɪfɪkəns əv faɪv ˈkʌlərz / 五色主病 wǔsèzhǔbìng

diarrhea / ˌdaɪəˈriə / 腹泻 fùxiè

diarrhea with undigested food / ˌdaɪəˈriə wɪð ˌʌndəˈdʒɛstɪd fud / 完谷不化 wángǔbùhuà

differentiation of symptoms and signs to identify etiology / ˌdɪfərenʃiˈeɪʃn əv ˈsɪmptəmz ənd saɪnz tə aɪˈdentɪfaɪ ˌitiˈɑlədʒi / 审症求因 shěnzhèngqiúyīn

difficulty and pain in micturition / ˈdɪfɪkəlti ənd peɪn ɪn ˌmɪktʃəˈrɪʃn / 小便涩痛 xiǎobiànsètòng

difficulty in defecation / ˈdɪfɪkəlti ɪn ˌdefəˈkeɪʃn / 大便艰难 dàbiànjiānnán

dim complexion / dɪm kəmˈplekʃn / 面色晦暗 miànsèhuìàn

dirty face / ˈdɜrti feɪs / 面垢 miàngòu

disabled wilted limbs / dɪsˈeɪbld ˈwɪltɪd lɪmz / 肢体痿废 zhītǐwěifèi

distal bleeding / ˈdɪstl ˈblidɪŋ / 近血 jìnxuè

distant anal bleeding / ˈdɪstənt ˈeɪnl ˈblidɪŋ / 远血 yuǎnxuè

distending pain / dɪˈstendɪŋ peɪn / 胀痛 zhàngtòng

distention and fullness / dɪsˈtenʃən ənd ˈfulnəs / 痞满 pǐmǎn

dizziness / ˈdɪzinəs / 目眩 mùxuàn

dizziness / ˈdɪzinəs / 头晕 tóuyūn

double tongue / ˈdʌbl tʌŋ / 重舌 chóngshé

double visual images / ˈdʌbl ˈvɪʒuəl ˈɪmɪdʒɪz / 视歧 shìqí

dragging pain / dræɡiŋ peɪn / 掣痛 chètòng

dreaminess / ˈdriminəs / 多梦 duōmèng

dribble of urine / ˈdrɪbl əv ˈjʊrɪn / 尿后余沥 niàohòu yúlì

dry and cracked fur / draɪ ənd krækt fɜr / 燥裂苔 zàolìètāi

dry and withered lips / draɪ ənd ˈwɪðərd lɪps / 口唇焦裂 kǒuchúnjiāoliè

dry cough / draɪ kɔf / 干咳 gānké

dry eye / draɪ aɪ / 目涩 mùsè

dry fur / draɪ fɜr / 燥苔 zàotāi

dry mouth / draɪ maʊθ / 口干 kǒugān

dry tongue / draɪ tʌŋ / 舌干 shégān

dull pain / dʌl peɪn / 隐痛 yǐntòng

dysphasia / dɪsˈfeɪziə / 重言 chóngyán

dysphasia / dɪsˈfeɪziə / 语言謇涩 yǔyánjiǎnsè

dysphoria / dɪsˈfɔriə / 烦躁 fánzào

dysphoria with feverish sensation in chest / dɪsˈfɔriə wɪð ˈfivərɪʃ senˈseɪʃn ɪn tʃest / 五心烦热 wǔxīn fánrè

dyspnea / dɪspˈniə / 喘 chuǎn

dysuria / dɪsˈjʊriə / 小便不利 xiǎobiànbùlì

＊**enuresis** / ˌenjʊˈrisɪs / 遗尿 yíniào

earache / ˈɪreɪk / 耳痛 ěrtòng

eating in morning but vomiting in evening / ˈitɪŋ ɪn ˈmɔrnɪŋ bət ˈvɑmɪtɪŋ ɪn ˈivnɪŋ / 朝食暮吐 zhāo shímùtǔ

ecchymosis on tongue / ˌɛkəˈmosɪs ɑn tʌŋ / 舌生瘀斑 shéshēngyūbān

ectopic radial pulse / ekˈtɑpɪk ˈreɪdiəl pʌls / 反关脉 fǎnguānmài

edema / iˈdimə / 浮肿 fúzhǒng

emaciation / ɪmeɪsiˈeɪʃn / 消瘦 xiāoshòu

emaciation and anorexia / ɪmeɪsiˈeɪʃn ənd ænəˈreksiə / 破䐃脱肉 pòjùntuōròu

empty pain / ˈempti peɪn / 空痛 kōngtòng

empty sensation in heart / ˈempti senˈseɪʃn ɪn hɑrt / 心中憺憺大动 xīnzhōngdàndàndàdòng

epigastric oppression / ˌepɪˈgæstrɪk əˈpreʃn / 心下痞 xīnxiàpǐ

epigastric throb / ˌepɪˈgæstrɪk θrɑb / 心下悸 xīnxiàjì

epistaxis / ˌɛpɪˈstæksɪs / 鼻衄 bínǜ

eroded fur / ɪˈroʊded fɜr / 剥苔 bōtāi

examining skin of forearm / ɪgˈzæmɪnɪŋ skɪn əv ˈfɔrɑm / 诊尺肤 zhěnchǐfū

examining xuli / ɪgˈzæmɪnɪŋ ˈʃwli / 诊虚里 zhěnxūlǐ

excess pulse / ɪkˈses pʌls / 实脉 shímài

expectoration / ɪkˌspektəˈreɪʃn / 咳痰 kétán

exterior syndrome / ɪkˈstɪriər ˈsɪndroʊm / 外证 wàizhèng

extreme emaciation / ɪkˈstrim ɪmeɪsiˈeɪʃn / 脱形 tuōxíng

eyelids swelling / ˈaɪlɪdz ˈswelɪŋ / 眼睑浮肿 yǎnjiǎn fúzhǒng

facial edema / ˈfeɪʃəl iˈdimə / 颜面浮肿 yánmiàn fúzhǒng

fading murmuring / ˈfedɪŋ ˈmɜrmərɪŋ / 郑声 zhèng shēng

failure of closure of fontanel / ˈfeɪljər əv ˈklouʒər əv ˌfɒntəˈnel / 囟门不合 xìnménbùhé

faint low voice / feɪnt lou vɔɪs / 语声低微 yǔshēng dīwēi

faint pulse / feɪnt pʌls / 微脉 wēimài

fainting / ˈfentɪŋ / 昏厥 hūnjué

false vitality / fɔls vaɪˈtæləti / 假神 jiǎshén

fear of cold / fɪr əv kould / 畏寒 wèihán

feeble pulse / ˈfibl pʌls / 虚脉 xūmài

feeling obstructed in epigastrium / ˈfilɪŋ əbˈstrʌktid ɪn ˌepɪˈgæstrɪəm / 心下支结 xīnxiàzhījié

fever / ˈfivər / 发热 fārè

fever aggravated at night / ˈfivər ˈægrəveɪtɪd ət naɪt / 身热夜甚 shēnrèyèshèn

fever without chill / ˈfivər wɪˈðaut tʃɪl / 但热不寒 dànrèbùhán

feverishness in palms and soles / ˈfivərɪʃnis ɪn pɑmz ənd souls / 手足心热 shǒuzúxīnrè

feverishness on dorsum of hand / ˈfivərɪʃnis ɑn ˈdɔrsəm əv hænd / 手背热 shǒubèirè

fifty beats / ˈfɪfti bits / 五十动 wǔshídòng

firm pulse / fɜrm pʌls / 牢脉 láomài

fissured tongue / ˈfɪʃərd tʌŋ / 裂纹舌 lièwénshé

fistula / ˈfɪstʃələ / 瘘管 lòuguǎn

fistula / ˈfɪstʃələ / 漏 lòu

five colors / faɪv ˈkʌlərz / 五色 wǔsè

fixed pain / fɪkst peɪn / 痛有定处 tòngyǒudìngchù

flaccid tongue / ˈflæsɪd tʌŋ / 舌痿 shéwěi

flapping of nasal wings / ˈflæpɪŋ əv ˈneɪzl wɪŋz / 鼻煽 bíshān

flatus / ˈfleɪtəs / 矢气 shǐqì

floating pulse / ˈfloʊtɪŋ pʌls / 浮脉 fúmài

flush face / flʌʃ feɪs / 泛红如妆 fànhóngrúzhuāng

foot pain / fʊt peɪn / 足痛 zútòng

four diagnostic methods / fɔr ˌdaɪəgˈnɑstɪk ˈmeθədz / 四诊 sìzhěn

frequent micturition / ˈfrikwənt ˌmɪktʃəˈrɪʃn / 小便频数 xiǎobiànpínshuò

frequent protrusion of tongue / ˈfrikwənt proʊˈtruʒn əv tʌŋ / 弄舌 nòngshé

frequent urination at night / ˈfrikwənt ˌjʊrɪˈneɪʃn ət naɪt / 夜尿多 yèniàoduō

fullness and discomfort in chest and hypochondrium / ˈfʊlnəs ənd dɪsˈkʌmfərt ɪn tʃest ənd ˌhaɪpəˈkɑndrɪəm / 胸胁苦满 xiōngxiékǔmǎn

fullness in head / ˈfʊlnəs ɪn hed / 头胀 tóuzhàng

fullness of vitality / ˈfʊlnəs əv vaɪˈtæləti / 得神 déshén

fur / fɜr / 舌苔 shétāi

fur character / fɜr ˈkærəktər / 苔质 tāizhì

fur color / fɜr ˈkʌlər / 苔色 tāisè

* **gastric upset** / ˈɡæstrɪk ʌpˈset / 嘈杂 cáozá

genuine visceral complexion / ˈdʒenjuɪn ˈvɪsərə kəmˈplekʃn / 真脏色 zhēnzàngsè

gingival atrophy / dʒɪnˈdʒaɪvl ˈætrəfi / 牙龈萎缩 yá yínwěisuō

going through passes to reach nails / ˈɡoʊɪŋ θru pæsiz tə ritʃ nels / 透关射甲 tòuguānshèjiǎ

gonorrhea / ˌɡɑnəˈriə / 白浊 báizhuó

governing complexion / ˈɡʌvərnɪŋ kəmˈplekʃn / 主色 zhǔsè

governing exterior to infer interior / ˈɡʌvərnɪŋ ɪkˈstɪriər tə ɪnˈfɜr ɪnˈtɪriər / 司外揣内 sīwài chuǎinèi

graphic tongue / ˈɡræfɪk tʌŋ / 地图舌 dìtúshé

gray fur / ɡreɪ fɜr / 灰苔 huītāi

greasy fur / ˈɡrisi fɜr / 腻苔 nìtāi

green fur / ɡrin fɜr / 绿苔 lǜtāi

greenish complexion / ˈɡrinɪʃ kəmˈplekʃn / 面色青 miànsèqīng

gum bleeding / ɡʌm ˈblidɪŋ / 齿衄 chǐnǜ

* **hypochondriac pain** / ˌhaɪpəˈkɑ ndriæk peɪn / 胁痛 xiétòng

halitosis / ˌhælɪˈtoʊsɪs / 口臭 kǒuchòu

hard and full in abdomen / hɑrd ənd fʊl ɪˈæbdəmən / 腹部硬满 fùbùyìngmǎn

head sweating / hed ˈswetɪŋ / 头汗 tóuhàn

head tremor / hed ˈtremər / 头摇 tóuyáo

head with binding sensation / hed wɪð ˈbaɪndɪŋ

sen'seɪʃn / 首如裹 shǒurúguǒ

healthy person / 'helθi 'pɜrsn / 平人 píngrén

hearing impairment / 'hɪrɪŋ ɪm'permənt / 重听 zhòng tīng

heartburn / 'hɑrtbɜrn / 心中懊恼 xīnzhōng'àonáo

heat fecaloma with watery discharge / hit fɪkæ'loʊmə wɪð 'wɔtəri dɪs'tʃɑrdʒ / 热结旁流 rèjiépángliú

heaviness in waist / 'hevinəs ɪn weɪst / 腰重 yāo zhòng

heavy body / 'hevi 'bɑdi / 身重 shēnzhòng

heavy pain / 'hevi peɪn / 重痛 zhòngtòng

heavy sensation of head / 'hevi sen'seɪʃn əv hed / 头重 tóuzhòng

hectic cheek / 'hektɪk tʃik / 颧红 quánhóng

hectic fever / 'hektɪk 'fivər / 骨蒸 gǔzhēng

heel pain / hil peɪn / 足跟痛 zúgēntòng

hemafecia / hemə'fisɪə / 便血 biànxiě

hematemesis / ˌhimə'tɛmɪsɪs / 吐血 tùxiě

hematohidrosis / hemætəʊ'hɪdroʊsɪs / 红汗 hónghàn

hematospermia / himətəʊ'spɜrmɪə / 血精 xuèjīng

hematuria / ˌhimə'tjʊrɪə / 尿血 niàoxiě

hemi-anhidrosis / 'hemɪˌænhaɪ'drəʊsɪs / 半身无汗 bàn shēnwúhàn

hemihidrosis / hemɪ'hɪdroʊsɪs / 半身汗出 bànshēn hànchū

hemiplegia / ˌhɛmɪ'plidʒɪə / 半身不遂 bànshēnbùsuí

hemoptysis / hɪ'mɑptəsɪs / 咯血 kǎxiě

hemoptysis / hɪ'mɑptəsɪs / 咳血 kéxiě

hesitant pulse / ˈhezɪtənt pʌls / 涩脉 sèmài

hiccough / ˈhɪkɔf / 呃逆 ènì

hiccup / ˈhɪkʌp / 呃逆 ènì

hiding fever / ˈhaɪdɪŋ ˈfivər / 身热不扬 shēnrèbù yáng

high fever / haɪ ˈfivər / 壮热 zhuàngrè

hoarseness / ˈhɔrsnəs / 声嘎 shēngshà

hollow pulse / ˈhɑloʊ pʌls / 芤脉 kōumài

hotness in back / ˈhɔtnis ɪn bæk / 背热 bèirè

hunger without desire to eat / ˈhʌŋgər wɪˈðaʊt dɪˈzaɪər tə it / 饥不欲食 jībùyùshí

hyperhidrosis / ˌhaɪpəhaɪˈdroʊsɪs / 多汗 duōhàn

* **impotence** / ˈɪmpətəns / 阳痿 yángwěi

* **lumbago** / lʌmˈbeɪgoʊ / 腰痛 yāotòng

inch bar and cubit / ɪntʃ bɑr ənd ˈkjubɪt / 寸关尺 cùn guānchǐ

incongruence of pulse with four seasons / ɪnˈkɑŋgruəns əv pʌls wɪð fɔr siznz / 脉逆四时 màinìsìshí

incontinence of feces / ɪnˈkɑntɪnəns əv ˈfisiz / 大便滑脱 dàbiànhuátuō

incontinence of urine / ɪnˈkɑntɪnəns əv ˈjʊrɪn / 小便失禁 xiǎobiànshījìn

infantile hand venule / ˈɪnfəntaɪl hænd ˈvɛnjʊl / 小儿指纹 xiǎoˈérzhǐwén

inquiry / ɪnˈkwaɪri / 问诊 wènzhěn

inquiry about sweating / ɪnˈkwaɪri əˈbaʊt ˈswetɪŋ / 问汗 wènhàn

inspection / ɪnˈspekʃn / 望诊 wàngzhěn

inspection of body statue and movements / ɪnˈspekʃn əv ˈbɑdi ˈstætʃu ənd ˈmuvmənts / 望形态 wàngxíngtài

inspection of collateral / ɪnˈspekʃn əv kəˈlætərəl / 望络脉 wàngluòmài

inspection of color / ɪnˈspekʃn əv ˈkʌlər / 望色 wàngsè

inspection of excreta / ɪnˈspekʃn əv ɪkˈskritə / 望排出物 wàngpáichūwù

inspection of eye spirit / ɪnˈspekʃn əv aɪ ˈspɪrɪt / 望眼神 wàngyǎnshén

inspection of five apertures / ɪnˈspekʃn əv faɪv ˈæpərtʃʊrz / 望五官 wàngwǔguān

inspection of menstrual blood / ɪnˈspekʃn əv ˈmenstruəl blʌd / 望经血 wàngjīngxuè

inspection of philtrum / ɪnˈspekʃn əv ˈfiltrəm / 望人中 wàngrénzhōng

inspection of skin / ɪnˈspekʃn əv skɪn / 望皮肤 wàng pífū

inspection of spirit / ɪnˈspekʃn əv ˈspɪrɪt / 望神 wàng shén

interior syndrome / ɪnˈtɪriər ˈsɪndroʊm / 内证 nèi zhèng

irregularly intermittent pulse / ɪˈregjələrli ˌɪntərˈmɪtənt pʌls / 结脉 jiémài

irregular-rapid pulse / ɪˈregjələr ˈræpɪd pʌls / 促脉 cùmài

itching in ear / ˈɪtʃɪŋ ɪn ɪr / 耳痒 ěryǎng

itching of eye / ˈɪtʃɪŋ əv aɪ / 目痒 mùyǎng

kyphosis / kaɪˈfosɪs / 腰背偻俯 yāobèilóufǔ

leukorrhea / ˌlukəˈriə / 带下 dàixià

life pass / laɪf pæs / 命关 mìngguān

limbs pain / lɪmz peɪn / 四肢疼痛 sìzhīténgtòng

listening / ˈlɪsənɪŋ / 听声音 tīngshēngyīn

listening and smelling / ˈlɪsənɪŋ ənd smelɪŋ / 闻诊 wénzhěn

lochia / ˈlokɪə / 恶露 èlù

locked jaw / lɔkt dʒɔ / 撮口 cuōkǒu

lockjaw / ˈlɑkˌdʒɔ / 口噤 kǒujìn

long pulse / lɔŋ pʌls / 长脉 chángmài

loose stool / lus stul / 便溏 biàntáng

loss of hair / lɔs əv her / 毛发脱落 máofàtuōluò

loss of smell / lɔs əv smel / 不闻香臭 bùwénxiāng chòu

loss of vitality / lɔs əv vaɪˈtæləti / 失神 shīshén

loss of voice / lɔs əv vɔɪs / 失音 shīyīn

lower abdominal pain / ˈloʊr æbˈdɑmɪnl peɪn / 小腹痛 xiǎofùtòng

lustrous tongue / ˈlʌstrəs tʌŋ / 荣舌 róngshé

lustrous-withered-tough-tender / ˈlʌstrəs ˈwɪðərd tʌf ˈtendər / 荣枯老嫩 róngkūlǎonèn

luxated teeth / ˈlʌkseɪted tiθ / 牙齿浮动 yáchǐfúdòng

∗ **migraine** / ˈmaɪgreɪn / 偏头痛 piāntóutòng

macula / ˈmækjʊlə / 癍 bān

malignant complexion / məˈlɪgnənt kəmˈplekʃn / 恶色 èsè

mass in abdomen / mæs ɪn ˈæbdəmən / 腹中痞块

fùzhōngpǐkuài

migratory pain / ˈmaɪɡrətɔri peɪn / 痛无定处 tòng wúdìngchù

mild fever / maɪld ˈfivər / 微热 wēirè

miliaria alba / ˌmɪliˈɛriə ˈælbə / 白㾦 báipēi

mirror-like tongue / ˈmɪrər laɪk tʌŋ / 镜面舌 jìng miànshé

moderate pulse / ˈmɑdərət pʌls / 缓脉 huǎnmài

moist fur / mɔɪst fɜr / 润苔 rùntāi

moistened tongue / ˈmɔɪsnd tʌŋ / 舌润 shérùn

morbid vaginal discharge / ˈmɔrbɪd vəˈdʒaɪnl dɪsˈtʃɑrdʒ / 带下 dàixià

mumps / mʌmps / 腮肿 sāizhǒng

muscular twitching and cramp / ˈmʌskjələr ˈtwitʃiŋ ənd kræmp / 筋惕肉瞤 jīntìròurún

mutual restriction between disease and complexion / ˈmjutʃuəl rɪˈstrɪkʃn bɪˈtwin dɪˈziz ənd kəmˈplekʃn / 病色相克 bìngsèxiāngkè

* **numbness** / ˈnʌmnəs / 麻木 mámù

nausea / ˈnɔziə / 恶心 ěxin

nearby anal bleeding / ˌnɪrˈbaɪ ˈeɪnl ˈblidɪŋ / 近血 jìnxuè

night emission / naɪt ɪˈmɪʃn / 滑精 huájīng

night fever abating at dawn / naɪt ˈfivər əˈbetɪŋ ət dɔn / 夜热早凉 yèrèzǎoliáng

night sweating / naɪt ˈswetɪŋ / 盗汗 dàohàn

nocturnal emission / nɑkˈtɜrnl ɪˈmɪʃn / 梦遗 mèngyí

non-smooth diarrhea / nɑn smuð ˌdaɪəˈriə / 泻下不

爽 xièxiàbùshuǎng

normal complexion / ˈnɔrml kəmˈplekʃn / 常色 chángsè

normal pulse / ˈnɔrml pʌls / 平脉 píngmài

normal respiration / ˈnɔrml ˌrespəˈreɪʃn / 平息 píngxī

normal sensation in mouth / ˈnɔrml senˈseɪʃn ɪn maʊθ / 口中和 kǒuzhōnghé

normal tongue manifestation / ˈnɔrml tʌŋ ˌmænɪfeˈsteɪʃn / 正常舌象 zhèngchángshéxiàng

numbness in mouth / ˈnʌmnəs ɪn maʊθ / 口麻 kǒumá

numbness of scalp / ˈnʌmnəs əv skælp / 头皮麻木 tóu pímámù

numbness of tongue / ˈnʌmnəs əv tʌŋ / 舌麻 shémá

obesity / oʊˈbisəti / 肥胖 féipàng

oblique flying pulse / əˈblik ˈflaɪɪŋ pʌls / 斜飞脉 xiéfēi mài

opisthotonus / əʊpɪsθəʊˈtʌnəs / 角弓反张 jiǎogōng fǎnzhāng

oppression in chest / əˈpreʃn ɪn tʃest / 胸闷 xiōng mèn

oral ulcer / ˈɔrəl ˈʌlsər / 口疮 kǒuchuāng

osteodynia / ˌɒstɪəʊˈdɪnɪə / 骨痛 gǔtòng

* **palpitation** / ˌpælpəˈteʃən / 心悸 xīnjì

pain at xuli / peɪn ət ˈʃuli / 虚里疼痛 xūlǐténgtòng

pain in lateral lower abdomen / peɪn ɪn ˈlætərəl ˈloʊər ˈæbdəmən / 少腹痛 shàofùtòng

pain in tongue / peɪn ɪn tʌŋ / 舌痛 shétòng

pain of eye / peɪn əv aɪ / 目痛 mùtòng

pale complexion / peɪl kəmˈplekʃn / 面色白 miàn

sèbái

pale complexion / peɪl kəm'plekʃn / 面色苍白 miàn sècāngbái

pale lips / peɪl lɪps / 口唇淡白 kǒuchúndànbái

pale tongue / peɪl tʌŋ / 淡白舌 dànbáishé

pale white complexion / peɪl waɪt kəm'plekʃn / 面色淡白 miànsèdànbái

pallid complexion / 'pælɪd kəm'plekʃn / 面色㿠白 miànsèhuàngbái

palms and soles / pɑms ənd 'soles / 五心烦热 wǔxīnfánrè

palpation and pulse taking / pæl'peɪʃn ənd pʌls 'tekɪŋ / 切诊 qièzhěn

palpitation / ˌpælpə'teʃən / 心慌 xīnhuāng

pantalgia / pæn'tældʒə / 身痛 shēntòng

papule / 'pæpjul / 丘疹 qiūzhěn

paradox pulse / 'pærədɑks pʌls / 怪脉 guàimài

parahidrosis / ˌpærədrousɪs / 半身汗出 bànshēnhànchū

paralysis / pə'ræləsɪs / 瘫痪 tānhuàn

paraphasia / ˌpærə'feziə / 错语 cuòyǔ

paroxysmal pain / ˌpærək'sɪzml peɪn / 阵发痛 zhènfātòng

passing stool with pus and blood / 'pæsɪŋ stul wɪð pʌs ənd blʌd / 便脓血 biànnóngxuè

peri-navel pain / 'piri 'neɪvl peɪn / 脐腹痛 qífùtòng

perineal sweating / peri'niəl 'swetɪŋ / 阴汗 yīnhàn

persistent pain / pər'sɪstənt peɪn / 持续痛 chíxùtòng

photophobia / ˌfotəˈfobɪə / 畏光 wèiguāng

pillow bald / ˈpɪlzoʊ bɔld / 枕秃 zhěntū

pink tongue / pɪŋk tʌŋ / 淡红舌 dànhóngshé

plump tongue / plʌmp tʌŋ / 胖大舌 pàngdàshé

polyp / ˈpɑlɪp / 息肉 xīròu

poor appetite / pʊr ˈæpɪtaɪt / 纳谷不香 nàgǔbùxiāng

powder-like fur / ˈpaʊdə laɪk fɜr / 积粉苔 jīfěntāi

precedence of pulse manifestation over symptoms / ˈpresɪdəns əv pʌls ˌmænɪfeˈsteɪʃn ˈoʊvər ˈsɪmptəms / 舍症从脉 shězhèngcóngmài

precedence of symptoms over pulse manifestation / ˈpresɪdəns əv ˈsɪmptəms ˈoʊvər pʌls ˌmænɪfeˈsteɪʃn / 舍脉从症 shěmàicóngzhèng

premature graying hair / ˌpriməˈtʃʊr ˈgreɪɪŋ her / 须发早白 xūfàzǎobái

prickly tongue / ˈprɪkli tʌŋ / 芒刺舌 mángcìshé

profuse spittle / prəˈfjus ˈspɪtl / 多唾 duōtuò

profuse sweating / prəˈfjus ˈswetɪŋ / 大汗 dàhàn

protracted tongue / prəˈtræktɪd tʌŋ / 舌纵 shézòng

proximal bleeding / ˈprɑksɪməl ˈblidɪŋ / 远血 yuǎnxuè

pruritus / prʊˈraɪtəs / 身痒 shēnyǎng

pruritus vulvae / prʊˈraɪtəs ˈvʌlvi / 阴痒 yīnyǎng

ptosis / ˈtosɪs / 眼睑下垂 yǎnjiǎnxiàchuí

pulse manifestation / pʌls ˌmænɪfeˈsteɪʃn / 脉象 màixiàng

pulse searching / pʌls ˈsɜrtʃɪŋ / 推寻 tuīxún

pulse taking / pʌls ˈtekɪŋ / 脉诊 màizhěn

purple macula / ˈpɜrpl ˈmækjʊlə / 紫癜 zǐbān

purplish tongue / ˈpɜrpəlɪʃ tʌŋ / 紫舌 zǐshé

purulent discharge in ear / ˈpjʊrələnt dɪsˈtʃɑrdʒ ɪn ɪr / 耳内流脓 ěrnèiliúnóng

purulent urine / ˈpjʊrələnt ˈjʊrɪn / 尿脓 niàonóng

putrid stool / ˈpjutrɪd stul / 肠垢 chánggòu

qi pass / tʃi pæs / 气关 qìguān

qi rushing upward to heart / tʃi ˈrʌʃɪŋ ˈʌpwərd tə hɑrt / 气上冲心 qìshàngchōngxīn

raised-shoulder breathing / reɪzd ˈʃoʊldər ˈbriðɪŋ / 肩息 jiānxī

rapid digestion of food and polyorexia / ˈræpɪd daɪˈdʒɛstʃən əv fud ənd pəʊlˈjɔreksiə / 消谷善饥 xiāo gǔshànjī

rapid pulse / ˈræpɪd pʌls / 数脉 shuòmài

rash / ræʃ / 疹 zhěn

raving / ˈreɪvɪŋ / 狂言 kuángyán

red and white vaginal discharge / red ənd waɪt vəˈdʒ aɪnl dɪsˈtʃɑrdʒ / 赤白带 chìbáidài

red complexion / red kəmˈplekʃn / 面色红 miànsè hóng

red eye / red aɪ / 目赤 mùchì

red tongue / red tʌŋ / 红舌 hóngshé

reddened and swollen lips / ˈrednd ənd ˈswoʊlən lɪps / 口唇红肿 kǒuchúnhóngzhǒng

redness and swelling of joints / ˈrednəs ənd ˈswelɪŋ əv dʒɔɪnts / 关节红肿 guānjiéhóngzhǒng

regularly intermittent pulse / ˈregjələrli ˌɪntərˈmɪtənt pʌls / 代脉 dàimài

regurgitation / rɪˌgɜrdʒɪˈteɪʃn / 反胃 fǎnwèi

renying / ˈrɛnyɪŋ / 人迎 rényíng

retching / ˈretʃiŋ / 干呕 gān'ǒu

rigidity of limbs / rɪˈdʒɪdəti əv lɪmz / 四肢强直 sìzhīqiángzhí

rigidity of nape and headache / rɪˈdʒɪdəti əv neɪp ənd ˈhedeɪk / 头项强痛 tóuxiàngjiàngtòng

root of pulse / rut əv pʌls / 根 gēn

rooted fur / ˈrutɪd fɜr / 有根苔 yǒugēntāi

rootless fur / ˈrutləs fɜr / 无根苔 wúgēntāi

rough fur / rʌf fɜr / 糙苔 cāotāi

＊**spasm** / ˈspæzəm / 转筋 zhuànjīn

＊**spermatorrhea** / spɜrmætoˈrɪr / 遗精 yíjīng

salivation / ˌsælɪˈveɪʃn / 流涎 liúxián

sallow complexion / ˈsælou kəmˈplekʃn / 面色萎黄 miànsèwěihuáng

salty taste in mouth / ˈsalti teɪst ɪn mauθ / 口咸 kǒuxián

sandy urine / ˈsændi ˈjʊrɪn / 尿中砂石 niàozhōng shāshí

scattered pulse / ˈskætərd pʌls / 散脉 sǎnmài

scurrying pain / ˈskɜriŋ peɪn / 窜痛 cuàntòng

semen in urine / ˈsimən ɪn ˈjʊrɪn / 小便夹精 xiǎobiàn jiájīng

severe pain / sɪˈvɪr peɪn / 剧痛 jùtòng

sexual intercourse in dream / ˈsekʃuəl ˈɪntərkɔrs ɪn drim / 梦交 mèngjiāo

sheeny complexion / ˈʃinɪ kəmˈplekʃn / 色泽 sèzé

shivering / ˈʃɪvərɪŋ / 寒战 hánzhàn

short pulse / ʃɔrt pʌls / 短脉 duǎnmài

shortened and contracted tongue / ˈʃɔrtned ənd kənˈtræktɪd tʌŋ / 舌短缩 shéduǎnsuō

shortness of breath / ˈʃɔrtnəs əv breθ / 短气 duǎnqì

shoulder pain / ˈʃoʊldər peɪn / 肩痛 jiāntòng

sick complexion / sɪk kəmˈplekʃn / 病色 bìngsè

sighing / saɪɪŋ / 太息 tàixī

simultaneous palpations with three fingers / ˌsaɪmlˈteɪnɪəs pælˈpeɪʃns wɪð θri ˈfɪŋgəs / 总按 zǒng'àn

single finger palpation / ˈsɪŋgl ˈfɪŋgər pælˈpeɪʃn / 单按 dānàn

site for taking carotid pulse / saɪt fər ˈtekɪŋ kəˈrɑtɪd pʌls / 人迎 rényíng

site for taking wrist pulse / saɪt fər ˈtekɪŋ rɪst pʌls / 寸口 cùnkǒu

slippery fur / ˈslɪpəri fɜr / 滑苔 huátāi

slippery pulse / ˈslɪpəri pʌls / 滑脉 huámài

slow pulse / sloʊ pʌls / 迟脉 chímài

snoring / ˈsnɔrɪŋ / 鼻鼾 bíhān

soft pulse / sɔft pʌls / 濡脉 rúmài

soliloquy / səˈlɪləkwi / 独语 dúyǔ

somnambulism / sɑmˈnæmbjəlɪzəm / 梦游 mèngyóu

sonorous voice / ˈsɑnərəs vɔɪs / 语声洪亮 yǔshēng hóngliàng

sore in mouth / sɔr ɪn maʊθ / 口中生疮 kǒuzhōng

shēngchuāng

soreness and weakness of waist and knees / ˈsɔrnəs ənd ˈwiknəs əv weɪst ənd niz / 腰膝酸软 yāoxīsuānruǎn

soreness of loins / ˈsɔrnəs əv lɔinz / 腰酸 yāosuān

sour pain / ˈsauər peɪn / 酸痛 suāntòng

sour taste in mouth / ˈsauər teɪst ɪn mauθ / 口酸 kǒusuān

spasm of fingers / ˈspæzəm əv ˈfɪŋɡəs / 手指挛急 shǒuzhǐluánjí

spasm of limbs / ˈspæzəm əv lɪmz / 四肢拘急 sìzhījūjí

spasm of nape and back / ˈspæzəm əv neɪp ənd bæk / 项背拘急 xiàngbèijūjí

spasmodic pain in lower abdomen / spæzˈmɑdɪk peɪn ɪn ˈlouər ˈæbdəmən / 少腹急结 shàofùjíjié

spirit of pulse / ˈspɪrɪt əv pʌls / 神 shén

spiritlessness / ˈspɪrɪtləsnəs / 神疲 shénpí

spitting blood / ˈspɪtɪŋ blʌd / 唾血 tuòxuè

spontaneous sweating / spɑnˈteɪniəs ˈswetɪŋ / 自汗 zìhàn

squamous and dry skin / ˈskweməs ənd draɪ skɪn / 肌肤甲错 jīfūjiǎcuò

stabbing pain / ˈstæbɪŋ peɪn / 刺痛 cìtòng

stained fur / steɪnd fɜr / 染苔 rǎntāi

sticky and greasy in mouth / ˈstɪki ænd ˈgrisi ɪn mauθ / 口黏腻 kǒuniánnì

sticky greasy fur / ˈstɪki ˈgrisi fɜr / 黏腻苔 niánnìtāi

sticky sweating / ˈstɪki ˈswetɪŋ / 油汗 yóuhàn

stiff neck / stɪf nek / 项强 xiàngjiàng

stiff tongue / stɪf tʌŋ / 舌强 shéjiàng

stomach pain / ˈstʌmək peɪn / 胃痛 wèitòng

stomach qi of pulse / ˈstʌmək tʃi əv pʌls / 胃脉气 wèimàiqì

stomach qi spirit and root of pulse / ˈstʌmək tʃi ˈspɪrɪt ənd rut əv pʌls / 胃神根 wèishéngēn

stopped pulse / ˌstɑpt pʌls / 歇止脉 xiēzhǐmài

stringy pulse / ˈstrɪŋi pʌls / 弦脉 xiánmài

stuffy nose / ˈstʌfi noʊz / 鼻塞 bísè

stuffy pain / ˈstʌfi peɪn / 闷痛 mēntòng

stutter / ˈstʌtər / 重言 chóngyán

sublingual vessel / sʌbˈlɪŋgwəl ˈvesl / 舌下络脉 shé xiàluòmài

suffocation / ˌsʌfəˈkeɪʃn / 憋气 biēqì

sunken fontanel in infant / ˈsʌŋkən ˌfɑntəˈnel ɪn ˈɪnfənt / 囟门下陷 xìnménxiàxiàn

surging pulse / sɛdʒɪŋ pʌls / 洪脉 hóngmài

sweating / ˈswetɪŋ / 有汗 yǒuhàn

sweating following shiver / ˈswetɪŋ ˈfɑloʊɪŋ ˈʃɪvər / 战汗 zhànhàn

sweating of dying / ˈswetɪŋ əv ˈdaɪɪŋ / 绝汗 juéhàn

sweating of dying / ˈswetɪŋ əv ˈdaɪɪŋ / 脱汗 tuōhàn

sweating of hands and feet / ˈswetɪŋ əv hænds ənd fit / 手足汗出 shǒuzúhànchū

sweating of palms and soles / ˈswetɪŋ əv pɑms ənd ˈsoles / 手足心汗 shǒuzúxīnhàn

sweet taste in mouth / swit teɪst ɪn maʊθ / 口甜 kǒutián

swelling and aching of gum / ˈswelɪŋ ənd ˈeɪkɪŋ əv gʌm / 牙龈肿痛 yáyínzhǒngtòng

swelling and pain in knee / ˈswelɪŋ ənd peɪn ɪn ni / 膝肿痛 xīzhǒngtòng

swelling and pain in throat / ˈswelɪŋ ənd peɪn ɪn θroʊt / 咽喉肿痛 yānhóuzhǒngtòng

swift pulse / swɪft pʌls / 疾脉 jímài

swollen tongue / ˈswoʊlən tʌŋ / 肿胀舌 zhǒngzhàngshé

symptom / ˈsɪmptəm / 症状 zhèngzhuàng

syncope with convulsion / ˈsɪŋkəpi wɪð kənˈvʌlʃn / 痉厥 jìngjué

∗ **tinnitus** / ˈtɪnɪtəs / 耳鸣 ěrmíng

taste / teɪst / 口味 kǒuwèi

tasteless of tongue / ˈteɪstləs əv tʌŋ / 舌不知味 shé bùzhīwèi

tastelessness / ˈteɪstləsnəs / 口淡 kǒudàn

teeth-printed tongue / tiθ ˈprɪntɪd tʌŋ / 齿痕舌 chǐhénshé

ten questions / ten ˈkwestʃənz / 十问 shíwèn

tender tongue / ˈtendər tʌŋ / 嫩舌 nènshé

tenderness of acupoints / ˈtendərnəs əv ˈækjʊpɒɪnts / 腧穴压痛 shùxuéyātòng

tenesmus / tɪˈnezməs / 里急后重 lǐjíhòuzhòng

thick fur / θɪk fɜr / 厚苔 hòutāi

thigh pain / θaɪ peɪn / 股阴痛 gǔyīntòng

thin and weak body / θɪn ənd wik ˈbɑdi / 身体尪羸 shēntǐwāngléi

thin fur / θɪn fɜr / 薄苔 báotāi

thin tongue / θɪn tʌŋ / 瘦薄舌 shòubáoshé

thirst / θɜrst / 口渴 kǒukě

thirst without desire to drink / θɜrst wɪˈðaʊt dɪˈzaɪər tə drɪŋk / 渴不欲饮 kěbùyùyǐn

thready pulse / ˈθrɛdi pʌls / 细脉 xìmài

three body parts and nine pulse taking sites / θri ˈbɑdi pɑts ənd naɪn pʌls ˈtekɪŋ saɪts / 三部九候 sānbù jiǔhòu

three passes at tiger-mouth / θri pæsiz ət ˈtaɪgər maʊθ / 虎口三关 hǔkǒusānguān

throbbing below umbilical region / ˈθrɒbɪŋ bɪˈlou ʌmˈbɪlɪkl ˈridʒən / 脐下悸动 qíxiàjìdòng

tidal fever / ˈtaɪdl ˈfivər / 潮热 cháorè

tidal fever in the afternoon / ˈtaɪdl ˈfivər ɪn ðə ˌæftərˈnun / 午后潮热 wǔhòucháorè

tight pulse / taɪt pʌls / 紧脉 jǐnmài

tongue biting / tʌŋ ˈbaɪtɪŋ / 啮舌 nièshé

tongue bleeding / tʌŋ ˈblidɪŋ / 舌衄 shénǜ

tongue color / tʌŋ ˈkʌlər / 舌色 shésè

tongue condition / tʌŋ kənˈdɪʃn / 舌态 shétài

tongue inspection / tʌŋ ɪnˈspekʃn / 舌诊 shézhěn

tongue manifestation / tʌŋ ˌmænifeˈsteɪʃn / 舌象 shéxiàng

tongue quality / tʌŋ ˈkwɑləti / 舌质 shézhì

tongue shape / tʌŋ ʃeɪp / 舌形 shéxíng

tongue sore / tʌŋ sor / 舌疮 shéchuāng

tongue spirit / tʌŋ ˈspɪrɪt / 舌神 shéshén

toothache / ˈtuθeɪk / 牙痛 yátòng

touching pressing and searching / ˈtʌtʃɪŋ ˈpresɪŋ ənd ˈsɜrtʃɪŋ / 举按寻 jǔànxún

tough tongue / tʌf tʌŋ / 老舌 lǎoshé

tranquil pulse / ˈtræŋkwɪl pʌls / 脉静 màijìng

trembling tongue / ˈtremblɪŋ tʌŋ / 舌颤 shéchàn

tremor of feet / ˈtremər əv fit / 足颤 zúchàn

tremor of hand / ˈtremər əv hænd / 手颤 shǒuchàn

tremor of lips / ˈtremər əv lɪps / 口唇颤动 kǒuchún chàndòng

tremulous pulse / ˈtremjələs pʌls / 动脉 dòngmài

tugging and slackening / ˈtʌgɪŋ ənd ˈslækənɪŋ / 瘈疭 chìzòng

turbid urine / ˈtɜrbɪd ˈjʊrɪn / 小便浑浊 xiǎobiàn húnzhuó

tympanic pulse / tɪmˈpænɪk pʌls / 革脉 gémài

tympanites / ˌtɪmpəˈnaɪtiz / 单腹胀大 dānfùzhàngdà

ulcer / ˈʌlsər / 溃疡 kuìyáng

ulcer of gums / ˈʌlsər əv gʌms / 牙龈溃烂 yáyínkuìlàn

unconsciousness / ʌnˈkɑnʃəsnɪs / 神昏 shénhūn

urinary smell / ˈjʊrɪneri smel / 尿臭 niàochòu

urinary stoppage / ˈjʊrɪneri ˈstɑpɪdʒ / 小便不通 xiǎo biànbùtōng

urticaria / ˌɜrtɪˈkeriə / 风团 fēngtuán

venous engorgement on abdomen / ˈvinəs ɪnˈgɔrdʒmənt ɑn ˈæbdəmən / 腹露青筋 fùlùqīngjīn

vertigo / ˈvɜrtɪgoʊ / 头昏 tóuhūn

visiting complexion / ˈvɪzɪtɪŋ kəmˈplekʃn / 客色 kèsè

vomit in the morning what eaten at last night / ˈvɑmɪt ɪn ðə ˈmɔrnɪŋ wʌt itn ət læst naɪt / 暮食朝吐 mù shízhāotǔ

vomiting / ˈvɑmɪtɪŋ / 呕吐 ǒutù

vomiting ascaris / ˈvɑmɪtɪŋ ˈæskərɪs / 吐蛔 tǔhuí

vomiting right after eating / ˈvɑmɪtɪŋ raɪt ˈæftər ˈitɪŋ / 食已则吐 shíyǐzétǔ

wagging tongue / ˈwægɪŋ tʌŋ / 吐舌 tǔshé

watery stool / ˈwɔtəri stul / 自利清水 zìlìqīngshuǐ

weak pulse / wik pʌls / 弱脉 ruòmài

weak teeth with aching / wik tiθ wɪð ˈeɪkɪŋ / 牙齿酸弱 yáchǐsuānruò

weakness / ˈwiknəs / 乏力 fálì

wheezing / wizɪŋ / 哮鸣 xiàomíng

wheezing due to retention of phlegm in throat / wizɪŋ du tə rɪˈtenʃn əv flem ɪn θroʊt / 喉中痰鸣 hóuzhōngtánmíng

white fur / waɪt fɜr / 白苔 báitāi

white vaginal discharge / waɪt vəˈdʒaɪnl dɪsˈtʃɑrdʒ / 白带 báidài

wind pass / wɪnd pæs / 风关 fēngguān

wind patches / wɪnd pætʃes / 风团 fēngtuán

withered auricle / ˈwɪðərd ˈɔrɪkl / 耳郭枯槁 ěrguō kūgǎo

withered skin and hair / ˈwɪðərd skɪn ənd hɜr / 毛悴色夭 máocuìsèyāo

withered tongue / ˈwɪðərd tʌŋ / 枯舌 kūshé

wriggling of limbs / ˈrɪglɪŋ əv lɪmz / 手足蠕动 shǒu

zúrúdòng

wry eye and mouth / raɪ aɪ ənd maʊθ / 口眼喎斜 kǒuyǎnwāixié

wry tongue / raɪ tʌŋ / 舌歪 shéwāi

yawning / ˈjɔnɪŋ / 呵欠 hēqiàn

yellow fur / ˈjelou fɜr / 黄苔 huángtāi

yellow skin and eye / ˈjelou skɪn ənd aɪ / 身目俱黄 shēnmùjùhuáng

yellow vaginal discharge / ˈjelou vəˈdʒaɪnl dɪsˈtʃɑrdʒ / 黄带 huángdài

yellowish sweating / ˈjelouɪʃ ˈswetɪŋ / 黄汗 huánghàn

Section 2　Syndrome Differentiations

第二节　辨　证

∗ **cold syndrome** / kould ˈsɪndroum / 寒证 hánzhèng

coagulated cold syndrome / kouˈægjuleɪtɪd kould ˈsɪndroum / 寒凝证 hánníngzhèng

cold transformation syndrome of Shaoyin / kould ˌtrænsfərˈmeɪʃn ˈsɪndroum əv ʃaʊjin / 少阴寒化证 shàoyīnhánhuàzhèng

cold-dampness syndrome / kould ˈdæmpnəs ˈsɪndroum / 寒湿证 hánshīzhèng

cold-dryness syndrome / kould ˈdraɪnəs ˈsɪndroum / 凉燥证 liángzàozhèng

cold-phlegm syndrome / kould flem ˈsɪndroum / 寒痰证 hántánzhèng

concurrent syndromes / kənˈkɜrənt ˈsɪndroums / 证候相兼 zhènghòuxiāngjiān

* **dampness-heat syndrome with predominant dampness** / ˈdæmpnəs hit ˈsɪndroʊm wɪð prɪˈdɑmɪnənt ˈdæmpnəs / 湿重于热证 shīzhòngyúrèzhèng

* **dampness-phlegm syndrome** / ˈdæmpnəs flem ˈsɪndroʊm / 湿痰证 shītánzhèng

* **dry-phlegm syndrome** / draɪ flem ˈsɪndroʊm / 燥痰证 zàotánzhèng

dampness [retention] syndrome / ˈdæmpnəs [rɪˈtenʃn] ˈsɪndroʊm / 湿阻证 shīzǔzhèng

dampness-heat syndrome with predominant heat / ˈdæmpnəs hit ˈsɪndroʊm wɪð prɪˈdɑmɪnənt hit / 热重于湿证 rèzhòngyúshīzhèng

deteriorated case / dɪˈtɪriəreɪted keɪs / 变证 biànzhèng

dryness syndrome / ˈdraɪnəs ˈsɪndroʊm / 燥证 zào zhèng

* **excessive cold syndrome** / ɪkˈsesɪv koʊld ˈsɪndroʊm / 实寒证 shíhánzhèng

eight principles / eɪt ˈprɪnsəplz / 八纲 bāgāng

excessive heat syndrome / ɪkˈsesɪv hit ˈsɪndroʊm / 实热证 shírèzhèng

exogenous dryness syndrome / ekˈsɑdʒənəs ˈdraɪnəs ˈsɪndroʊm / 外燥证 wàizàozhèng

exogenous wind syndrome / ekˈsɑdʒənəs wɪnd ˈsɪndroʊm / 外风证 wàifēngzhèng

fire syndrome / ˈfaɪər ˈsɪndroʊm / 火证 huǒzhèng

fire-toxicity syndrome / ˈfaɪər tɑkˈsɪsəti ˈsɪndroʊm / 火毒证 huǒdúzhèng

fluid retention syndrome / ˈfluɪd rɪˈtenʃn ˈsɪndroʊm /

饮证 yǐnzhèng

* **heat syndrome** / hit ˈsɪndroʊm / 热证 rèzhèng

heat transformation syndrome of Shaoyin / hit ˌtrænsfərˈmeɪʃn ˈsɪndroʊm əv ʃɑʊjɪn / 少阴热化证 shào yīnrèhuàzhèng

heat-phlegm syndrome / hit flem ˈsɪndroʊm / 热痰证 rètánzhèng

* [**interior**] **excess syndrome** / ɪnˈtɪriər ɪkˈses ˈsɪndroʊm / [里]实证 [lǐ]shízhèng

* **interior cold syndrome** / ɪnˈtɪriər koʊld ˈsɪndroʊm / 里寒证 lǐhánzhèng

* **interior heat syndrome** / ɪnˈtɪriər hit ˈsɪndroʊm / 里热证 lǐrèzhèng

* **interior syndrome** / ɪnˈtɪriər ˈsɪndroʊm / 里证 lǐzhèng

[**interior**] **deficiency syndrome** / ɪnˈtɪriər dɪˈfɪʃənsi ˈsɪndroʊm / [里]虚证 [lǐ]xūzhèng

intermingling syndrome / ˌɪntəˈmɪŋglɪŋ ˈsɪndroʊm / 证候错杂 zhènghòucuòzá

mistreated disease / ˌmɪsˈtrited dɪˈziz / 坏病 huàibìng

pattern / ˈpætərn / 证 zhèng

phlegm syndrome / flem ˈsɪndroʊm / 痰证 tánzhèng

* **qifen syndrome** / tʃifen ˈsɪndroʊm / 气分证 qìfēn zhèng

* **Shaoyang syndrome** / ʃɑʊjæŋ ˈsɪndroʊm / 少阳病证 shàoyángbìngzhèng

* **Shaoyin syndrome** / ʃɑʊjɪn ˈsɪndroʊm / 少阴病证 shàoyīnbìngzhèng

* **superficies syndrome** / ˌsʊpəˈfiʃiˌiz ˈsɪndroʊm / 表证 biǎozhèng

* **syndrome of accumulated heat due to fetal toxicity** / ˈsɪndroʊm əv əˈkjʊmjəˈletɪd hit du tə ˈfitl tɑkˈsɪsəti / 胎毒蕴热证 tāidúyùnrèzhèng

* **syndrome of adverse rising of stomach qi** / ˈsɪndroʊm əv ədˈvɜrs ˈraɪzɪŋ əv ˈstʌmək tʃi / 胃气上逆证 wèiqìshàngnìzhèng

* **syndrome of blood deficiency** / ˈsɪndroʊm əv blʌd dɪˈfiʃnsi / 血虚证 xuèxūzhèng

* **syndrome of blood stasis** / ˈsɪndroʊm əv blʌd ˈsteɪsɪs / 血瘀证 xuèyūzhèng

* **syndrome of channel hit by wind** / ˈsɪndroʊm əv ˈtʃænl hɪt baɪ wɪnd / 风中经络证 fēngzhòngjīngluòzhèng

* **syndrome of coagulated cold in uterus** / ˈsɪndroʊm əv koʊˈægjuleɪtɪd koʊld ɪn ˈjutərəs / 寒凝胞宫证 hánníngbāogōngzhèng

* **syndrome of cold in blood** / ˈsɪndroʊm əv koʊld ɪn blʌd / 血寒证 xuèhánzhèng

* **syndrome of cold in both superficies and interior** / ˈsɪndroʊm əv koʊld ɪn boʊθ ˌsʊpəˈfiʃiˌiz ənd ɪnˈtɪriər / 表里俱寒证 biǎolǐjùhánzhèng

* **syndrome of cold pathogen attacking stomach** / ˈsɪndroʊm əv koʊld ˈpæθədʒən əˈtækɪŋ ˈstʌmək / 寒邪犯胃证 hánxiéfànwèizhèng

* **syndrome of cold pathogen of Taiyang** / ˈsɪndroʊm əv koʊld ˈpæθədʒən əv taɪjæŋ / 太阳伤寒证 tàiyángshānghánzhèng

* **syndrome of cold-dampness disturbing spleen**
/ ˈsɪndroʊm əv koʊld ˈdæmpnəs dɪˈstɜrbɪŋ splin / 寒湿困脾证 hánshīkùnpízhèng

* **syndrome of dampness stagnancy due to spleen deficiency** / ˈsɪndroʊm əv ˈdæmpnəs ˈstægnənsi du tə splin dɪˈfɪʃnsi / 脾虚湿困证 píxūshīkùnzhèng

* **syndrome of dampness-heat due to spleen deficiency**
/ ˈsɪndroʊm əv ˈdæmpnəs hit du tə splin dɪˈfɪʃnsi / 脾虚湿热证 píxūshīrèzhèng

* **syndrome of dampness-heat in large intestine**
/ ˈsɪndroʊm əv ˈdæmpnəs hit ɪn lɑrdʒ ɪnˈtestɪn / 大肠湿热证 dàchángshīrèzhèng

* **syndrome of dampness-heat in lower jiao**
/ ˈsɪndroʊm əv ˈdæmpnəs hit ɪn ˈloə dʒjɑʊ / 下焦湿热证 xiàjiāoshīrèzhèng

* **syndrome of dampness-heat in middle jiao**
/ ˈsɪndroʊm əv ˈdæmpnəs hit ɪn ˈmɪdl dʒjɑʊ / 中焦湿热证 zhōngjiāoshīrèzhèng

* **syndrome of dampness-heat in qifen** / ˈsɪndroʊm əv ˈdæmpnəs hit ɪn tʃifen / 气分湿热证 qìfēnshīrèzhèng

* **syndrome of dampness-heat in upper jiao**
/ ˈsɪndroʊm əv ˈdæmpnəs hit ɪn ˈʌpər dʒjɑʊ / 上焦湿热证 shàngjiāoshīrèzhèng

* **syndrome of dampness-heat in uterus** / ˈsɪndroʊm əv ˈdæmpnəs hit ɪn ˈjutərəs / 胞宫湿热证 bāogōng shī rèzhèng

* **syndrome of dampness-heat in womb** / ˈsɪndrəm əv ˈdæmpnəs hit ɪn wum / 胞宫湿热证 bāogōngshī

rèzhèng

* **syndrome of dampness-heat of bladder** / ˈsɪndroʊm əv ˈdæmpnəs hit əv ˈblædə / 膀胱湿热证 pángguāngshīrèzhèng

* **syndrome of dampness-heat of liver and gallbladder** / ˈsɪndroʊm əv ˈdæmpnəs hit əv ˈlɪvə ənd ˈgɔlˌblædə / 肝胆湿热证 gāndǎnshīrèzhèng

* **syndrome of dampness-heat of liver channel** / ˈsɪndroʊm əv ˈdæmpnəs hit əv ˈlɪvə ˈtʃænl / 肝经湿热证 gānjīngshīrèzhèng

* **syndrome of dampness-heat of spleen and stomach** / ˈsɪndroʊm əv ˈdæmpnəs hit əv splin ənd ˈstʌmək / 脾胃湿热证 píwèishīrèzhèng

* **syndrome of dampness-heat stagnating in spleen** / ˈsɪndroʊm əv ˈdæmpnəs hit ˈstægneɪtɪŋ ɪn splin / 湿热蕴脾证 shīrèyùnpízhèng

* **syndrome of deficiency of both heart and spleen** / ˈsɪndroʊm əv dɪˈfɪʃnsi əv boʊθ hɑrt ənd splin / 心脾两虚证 xīnpíliǎngxūzhèng

* **syndrome of deficiency of both qi and blood of heart** / ˈsɪndroʊm əv dɪˈfɪʃnsi əv boʊθ tʃi ənd blʌd əv hɑrt / 心气血两虚证 xīnqìxuèliǎngxūzhèng

* **syndrome of deficiency of both qi and yin of heart** / ˈsɪndroʊm əv dɪˈfɪʃnsi əv boʊθ tʃi ənd jɪn əv hɑrt / 心气阴两虚证 xīnqìyīnliǎngxūzhèng

* **syndrome of deficiency of both qi and yin of lung** / ˈsɪndroʊm əv dɪˈfɪʃnsi əv boʊθ tʃi ənd jɪn əv lʌŋ / 肺气阴两虚证 fèiqìyīnliǎngxūzhèng

* **syndrome of deficiency of fluid** / ˈsɪndroʊm əv

dɪˈfɪʃnsi əv ˈfluɪd / 津液亏虚证 jīnyèkuīxūzhèng

* **syndrome of deficiency of heart blood** / ˈsɪndroʊm əv dɪˈfɪʃnsi əv hɑrt blʌd / 心血虚证 xīnxuèxū zhèng

* **syndrome of deficiency of heart qi** / ˈsɪndroʊm əv dɪˈfɪʃnsi əv hɑrt tʃi / 心气虚证 xīnqìxūzhèng

* **syndrome of deficiency of heart yang** / ˈsɪndroʊm əv dɪˈfɪʃnsi əv hɑrt jæŋ / 心阳虚证 xīnyángxū zhèng

* **syndrome of deficiency of heart yin** / ˈsɪndroʊm əv dɪˈfɪʃnsi əv hɑrt jɪn / 心阴虚证 xīnyīnxūzhèng

* **syndrome of deficiency of kidney essence** / ˈsɪndroʊm əv dɪˈfɪʃnsi əv ˈkɪdni ˈesns / 肾精亏虚证 shènjīng kuīxūzhèng

* **syndrome of deficiency of kidney qi** / ˈsɪndroʊm əv dɪˈfɪʃnsi əv ˈkɪdni tʃi / 肾气虚证 shènqìxūzhèng

* **syndrome of deficiency of kidney yang** / ˈsɪndroʊm əv dɪˈfɪʃnsi əv ˈkɪdni jæŋ / 肾阳虚证 shènyáng xūzhèng

* **syndrome of deficiency of kidney yin** / ˈsɪndroʊm əv dɪˈfɪʃnsi əv ˈkɪdni jɪn / 肾阴虚证 shènyīnxūzhèng

* **syndrome of deficiency of liver blood** / ˈsɪndroʊm əv dɪˈfɪʃnsi əv ˈlɪvər blʌd / 肝血虚证 gānxuèxūzhèng

* **syndrome of deficiency of liver qi** / ˈsɪndroʊm əv dɪˈfɪʃnsi əv ˈlɪvər tʃi / 肝气虚证 gānqìxūzhèng

* **syndrome of deficiency of liver yang** / ˈsɪndroʊm əv dɪˈfɪʃnsi əv ˈlɪvər jæŋ / 肝阳虚证 gānyángxūzhèng

* **syndrome of deficiency of liver yin** / ˈsɪndroʊm əv

dɪˈfɪʃnsi əv ˈlɪvər jɪn / 肝阴虚证 gānyīnxūzhèng

* **syndrome of deficiency of lung qi** / ˈsɪndroʊm əv
dɪˈfɪʃnsi əv lʌŋ tʃi / 肺气虚证 fèiqìxūzhèng

* **syndrome of deficiency of lung yin** / ˈsɪndroʊm əv
dɪˈfɪʃnsi əv lʌŋ jɪn / 肺阴虚证 fèiyīnxūzhèng

* **syndrome of deficiency of spleen qi** / ˈsɪndroʊm əv
dɪˈfɪʃnsi əv splin tʃi / 脾气虚证 píqìxūzhèng

* **syndrome of deficiency of spleen yang** / ˈsɪndroʊm əv
dɪˈfɪʃnsi əv splin jæŋ / 脾阳虚 píyángxū
zhèng

* **syndrome of deficiency of spleen yin** / ˈsɪndroʊm əv
dɪˈfɪʃnsi əv splin jɪn / 脾阴虚证 píyīnxūzhèng

* **syndrome of deficiency of stomach qi** / ˈsɪndroʊm əv
dɪˈfɪʃnsi əv ˈstʌmək tʃi / 胃气虚证 wèiqìxū
zhèng

* **syndrome of deficiency of stomach yin** / ˈsɪndroʊm
əv dɪˈfɪʃnsi əv ˈstʌmək jɪn / 胃阴虚证 wèiyīnxū
zhèng

* **syndrome of deficient cold in uterus** / ˈsɪndroʊm əv
dɪˈfɪʃnt koʊld ɪn ˈjutərəs / 胞宫虚寒证 bāogōng
xūhánzhèng

* **syndrome of deficient cold in womb** / ˈsɪndroʊm əv
dɪˈfɪʃnt koʊld ɪn wum / 胞宫虚寒证 bāogōngxū
hánzhèng

* **syndrome of deficient cold of bladder** / ˈsɪndroʊm əv
dɪˈfɪʃnt koʊld əv ˈblædə / 膀胱虚寒证 pángguāng
xūhánzhèng

* **syndrome of deficient cold of spleen and stomach**

/ ˈsɪndroʊm əv dɪˈfɪʃnt koʊld əv splin ənd ˈstʌmək /
脾胃虚寒证 píwèixūhánzhèng

* **syndrome of disharmony between heart and kidney**
/ ˈsɪndroʊm əv dɪsˈhɑrməni bɪˈtwin hɑrt ənd ˈkɪdni /
心肾不交证 xīnshènbùjiāozhèng

* **syndrome of endogenous heat due to yin deficiency**
/ ˈsɪndroʊm əv enˈdɑdʒənəs hit du tə jɪn dɪˈfɪʃnsi /
阴虚内热证 yīnxūnèirèzhèng

* **syndrome of excessive heat in middle jiao**
/ ˈsɪndroʊm əv ɪkˈsesɪv hit ɪn ˈmɪdl dʒjɑʊ / 中焦
实热证 zhōngjiāoshírèzhèng

* **syndrome of excessive heat of small intestine**
/ ˈsɪndroʊm əv ɪkˈsesɪv hit əv smɔl ɪnˈtestɪn / 小
肠实热证 xiǎochángshírèzhèng

* **syndrome of exogenous disease due to qi deficiency**
/ ˈsɪndroʊm əv enˈdsɑdʒənəs dɪˈziz du tə tʃi
dɪˈfɪʃnsi / 气虚外感证 qìxūwàigǎnzhèng

* **syndrome of exuberance of lung heat** / ˈsɪndroʊm əv
ɪgˈzubərəns əv lʌŋ hit / 肺热炽盛证 fèirèchì
shèngzhèng

* **syndrome of fever due to qi deficiency** / ˈsɪndroʊm əv
ˈfivər du tə tʃi dɪˈfɪʃnsi / 气虚发热证 qìxūfārè
zhèng

* **syndrome of flaring up of heart fire** / ˈsɪndroʊm əv
ˈflɛrɪŋ ʌp əv hɑrt ˈfaɪər / 心火上炎证 xīnhuǒ
shàngyánzhèng

* **syndrome of food retention due to spleen deficiency**
/ ˈsɪndroʊm əv fud rɪˈtenʃn du tə splin dɪˈfɪʃnsi /
脾虚食积证 píxūshíjīzhèng

* **syndrome of heat in both superficies and interior** / ˈsɪndroʊm əv hit ɪn boʊθ ˌsupəˈfɪʃɪ ˌiz ənd ɪnˈtɪriər / 表里俱热证 biǎolǐjùrèzhèng

* **syndrome of heat transformed from wind-cold** / ˈsɪndroʊm əv hit trænsˈfɔrmd frəm wɪnd koʊld / 风寒化热证 fēnghánhuàrèzhèng

* **syndrome of heat transformed from wind-dampness** / ˈsɪndroʊm əv hit trænsˈfɔrmd frə mwɪnd ˈdæmpnəs / 风湿化热证 fēngshīhuàrèzhèng

* **syndrome of hyperactivity of fire due to deficiency of kidney yin** / ˈsɪndroʊm əv ˌhaɪpərækˈtɪvəti əv ˈfaɪər du tə dɪˈfɪʃnsi əv ˈkɪdni jɪn / 肾阴虚火旺证 shènyīnxūhuǒwàngzhèng

* **syndrome of incoordination between liver and stomach** / ˈsɪndroʊm əv ˌɪnkoˌɔrdnˈeʃən bɪˈtwin ˈlɪvər ənd ˈstʌmək / 肝胃不和证 gānwèibùhézhèng

* **syndrome of intermingled heat and cold** / ˈsɪndroʊm əv ˌɪntərˈmɪŋgld hit ənd koʊld / 寒热错杂证 hánrècuòzázhèng

* **syndrome of liver fire flaring up** / ˈsɪndroʊm əv ˈlɪvər ˈfaɪər ˈflɛrɪŋ ʌp / 肝火上炎证 gānhuǒshàngyánzhèng

* **syndrome of liver fire invading lung** / ˈsɪndroʊm əv ˈlɪvər ˈfaɪər ɪnˈvedɪŋ lʌŋ / 肝火犯肺证 gānhuǒfànfèizhèng

* **syndrome of marrow depletion due to kidney deficiency** / ˈsɪndroʊm əv ˈmæroʊ dɪˈpliʃn du tə ˈkɪdni dɪˈfɪʃnsi / 肾虚髓亏证 shènxūsuǐkuīzhèng

* **syndrome of qi deficiency** / ˈsɪndroʊm əv tʃi dɪˈfɪʃnsi /

气虚证 qìxūzhèng

* **syndrome of qi deficiency of heart and lung** / ˈsɪndroʊm əv tʃi dɪˈfɪʃnsi əv hɑrt ənd lʌŋ / 心肺气虚证 xīnfèiqìxūzhèng

* **syndrome of qi deficiency of spleen and lung** / ˈsɪndroʊm əv tʃi dɪˈfɪʃnsi əv splin ənd lʌŋ / 脾肺气虚证 pífèiqìxūzhèng

* **syndrome of qi desertion** / ˈsɪndroʊm əv tʃi dɪˈzɜrʃn / 气脱证 qìtuōzhèng

* **syndrome of qi sinking** / ˈsɪndroʊm əv tʃi ˈsɪŋkɪŋ / 气陷证 qìxiànzhèng

* **syndrome of qi stagnation** / ˈsɪndroʊm əv tʃi stæɡˈneɪʃn / 气滞证 qìzhìzhèng

* **syndrome of reversed flow of qi** / ˈsɪndroʊm əv rɪˈvɜst floʊ əv tʃi / 气逆证 qìnìzhèng

* **syndrome of sinking of qi due to spleen deficiency** / ˈsɪndroʊm əv ˈsɪŋkɪŋ əv tʃi du tə splin dɪˈfɪʃnsi / 脾虚气陷证 píxūqìxiànzhèng

* **syndrome of spleen failing to manage blood** / ˈsɪndroʊm əv splin ˈfeɪlɪŋ tə ˈmænɪdʒ blʌd / 脾不统血证 píbùtǒngxuèzhèng

* **syndrome of stagnation of liver qi and blood deficiency** / ˈsɪndroʊm əv stæɡˈneɪʃn əv ˈlɪvər tʃi ənd blʌd dɪˈfɪʃnsi / 肝郁血虚证 gānyùxuèxūzhèng

* **syndrome of superficies cold and interior heat** / ˈsɪndroʊm əv ˌsʊpəˈfɪʃɪˌiz koʊld ənd ɪnˈtɪriər hit / 表寒里热证 biǎohánlǐrèzhèng

* **syndrome of superficies heat and interior cold** / ˈsɪndroʊm əv ˌsʊpəˈfɪʃɪˌiz hit ənd ɪnˈtɪriər koʊld /

表热里寒证 biǎorèlǐhánzhèng

* **syndrome of true cold disease with false heat manifestation** / ˈsɪndroʊm əv tru koʊld dɪˈziz wɪð fɔls hit ˌmænɪfeˈsteɪʃn / 真寒假热证 zhēnhánjiǎrèzhèng

* **syndrome of true heat disease with false cold manifestation** / ˈsɪndroʊm əv tru hit dɪˈziz wɪð fɔls koʊld ˌmænɪfeˈsteɪʃn / 真热假寒证 zhēnrèjiǎhánzhèng

* **syndrome of upper cold and lower heat** / ˈsɪndroʊm əv ˈʌpə koʊld ənd ˈloə hit / 上寒下热证 shànghánxiàrèzhèng

* **syndrome of upper heat and lower cold** / ˈsɪndroʊm əv ˈʌpə hit ənd ˈloə koʊld / 上热下寒证 shàngrèxiàhánzhèng

* **syndrome of upper hyperactivity of liver yang** / ˈsɪndroʊm əv ˈʌpər ˌhaɪpərækˈtɪvəti əv ˈlɪvə jæŋ / 肝阳上亢证 gānyángshàngkàngzhèng

* **syndrome of water diffusion due to spleen deficiency** / ˈsɪndroʊm əv ˈwɔtər dɪˈfjuʒn du tə splin dɪˈfɪʃnsi / 脾虚水泛证 píxūshuǐfànzhèng

* **syndrome of wind-heat invading lung** / ˈsɪndroʊm əv wɪnd hit ɪnˈvedɪŋ lʌŋ / 风热犯肺证 fēngrèfànfèizhèng

* **syndrome of yang deficiency of heart and kidney** / ˈsɪndroʊm əv jæŋ dɪˈfɪʃnsi əv hɑrt ənd ˈkɪdni / 心肾阳虚证 xīnshènyángxūzhèng

* **syndrome of yang deficiency of spleen and kidney** / ˈsɪndroʊm əv jæŋ dɪˈfɪʃnsi əv splin ənd ˈkɪdni / 脾肾阳虚证 píshènyángxūzhèng

* **syndrome of yin deficiency and blood heat**

/ ˈsɪndroʊm əv jɪn dɪˈfɪʃnsi ənd blʌd hit / 阴虚血热证 yīnxūxuèrèzhèng

* **syndrome of yin deficiency and dampness-heat** / ˈsɪndroʊm əv jɪn dɪˈfɪʃnsi ənd ˈdæmpnəs hit / 阴虚湿热证 yīnxūshīrèzhèng

* **syndrome of yin deficiency of liver and kidney** / ˈsɪndroʊm əv jɪn dɪˈfɪʃnsi əv ˈlɪvər ənd ˈkɪdni / 肝肾阴虚证 gānshènyīnxūzhèng

* **syndrome of yin deficiency of lung and kidney** / ˈsɪndroʊm əv jɪn dɪˈfɪʃnsi əv lʌŋ ənd ˈkɪdni / 肺肾阴虚证 fèishènyīnxūzhèng

stagnated blood syndrome / ˈstægneɪtɪd blʌd ˈsɪndroʊm / 蓄血证 xùxuèzhèng

stagnated fluid syndrome / ˈstægneɪtɪd ˈfluɪd ˈsɪndroʊm / 蓄水证 xùshuǐzhèng

summer-heat[-heat] syndrome / ˈsʌmər hit [hit] ˈsɪndroʊm / 暑[热]证 shǔ[rè]zhèng

superficies deficiency syndrome / ˌsʊpəˈfɪʃiˌiz dɪˈfɪʃənsi ˈsɪndroʊm / 表虚证 biǎoxūzhèng

superficies excess syndrome / ˌsʊpəˈfɪʃiˌiz ɪkˈses ˈsɪndroʊm / 表实证 biǎoshízhèng

syndrome / ˈsɪndroʊm / 证候 zhènghòu

syndrome differentiation of channel theory / ˈsɪndroʊm ˌdɪfəˌrenʃiˈeɪʃn əv ˈtʃænl ˈθiəri / 经络辨证 jīngluò biànzhèng

syndrome differentiation of concurrent visceral manifestation / ˈsɪndroʊm ˌdɪfəˌrenʃiˈeɪʃn əv kənˈkɜrənt ˈvɪsərəl ˌmænɪfeˈsteɪʃn / 脏腑兼病辨证 zàngfǔ jiānbìngbiànzhèng

syndrome differentiation of defense tier qi tier, nutrient tier and blood tier / ˈsɪndroʊm ˌdɪfəˌrenʃiˈeɪʃn əv dɪˈfɛns tɪr tʃi tɪr ˈnutriənt tɪr ənd blʌd tɪr / 卫气营血辨证 wèiqìyíngxuèbiànzhèng

syndrome differentiation of eight principles / ˈsɪndroʊm ˌdɪfəˌrenʃiˈeɪʃn əv eɪt ˈprɪnsəplz / 八纲辨证 bāgāngbiànzhèng

syndrome differentiation of etiology / ˈsɪndroʊm ˌdɪfəˌrenʃiˈeɪʃn əv ˌitiˈɑlədʒi / 病因辨证 bìngyīnbiànzhèng

syndrome differentiation of excess and deficiency / ˈsɪndroʊm ˌdɪfəˌrenʃiˈeɪʃn əv ɪkˈses ənd dɪˈfɪʃnsi / 虚实辨证 xūshíbiànzhèng

syndrome differentiation of heart and small intestine / ˈsɪndroʊm ˌdɪfəˌrenʃiˈeɪʃn əv hɑrt ənd smɔl ɪnˈtestɪn / 心及小肠辨证 xīnjíxiǎochángbiànzhèng

syndrome differentiation of kidney and bladder / ˈsɪndroʊm ˌdɪfəˌrenʃiˈeɪʃn əv ˈkɪdni ənd ˈblædər / 肾及膀胱辨证 shènjípángguāngbiànzhèng

syndrome differentiation of liver and gallbladder / ˈsɪndroʊm ˌdɪfəˌrenʃiˈeɪʃn əv ˈlɪvər ənd ˈgɔlˌblædə / 肝胆辨证 gāndǎnbiànzhèng

syndrome differentiation of lung and large intestine / ˈsɪndroʊm ˌdɪfəˌrenʃiˈeɪʃn əv lʌŋ ənd lɑrdʒ ɪnˈtestɪn / 肺及大肠辨证 fèijídàchángbiànzhèng

syndrome differentiation of sanjiao theory / ˈsɪndroʊm ˌdɪfəˌrenʃiˈeɪʃn əv sɑnˈdʒjau ˈθiəri / 三焦辨证 sānjiāobiànzhèng

syndrome differentiation of six channels theory

/ ˈsɪndroʊm ˌdɪfəˌrenʃiˈeɪʃn əv sɪks ˈtʃænlz ˈθiəri /
六经辨证 liùjīngbiànzhèng

syndrome differentiation of spleen and stomach
/ ˈsɪndroʊm ˌdɪfəˌrenʃiˈeɪʃn əv splin ənd ˈstʌmək /
脾胃辨证 píwèibiànzhèng

syndrome differentiation of superficies and interior
/ ˈsɪndroʊm ˌdɪfəˌrenʃiˈeɪʃn əv ˌsupəˈfɪʃɪˌiz ənd
ɪnˈtɪriər / 表里辨证 biǎolǐbiànzhèng

**syndrome differentiation of weifen, qifen, yingfen and
xuefen** / ˈsɪndroʊm ˌdɪfəˌrenʃiˈeɪʃn əv weɪˌfen
tʃiˌfen yɪŋˌfen ənd ˈʃuɛˌfen / 卫气营血辨证 wèiqì
yīngxuèbiànzhèng

syndrome differentiation of yin-yang / ˈsɪndroʊm
ˌdɪfəˌrenʃiˈeɪʃn əv jɪn jæŋ / 阴阳辨证 yīnyáng
biànzhèng

syndrome differentiation of Zang-Fu viscera
/ ˈsɪndroʊm ˌdɪfəˌrenʃiˈeɪʃn əv zæŋ fu ˈvɪsərə /
脏腑辨证 zàngfǔbiànzhèng

syndrome differentiation / ˈsɪndroʊm ˌdɪfəˌrenʃiˈeɪʃn /
辨证 biànzhèng

syndrome of [accumulated] dampness-heat / ˈsɪndroʊm
əv [əˈkjʊmjəˌletɪd] ˈdæmpnəs hit / 湿热[蕴结]证
shīrè[yùnjié]zhèng

syndrome of accumulated dampness-toxicity / ˈsɪndroʊm
əv əˈkjʊmjəˌletɪd ˈdæmpnəs tɑkˈsɪsəti / 湿毒蕴结
证 shīdúyùnjiézhèng

syndrome of affection of Taiyang by wind / ˈsɪndroʊm
əv əˈfekʃn əv taɪjæŋ baɪ wɪnd / 太阳中风证 tài
yángzhòngfēngzhèng

syndrome of ascariasis of small intestine / ˈsɪndroʊm əv ˌæskəˈraɪəsɪs əv smɔl ɪnˈtestɪn / 虫积小肠证 chóngjīxiǎochángzhèng

syndrome of bleeding due to collateral injury / ˈsɪndroʊm əv ˈblidɪŋ du tə kəˈlætərəl ˈɪndʒəri / 络伤出血证 luòshāngchūxuèzhèng

syndrome of blockade of dampness due to qi stagnation / ˈsɪndroʊm əv blɑˈkeɪd əv ˈdæmpnəs du tə tʃi stægˈneɪʃn / 气滞湿阻证 qìzhìshīzǔzhèng

syndrome of blood deficiency and depleted fluid / ˈsɪndroʊm əv blʌd dɪˈfɪʃnsi ənd diˈplitid ˈfluɪd / 血虚津亏证 xuèxūjīnkuīzhèng

syndrome of blood depletion / ˈsɪndroʊm əv blʌd dɪˈpliʃn / 血脱证 xuètuōzhèng

syndrome of blood stasis and stagnant qi / ˈsɪndroʊm əv blʌd ˈsteɪsɪs ənd ˈstægnənt tʃi / 血瘀气滞证 xuèyūqìzhìzhèng

syndrome of blood stasis due to lung heat / ˈsɪndroʊm əv blʌd ˈsteɪsɪs du tə lʌŋ hit / 肺热血瘀证 fèirèxuèyūzhèng

syndrome of blood stasis due to qi deficiency / ˈsɪndroʊm əv blʌd ˈsteɪsɪs du tə tʃi dɪˈfɪʃnsi / 气虚血瘀证 qìxūxuèyūzhèng

syndrome of blood stasis in ear / ˈsɪndroʊm əv blʌd ˈsteɪsɪs ɪn ɪr / 血瘀耳窍证 xuèyūěrqiàozhèng

syndrome of chest and diaphragm disturbed by heat / ˈsɪndroʊm əv tʃest ənd ˈdaɪəfræm dɪˈstɜrbd baɪ hit / 热扰胸膈证 rèrǎoxiōnggézhèng

syndrome of coagulated cold in womb / ˈsɪndroʊm əv

kou'ægjuleɪtɪd kould ɪn wum / 寒凝胞宫证 hán níngbāogōngzhèng

syndrome of coagulation cold due to blood deficiency / 'sɪndroum əv kou‚ægju'leɪʃn kould du tə blʌd dɪ'fɪʃnsi / 血虚寒凝证 xuèxūhánníngzhèng

syndrome of cold accumulated in channels / 'sɪndroum əv kould ə'kjumjə‚leɪtɪd ɪn 'tʃænlz / 寒滞经脉证 hánzhìjīngmàizhèng

syndrome of cold fluid retained in lung / 'sɪndroum əv kould 'fluɪd rɪ'teɪnd ɪn lʌŋ / 寒饮停肺证 hán yǐntíngfèizhèng

syndrome of cold-dampness blocking collaterals / 'sɪndroum əv kould 'dæmpnəs 'blɑkɪŋ kə'lætərəlz / 寒湿阻络证 hánshīzǔluòzhèng

syndrome of cold-dampness due to kidney deficiency / 'sɪndroum əv kould 'dæmpnəs du tə 'kɪdni dɪ'fɪʃnsi / 肾虚寒湿证 shènxūhánshīzhèng

syndrome of dampness-heat blocking collaterals / 'sɪndroum əv 'dæmpnəs hit 'blɑkɪŋ kə'lætərəlz / 湿热阻络证 shīrèzǔluòzhèng

syndrome of dampness-heat diffusing downward / 'sɪndroum əv 'dæmpnəs hit dɪ'fjuzɪŋ 'daunwərd / 湿热下注证 shīrèxiàzhùzhèng

syndrome of dampness-heat invading ear / 'sɪndroum əv 'dæmpnəs hit ɪn'vedɪŋ ɪr / 湿热犯耳证 shīrè fàn'ěrzhèng

syndrome of decline of vital gate fire / 'sɪndroum əv dɪ'klaɪn əv 'vaɪtl geɪt 'faɪər / 命门火衰证 mìng ménhuǒshuāizhèng

syndrome of deficiency of both qi and blood
／ˈsɪndroʊm əv dɪˈfɪʃnsi əv boʊθ tʃi ənd blʌd／
气血两虚证 qìxuèliǎngxūzhèng

syndrome of deficiency of both qi and yin ／ˈsɪndroʊm
əv dɪˈfɪʃnsi əv boʊθ tʃi ənd jɪn／气阴两虚证
qìyīnliǎngxūzhèng

syndrome of deficiency of both yin and yang ／ˈsɪndroʊm
əv dɪˈfɪʃənsi əv boʊθ jɪn ənd jæŋ／阴阳两虚证
yīnyángliǎngxūzhèng

syndrome of deficiency of both yin and yang of heart
／ˈsɪndroʊm əv dɪˈfɪʃnsi əv boʊθ jɪn ənd jæŋ əv
hɑrt／心阴阳两虚证 xīnyīnyángliǎngxūzhèng

syndrome of deficiency of both yin and yang of kidney
／ˈsɪndroʊm əv dɪˈfɪʃnsi əv boʊθ jɪn ənd jæŋ əv
ˈkɪdni／肾阴阳两虚证 shènyīnyángliǎngxūzhèng

syndrome of deficiency of fluid and qi ／ˈsɪndroʊm əv
dɪˈfɪʃnsi əv ˈfluɪd ənd tʃi／津气亏虚证 jīnqìkuīxū
zhèng

syndrome of deficiency of heart qi and blood stasis
／ˈsɪndroʊm əv dɪˈfɪʃnsi əv hɑrt tʃi ənd blʌd ˈsteɪsɪs／
心气虚血瘀证 xīnqìxūxuèyūzhèng

**syndrome of deficiency of liver yin and hyperactivity of
liver yang** ／ˈsɪndroʊm əv dɪˈfɪʃnsi əv ˈlɪvə jɪn ənd
ˌhaɪpərækˈtɪvəti əv ˈlɪvə jæŋ／肝阴虚阳亢证
gānyīnxūyángkàngzhèng

syndrome of deficiency of spleen qi and stomach qi
／ˈsɪndroʊm əv dɪˈfɪʃnsi əv splin tʃi ənd ˈstʌmək tʃi／
脾胃气虚证 píwèiqìxūzhèng

syndrome of deficiency of vital essence ／ˈsɪndroʊm əv

dɪˈfɪʃnsi əv ˈvaɪtl ˈesns / 精气亏虚证 jīngqìkuīxū zhèng

syndrome of depletion of yang involving yin / ˈsɪndroʊm əv dɪˈpliʃn əv jæŋ ɪnˈvɑlvɪŋ jɪn / 阳亡阴竭证 yángwángyīnjiézhèng

syndrome of depletion of yin causing yang collapse / ˈsɪndroʊm əv dɪˈpliʃn əv jɪn kɔzɪŋ jæŋ kəˈlæps / 阴竭阳脱证 yīnjiéyángtuōzhèng

syndrome of diffusive dampness-heat in sanjiao / ˈsɪndroʊm əv dɪˈfjʊsɪv ˈdæmpnəs hit ɪn sanˌdʒjɑʊ / 湿热弥漫三焦证 shīrèmímànsānjiāozhèng

syndrome of disease involving weifen and qifen / ˈsɪndroʊm əv dɪˈziz ɪnˈvɑlvɪŋ weɪˌfen ənd tʃiˌfen / 卫气同病证 wèiqìtóngbìngzhèng

syndrome of endogenous dryness / ˈsɪndroʊm əv enˈdɑdʒənəs ˈdraɪnəs / 内燥证 nèizàozhèng

syndrome of epidemic toxin blocked internally / ˈsɪndroʊm əv ˌepɪˈdemɪk ˈtɑksɪn blɑkt ɪnˈtɜrnəli / 疫毒内闭证 yìdúnèibìzhèng

syndrome of epidemic toxin invasion / ˈsɪndroʊm əv ˌepɪˈdemɪk ˈtɑksɪn ɪnˈveɪʒn / 疫毒侵袭证 yìdúqīnxízhèng

syndrome of excessive dampness-heat / ˈsɪndroʊm əv ɪkˈsesɪv ˈdæmpnəs hit / 湿热浸淫证 shīrèjìnyínzhèng

syndrome of exogenous disease due to yang deficiency / ˈsɪndroʊm əv ekˈsɑdʒənəs dɪˈziz du tə jæŋ dɪˈfɪʃnsi / 阳虚外感证 yángxūwàigǎnzhèng

syndrome of exogenous disease due to yin deficiency / ˈsɪndroʊm əv ekˈsɑdʒənəs dɪˈziz du tə jɪn dɪˈfɪʃnsi / 阴虚外感证 yīnxūwàigǎnzhèng

syndrome of exuberance of heart fire / ˈsɪndroʊm əv ɪgˈzubərəns əv hɑrt ˈfaɪər / 心火炽盛证 xīnhuǒ chìshèngzhèng

syndrome of exuberance of liver fire / ˈsɪndroʊm əv ɪgˈzubərəns əv ˈlɪvər ˈfaɪər / 肝火炽盛证 gānhuǒ chìshèngzhèng

syndrome of exuberance of stomach fire / ˈsɪndroʊm əv ɪgˈzubərəns əv ˈstʌmək ˈfaɪər / 胃火炽盛证 wèi huǒchìshèngzhèng

syndrome of fighting of wind with water / ˈsɪndroʊm əv ˈfaɪtɪŋ əv wɪnd wɪð ˈwɔtər / 风水相搏证 fēng shuǐxiāngbózhèng

syndrome of flaring heat in qifen and xuefen / ˈsɪndroʊm əv ˈflɛrɪŋ hit ɪn tʃiˌfen ənd ʃuɛˌfən / 气血两燔证 qìxuèliǎngfánzhèng

syndrome of flaring heat in qifen and yingfen / ˈsɪndroʊm əv ˈflɛrɪŋ hit ɪn tʃiˌfen ənd yɪŋˌfen / 气营两燔证 qìyíngliǎngfánzhèng

syndrome of flaring up of deficient fire / ˈsɪndroʊm əv ˈflɛrɪŋ ʌp əv dɪˈfɪʃnt ˈfaɪər / 虚火上炎证 xūhuǒ shàngyánzhèng

syndrome of fluid injury due to stomach dryness / ˈsɪndroʊm əv ˈfluɪd ˈɪndʒəri du tə ˈstʌmək ˈdraɪnəs / 胃燥津伤证 wèizàojīnshāngzhèng

syndrome of Fu-viscera of Yangming / ˈsɪndroʊm əv fu

ˌvɪsərə əv jæŋmɪŋ / 阳明腑证 yángmíngfǔzhèng

syndrome of heat accumulated in large intestine
/ ˈsɪndroʊm əv hit əˈkjʊmjəˌletɪd ɪn lɑrdʒ ɪnˈtestɪn / 大肠热结证 dàchángrèjiézhèng

syndrome of heat invading blood chamber / ˈsɪndroʊm əv hit ɪnˈvedɪŋ blʌd ˈtʃeɪmbər / 热入血室证 rè rùxuèshìzhèng

syndrome of heat-toxicity invading throat / ˈsɪndroʊm əv hit tɑkˈsɪsəti ɪnˈvedɪŋ θroʊt / 热毒攻喉证 rè dúgōnghóuzhèng

syndrome of heat-toxicity invading tongue / ˈsɪndroʊm əv hit tɑkˈsɪsəti ɪnˈvedɪŋ tʌŋ / 热毒攻舌证 rèdú gōngshézhèng

syndrome of hyperactivity of fire due to yin deficiency / ˈsɪndroʊm əv ˌhaɪpərækˈtɪvəti əv ˈfaɪər du tə jɪn dɪˈfɪʃnsi / 阴虚火旺证 yīnxūhuǒwàngzhèng

syndrome of hyperactivity of yang due to yin deficiency / ˈsɪndroʊm əv ˌhaɪpərækˈtɪvəti əv jæŋ du tə jɪn dɪˈfɪʃnsi / 阴虚阳亢证 yīnxūyángkàngzhèng

syndrome of incoordination between spleen and stomach / ˈsɪndroʊm əv ˌɪnkoˌɔrdnˈeʃən bɪˈtwin splin ənd ˈstʌmək / 脾胃不和证 píwèibùhézhèng

syndrome of interior invaded by heat-toxicity / ˈsɪndroʊm əv ɪnˈtɪriər ɪnˈveɪd baɪ hit tɑkˈsɪsəti / 热毒内陷证 rèdúnèixiànzhèng

syndrome of intermingled deficiency and excess / ˈsɪndroʊm əv ˌɪntərˈmɪŋgld dɪˈfɪʃənsi ənd ɪkˈses / 虚实夹杂证 xūshíjiāzázhèng

syndrome of intestine dryness due to blood deficiency

/ ˈsɪndroʊm əv ɪnˈtestɪn ˈdraɪnəs du tə blʌd dɪˈfɪʃnsi /
血虚肠燥证 xuèxūchángzàozhèng

syndrome of intestine dryness due to blood heat
/ ˈsɪndroʊm əv ɪnˈtestɪn ˈdraɪnəs du tə blʌd hit /
血热肠燥证 xuèrèchángzàozhèng

syndrome of intestine dryness due to yin deficiency
/ ˈsɪndroʊm əv ɪnˈtestɪn ˈdraɪnəs du tə jɪn dɪˈfɪʃnsi /
阴虚肠燥证 yīnxūchángzàozhèng

syndrome of lingering heat / ˈsɪndroʊm əv ˈlɪŋgərɪŋ hit /
余热未清证 yúrèwèiqīngzhèng

syndrome of lingering pathogen due to deficient vital Qi
/ ˈsɪndroʊm əv ˈlɪŋgərɪŋ ˈpæθədʒən du tə dɪˈfɪʃnt
ˈvaɪtl tʃi / 正虚邪恋证 zhèngxūxiéliànzhèng

syndrome of liver fire invading ear / ˈsɪndroʊm əv
ˈlɪvər ˈfaɪər ɪnˈvedɪŋ ɪr / 肝火燔耳证 gānhuǒ
fán'ěrzhèng

syndrome of loss of control due to spleen deficiency
/ ˈsɪndroʊm əv lɔs əv kənˈtroʊ du tə splin dɪˈfɪʃnsi /
脾虚不固证 píxūbùgùzhèng

syndrome of lung collaterals injured by heat / ˈsɪndroʊm
əv lʌŋ kəˈlætərəlz ˈɪndʒərd baɪ hit / 热伤肺络证
rèshāngfèiluòzhèng

syndrome of lung collaterals injured by summer-heat
/ ˈsɪndroʊm əv lʌŋ kəˈlætərəlz ˈɪndʒərd baɪ ˈsʌmə
hit / 暑伤肺络证 shǔshāngfèiluòzhèng

syndrome of lung dryness due to yin deficiency
/ ˈsɪndroʊm əv lʌŋ ˈdraɪnəs du tə jɪn dɪˈfɪʃnsi /
阴虚肺燥证 yīnxūfèizàozhèng

syndrome of marrow deficiency / ˈsɪndroʊm əv

ˈmærou dɪˈfɪʃnsi / 髓亏证 suǐkuīzhèng

syndrome of non-consolidation of kidney qi / ˈsɪndroʊm əv nɒn kənˌsɑlɪˈdeɪʃn əv ˈkɪdni tʃi / 肾气不固证 shènqìbùgùzhèng

syndrome of pathogen hidden in interpleuro-diaphra-matic space / ˈsɪndroʊm əv ˈpæθədʒən ˈhɪdən ɪn ˌɪntə'pluərəl ˌdaiəfræ'mætɪk speɪs / 邪伏膜原证 xiéfúmóyuánzhèng

syndrome of pathogen hidden in moyuan / ˈsɪndroʊm əv ˈpæθədʒən ˈhɪdn ɪn moʊjuɑn / 邪伏膜原证 xiéfúmóyuánzhèng

syndrome of pestilential toxicity invading downward / ˈsɪndroʊm əv ˌpestɪˈlenʃl tɑkˈsɪsəti ɪnˈvedɪŋ ˈdaʊnwərd / 瘟毒下注证 wēndúxiàzhùzhèng

syndrome of phlegm-dampness blocking collaterals / ˈsɪndroʊm əv flem ˈdæmpnəs ˈblɑkɪŋ kəˈlætərəlz / 痰湿阻络证 tánshīzǔluòzhèng

syndrome of phlegm-dampness due to spleen deficiency / ˈsɪndroʊm əv flem ˈdæmpnəs du tə splin dɪˈfɪʃnsi / 脾虚痰湿证 píxūtánshīzhèng

syndrome of phlegm-dampness invading ear / ˈsɪndroʊm əv flem ˈdæmpnəs ɪnˈvedɪŋ ɪr / 痰湿泛耳证 tánshī fàn'ěrzhèng

syndrome of qi blockade / ˈsɪndroʊm əv tʃi blɑˈkeɪd / 气闭证 qìbìzhèng

syndrome of qi deficiency of lung and kidney / ˈsɪndroʊm əv tʃi dɪˈfɪʃnsi əv lʌŋ ənd ˈkɪdni / 肺肾气虚证 fèishènqìxūzhèng

syndrome of qi depression transforming into fire /

ˈsɪndroʊm əv tʃi dɪˈpreʃn trænsˈfɔrmɪŋ ˈɪntə ˈfaɪər / 气郁化火证 qìyùhuàhuǒzhèng

syndrome of qi failing to control blood / ˈsɪndroʊm əv tʃi ˈfeɪlɪŋ tə kənˈtroʊl blʌd / 气不摄血证 qìbù shèxuèzhèng

syndrome of qi stagnation and blood stasis / ˈsɪndroʊm əv tʃi stægˈneɪʃn ənd blʌd ˈsteɪsɪs / 气滞血瘀证 qìzhìxuèyūzhèng

syndrome of qi stagnation in ear / ˈsɪndroʊm əv tʃi stægˈneɪʃn ɪn ɪr / 气滞耳窍证 qìzhì'ěrqiàozhèng

syndrome of remained toxicity / ˈsɪndroʊm əv rɪˈmeɪnd tɑkˈsɪsəti / 余毒未清证 yúdúwèiqīngzhèng

syndrome of retention of food in stomach / ˈsɪndroʊm əv rɪˈtenʃn əv fud ɪn ˈstʌmək / 食滞胃肠证 shízhì wèichángzhèng

syndrome of spleen deficiency / ˈsɪndroʊm əv splin dɪˈfɪʃnsi / 脾虚证 píxūzhèng

syndrome of stagnant and jamming dampness-heat / ˈsɪndroʊm əv ˈstægnənt ənd ˈdʒæmɪŋ ˈdæmpnəs hit / 湿热壅滞证 shīrèyōngzhìzhèng

syndrome of stagnant dampness heat / ˈsɪndroʊm əv ˈstægnənt ˈdæmpnəs hit / 湿热瘀阻证 shīrèyūzǔzhèng

syndrome of stagnant-heat invading collaterals / ˈsɪndroʊm əv ˈstægnənt hit ɪnˈvedɪŋ kəˈlætərəlz / 瘀热入络证 yūrèrùluòzhèng

syndrome of stagnation of liver qi / ˈsɪndroʊm əv stægˈneɪʃn əv ˈlɪvər tʃi / 肝气郁结证 gānqìyùjié zhèng

syndrome of stagnation of liver qi and blood stasis / ˈsɪndroʊm əv stægˈneɪʃn əv ˈlɪvər tʃi ənd blʌd ˈsteɪsɪs / 肝郁血瘀证 gānyùxuèyūzhèng

syndrome of stagnation of liver qi and spleen deficiency / ˈsɪndroʊm əv stægˈneɪʃn əv ˈlɪvər tʃi ənd splin dɪˈfɪʃnsi / 肝郁脾虚证 gānyùpíxūzhèng

syndrome of static blood blocking collaterals / ˈsɪndroʊm əv ˈstætɪk blʌd ˈblɑkɪŋ kəˈlætərəlz / 瘀血阻络证 yūxuèzǔluòzhèng

syndrome of static blood in stomach collaterals / ˈsɪndroʊm əv ˈstætɪk blʌd ɪn ˈstʌmək kəˈlætərəlz / 瘀阻胃络证 yūzǔwèiluòzhèng

syndrome of stirring blood due to yin deficiency / ˈsɪndroʊm əv ˈstɜrɪŋ blʌd du tə jɪn dɪˈfɪʃnsi / 阴虚动血证 yīnxūdòngxuèzhèng

syndrome of stirring wind due to yin deficiency / ˈsɪndroʊm əv ˈstɜrɪŋ wɪnd du tə jɪn dɪˈfɪʃnsi / 阴虚动风证 yīnxūdòngfēngzhèng

syndrome of sublingual blood stasis / ˈsɪndroʊm əv sʌbˈlɪŋgwəl blʌd ˈsteɪsɪs / 血瘀舌下证 xuèyūshéxià zhèng

syndrome of sudden yang collapse / ˈsɪndroʊm əv ˈsʌdn jæŋ kəˈlæps / 阳气暴脱证 yángqìbàotuō zhèng

syndrome of summer-heat-dampness [**accumulated in interior**] / ˈsɪndroʊm əv ˈsʌmər hit ˈdæmpnəs [əˈkjumjəˌleɪtɪd ɪn ɪnˈtɪriər] / 暑湿[内蕴]证 shǔshī [nèiyùn]zhèng

syndrome of superficies attacked by wind-heat / ˈsɪndroʊm əv ˌsupəˈfɪʃɪiz əˈtækt baɪ wɪnd hit / 风热袭表证 fēngrèxíbiǎozhèng

syndrome of superficies tightened by wind-cold / ˈsɪndroʊm əv ˌsupəˈfɪʃɪiz ˈtaɪtnd baɪ wɪnd koʊld / 风寒束表证 fēnghánshùbiǎozhèng

syndrome of timidity due to deficiency of heart Qi / ˈsɪndroʊm əv tɪˈmɪdəti du tə dɪˈfɪʃnsi əv hɑrt tʃi / 心虚胆怯证 xīnxūdǎnqièzhèng

syndrome of toxic fire invading ear / ˈsɪndroʊm əv ˈtɑksɪk ˈfaɪər ɪnˈvedɪŋ ɪr / 毒火犯耳证 dúhuǒ fàn'ěrzhèng

syndrome of true deficiency disease with false excessive manifestation / ˈsɪndroʊm əv tru dɪˈfɪʃnsi dɪˈziz wɪð fɔls ɪkˈsesɪv ˌmænɪfeˈsteɪʃn / 真虚假实证 zhēnxūjiǎshízhèng

syndrome of true excess disease with false deficient manifestation / ˈsɪndroʊm əv tru ɪkˈses dɪˈziz wɪð fɔls dɪˈfɪʃnt ˌmænɪfeˈsteɪʃn / 真实假虚证 zhēnshí jiǎxūzhèng

syndrome of turbid fluid depletion / ˈsɪndroʊm əv ˈtɜrbɪd ˈfluɪd dɪˈpliʃn / 液脱证 yètuōzhèng

syndrome of upper excess and lower deficiency / ˈsɪndroʊm əv ˈʌpə ɪkˈses ənd ˈloə dɪˈfɪʃənsi / 上盛下虚证 shàngshèngxiàxūzhèng

syndrome of water diffusion due to deficiency of kidney yang / ˈsɪndroʊm əv ˈwɔtər dɪˈfjuʒn du tə dɪˈfɪʃnsi əv ˈkɪdni jæŋ / 肾阳虚水泛证 shènyángxūshuǐ fànzhèng

syndrome of water overflowing due to yang deficiency
/ ˈsɪndroʊm əv ˈwɔtər ˌəʊvəˈfləʊɪŋ du tə jæŋ dɪˈfɪʃnsi / 阳虚水泛证 yángxūshuǐfànzhèng

syndrome of wind and dryness due to blood deficiency
/ ˈsɪndroʊm əv wɪnd ənd ˈdraɪnəs du tə blʌd dɪˈfɪʃnsi / 血虚风燥证 xuèxūfēngzàozhèng

syndrome of wind-cold attacking lung / ˈsɪndroʊm əv wɪnd koʊld əˈtækɪŋ lʌŋ / 风寒袭肺证 fēnghán xífèizhèng

syndrome of wind-cold invading head / ˈsɪndroʊm əv wɪnd koʊld ɪnˈvedɪŋ hed / 风寒犯头证 fēnghán fàntóuzhèng

syndrome of wind-cold invading nose / ˈsɪndroʊm əv wɪnd koʊld ɪnˈvedɪŋ noʊz / 风寒袭鼻证 fēnghán xíbízhèng

syndrome of wind-dampness invading eye / ˈsɪndroʊm əv wɪnd ˈdæmpnəs ɪnˈvedɪŋ aɪ / 风湿凌目证 fēng shīlíngmùzhèng

syndrome of wind-dampness invading head / ˈsɪndroʊm əv wɪnd ˈdæmpnəs ɪnˈvedɪŋ hed / 风湿犯头证 fēngshīfàntóuzhèng

syndrome of wind-dampness with toxicity / ˈsɪndroʊm əv wɪnd ˈdæmpnəs wɪð tɑkˈsɪsəti / 风湿夹毒证 fēngshījiādúzhèng

syndrome of wind-fire and heat-toxicity / ˈsɪndroʊm əv wɪnd ˈfaɪər ənd hit tɑkˈsɪsəti / 风火热毒证 fēng huǒrèdúzhèng

syndrome of wind-fire invading teeth / ˈsɪndroʊm əv

116

wind 'faɪər ɪn'vedɪŋ tiθ / 风火犯齿证 fēnghuǒ fànchǐzhèng

syndrome of wind-heat blocking collaterals / 'sɪndroʊm əv wɪnd hit 'blɑkɪŋ kə'lætərəlz / 风热阻络证 fēngrèzǔluòzhèng

syndrome of wind-heat invading ear / 'sɪndroʊm əv wɪnd hit ɪn'vedɪŋ ɪr / 风热犯耳证 fēngrèfàn'ěrzhèng

syndrome of wind-heat invading eye / 'sɪndroʊm əv wɪnd hit ɪn'vedɪŋ aɪ / 风热犯目证 fēngrèfànmùzhèng

syndrome of wind-heat invading head / 'sɪndroʊm əv wɪnd hit ɪn'vedɪŋ hed / 风热犯头证 fēngrèfàntóuzhèng

syndrome of wind-heat invading nose / 'sɪndroʊm əv wɪnd hit ɪn'vedɪŋ noʊz / 风热犯鼻证 fēngrèfànbízhèng

syndrome of wind-heat invading throat / 'sɪndroʊm əv wɪnd hit ɪn'vedɪŋ θroʊt / 风热侵[咽]喉证 fēngrèqīn[yān]hóuzhèng

syndrome of wind-phlegm invading collaterals / 'sɪndroʊm əv wɪnd flem ɪn'vedɪŋ kə'lætərəlz / 风痰入络证 fēngtánrùluòzhèng

syndrome of wind-toxicity invading collaterals / 'sɪndroʊm əv wɪnd tɑk'sɪsəti ɪn'vedɪŋ kə'lætərəlz / 风毒入络证 fēngdúrùluòzhèng

syndrome of yang deficiency and blood stasis / 'sɪndroʊm əv jæŋ dɪ'fɪʃnsi ənd blʌd 'steɪsɪs / 阳虚血瘀证

yángxūxuèyūzhèng

syndrome of yang deficiency and coagulated cold / ˈsɪndroʊm əv jæŋ dɪˈfɪʃnsi ənd koʊˈægjuleɪtɪd koʊld / 阳虚寒凝证 yángxūhánníngzhèng

syndrome of yang deficiency and coagulated phlegm / ˈsɪndroʊm əv jæŋ dɪˈfɪʃnsi ənd koʊˈægjuleɪtɪd flem / 阳虚痰凝证 yángxūtánníngzhèng

syndrome of yang deficiency and qi stagnation / ˈsɪndroʊm əv jæŋ dɪˈfɪʃnsi ənd tʃi stægˈneɪʃn / 阳虚气滞证 yángxūqìzhìzhèng

syndrome of yang deficiency due to yin excess / ˈsɪndroʊm əv jæŋ dɪˈfɪʃnsi du tə jɪn ɪkˈses / 阴盛阳衰证 yīnshèngyángshuāizhèng

syndrome of yang deficiency involving yin / ˈsɪndroʊm əv jæŋ dɪˈfɪʃnsi ɪnˈvɑlvɪŋ jɪn / 阳损及阴证 yángsǔnjíyīnzhèng

syndrome of yin deficiency and blood dryness / ˈsɪndroʊm əv jɪn dɪˈfɪʃnsi ənd blʌd ˈdraɪnəs / 阴虚血燥证 yīnxūxuèzàozhèng

syndrome of yin deficiency and blood stasis / ˈsɪndroʊm əv jɪn dɪˈfɪʃnsi ənd blʌd ˈsteɪsɪs / 阴虚血瘀证 yīnxūxuèyūzhèng

syndrome of yin deficiency and depletion of fluid / ˈsɪndroʊm əv jɪn dɪˈfɪʃnsi ənd dɪˈpliʃn əv ˈfluɪd / 阴虚津亏证 yīnxūjīnkuīzhèng

syndrome of yin deficiency due to lung heat / ˈsɪndroʊm əv jɪn dɪˈfɪʃnsi du tə lʌŋ hit / 肺热阴虚证 fèirèyīnxūzhèng

syndrome of yin deficiency involving yang / ˈsɪndroʊm

əv jɪn dɪˈfɪʃənsi ɪnˈvɑlvɪŋ jæŋ / 阴损及阳证 yīn sǔnjíyángzhèng

syndrome of yin deficiency of heart and kidney / ˈsɪndroʊm əv jɪn dɪˈfɪʃnsi əv hɑrt ənd ˈkɪdni / 心肾阴虚证 xīnshènyīnxūzhèng

syndrome of yin deficiency of spleen and stomach / ˈsɪndroʊm əv jɪn dɪˈfɪʃnsi əv splin ənd ˈstʌmək / 脾胃阴虚证 píwèiyīnxūzhèng

syndrome of yin injured by heat-toxicity / ˈsɪndroʊm əv jɪn ˈɪndʒərəd baɪ hit tɑkˈsɪsəti / 热毒伤阴证 rèdúshāngyīnzhèng

syndrome of yingfen and xuefen invaded by toxin / ˈsɪndroʊm əv yiŋˌfen ənd ʃuɛˌfen ɪnˈveɪdɪd baɪ ˈtɑksɪn / 毒入营血证 dúrùyíngxuèzhèng

syndrome with good prognosis / ˈsɪndroʊm wɪð gʊd prɑgˈnoʊsɪs / 顺证 shùnzhèng

syndrome with unfavorable prognosis / ˈsɪndroʊm wɪð ʌnˈfevərəbl prɑgˈnoʊsɪs / 逆证 nìzhèng

syndrome / ˈsɪndroʊm / 证 zhèng

* **Taiyang syndrome** / taɪjæŋ ˈsɪndroʊm / 太阳病证 tàiyángbìngzhèng

* **Taiyin syndrome** / taɪjɪn ˈsɪndroʊm / 太阴病证 tàiyīnbìngzhèng

treatment based on disease differentiation / ˈtritmənt beɪst ɑn dɪˈziz ˌdɪfəˌrenʃiˈeɪʃn / 辨病论治 biànbìnglùnzhì

true-false of syndrome / tru fɔls əv ˈsɪndroʊm / 证候真假 zhènghòuzhēnjiǎ

* **weifen syndrome** / weɪfen ˈsɪndroʊm / 卫分证 wèi

fēnzhèng

* **wind-phlegm syndrome** / wɪnd flem ˈsɪndroʊm / 风痰证 fēngtánzhèng

warm-dryness syndrome / wɔrm ˈdraɪnəs ˈsɪndroʊm / 温燥证 wēnzàozhèng

wind syndrome / wɪnd ˈsɪndroʊm / 风证 fēngzhèng

wind-toxicity syndrome / wɪnd tɑkˈsɪsəti ˈsɪndroʊm / 风毒证 fēngdúzhèng

* **xuefen syndrome** / ʃuɛˈfen ˈsɪndroʊm / 血分证 xuèfēnzhèng

* **yang syndrome** / jæŋ ˈsɪndroʊm / 阳证 yángzhèng

* **yangming syndrome** / jæŋmɪŋ ˈsɪndroʊm / 阳明病证 yángmíngbìngzhèng

* **yin syndrome** / jɪn ˈsɪndroʊm / 阴证 yīnzhèng

* **yingfen syndrome** / yɪŋˈfen ˈsɪndroʊm / 营分证 yíngfēnzhèng

yang deficiency syndrome / jæŋ dɪˈfɪʃnsi ˈsɪndroʊm / 阳虚证 yángxūzhèng

yang depletion syndrome / jæŋ dɪˈpliʃən ˈsɪndroʊm / 亡阳证 wángyángzhèng

Yangming channel syndrome / jæŋmɪŋ ˈtʃænl ˈsɪndroʊm / 阳明经证 yángmíngjīngzhèng

yin deficiency syndrome / jɪn dɪˈfɪʃnsi ˈsɪndroʊm / 阴虚证 yīnxūzhèng

Yin depletion syndrome / jɪn dɪˈpliʃən ˈsɪndroʊm / 亡阴证 wángyīnzhèng

Chapter 4   Chinese Materia Medica

第四章　中　药　学

Section 1   General Introduction

第一节　概　　论

antagonism / æn'tægənɪzəm / 相反 xiāngfǎn

ascending and descending / ə'sɛndɪŋ ənd dɪ'sɛndɪŋ / 升降 shēngjiàng

astringent / ə'strɪndʒənt / 涩 sè

bark / bɑrk / 皮 pí

bioassay / ˌbaɪəəˌse / 生物检定 shēngwùjiǎndìng

biological identification / ˌbaɪə'lɑdʒɪkl aɪˌdentɪfɪ'keɪʃn / 生物检定 shēngwùjiǎndìng

bitter / 'bɪtər / 苦 kǔ

calm / kɑm / 平 píng

channel affinity / 'tʃænl ə'fɪnəti / 引经 yǐnjīng

channel tropism / 'tʃænl 'troʊpɪzəm / 归经 guījīng

channel ushering / 'tʃænl 'ʌʃərɪŋ / 引经 yǐnjīng

clash / klæʃ / 相反 xiāngfǎn

cold / koʊld / 寒 hán

collection and preparation / kə'lekʃn ənd ˌprepə'reɪʃn / 采制 cǎizhì

collection period / kə'lekʃn 'pɪriəd / 采收期 cǎishōuqī

color and luster / 'kʌlər ənd 'lʌstər / 色泽 sèzé

compound / kɑm'paʊnd / 调剂 tiáojì

concerted application / kən'sɜrtɪd ˌæplɪ'keɪʃn / 配伍 pèiwǔ

contraindications / ˌkɑntrəˌɪndɪˈkeɪʃns / 禁忌 jìnjì

contraindications during pregnancy / ˌkɑntrəˌɪndɪˈkeɪʃns ˈdʊrɪŋ ˈpregnənsi / 妊娠禁忌[药] rènshēn jìnjì[药]

cool / kul / 凉 liáng

counteract toxicity of another drug / ˌkaʊntərˈækt tɑkˈsɪsəti əv əˈnʌðər drʌg / 相杀 xiāngshā

crude drug / krud drʌg / 药材 yàocái

crude medicine / krud ˈmedɪsn / 药材 yàocái

cut surface character / kʌt ˈsɜrfɪs ˈkærəktər / 断面特征 duànmiàntèzhēng

description / dɪˈskrɪpʃn / 性状描述 xìngzhuàngmiáoshù

dosage / ˈdoʊsɪdʒ / 剂量 jìliàng

drug used singly / drʌg juzd ˈsɪŋgli / 单行 dānxíng

drying / ˈdraɪɪŋ / 干燥 gānzào

drying by baking / ˈdraɪɪŋ baɪ ˈbeɪkɪŋ / 烘干 hōnggān

drying in shade / ˈdraɪɪŋ ɪn ʃeɪd / 阴干 yīngān

drying in sunshine / ˈdraɪɪŋ ɪn ˈsʌnʃaɪn / 晒干 shàigān

eighteen clash / ˌeɪˈtin klæʃ / 十八反 shíbāfǎn

extensive diffusion of oil / ɪkˈstensɪv dɪˈfjuʒn əv ɔɪl / 泛油 fànyóu

five flavours / faɪv ˈfleɪvərz / 五味 wǔwèi

floating and sinking / ˈfloʊtɪŋ ənd ˈsɪŋkɪŋ / 浮沉 fúchén

flower / ˈflaʊər / 花 huā

food taboo in drug application / fud təˈbu ɪn drʌg ˌæplɪˈkeɪʃn / 服药食忌 fúyàoshíjì

form / fɔrm / 形状 xíngzhuàng

four nature of drugs / fɔr ˈneɪtʃər əv drʌgz / 四气 sìqì

fracture surface / ˈfræktʃər ˈsɜrfɪs / 折断面 zhéduàn miàn

fresh crude drug / freʃ krud drʌg / 鲜药 xiānyào

fresh medicine / freʃ ˈmedɪsn / 鲜药 xiānyào

fruit / frut / 果实 guǒshí

genuine regional drug / ˈdʒenjuɪn ˈridʒənl drʌg / 道地药材 dàodìyàocái

germination period / ˌdʒɜrmɪˈneɪʃn ˈpɪriəd / 萌发期 méngfāqī

herb / hɜrb / 草药 cǎoyào

hot / hɑt / 热 rè

identification of origin / aɪˌdentɪfɪˈkeɪʃn əv ˈɔridʒɪn / 基源鉴定 jīyuánjiàndìng

identification of original animal / aɪˌdentɪfɪˈkeɪʃn əv əˈridʒənl ˈænɪml / 原动物鉴定 yuándòngwùjiàndìng

identification of original mineral / aɪˌdentɪfɪˈkeɪʃn əv əˈridʒənl ˈmɪnərəl / 原矿物鉴定 yuánkuàngwù jiàndìng

identification of original plant / aɪˌdentɪfɪˈkeɪʃn əv əˈridʒənl plænt / 原植物鉴定 yuánzhíwùjiàndìng

incompatibility / ˌɪnkəmˌpætəˈbɪləti / 相畏 xiāngwèi

incompatibility of drugs in pattern / ˌɪnkəmˌpætəˈbɪləti əv drʌgz ɪn ˈpætərn / 证候禁忌 zhènghòujìnjì

incompatibility of drugs in prescription / ˌɪnkəmˌpætəˈbɪləti əv drʌgz ɪn prɪˈskrɪpʃn / 配伍禁忌 pèiwǔjìnjì

leaf / lif / 叶 yè

microscopical identification / ˌmaɪkrə'skɑpɪkl aɪˌdentɪfɪ'keɪʃn / 显微鉴定 xiǎnwēijiàndìng

mildew and rot / 'mɪldu ənd rɑt / 霉变 méibiàn

milliliter / 'mɪlɪˌlitər / 毫升 háoshēng

mutual enhancement / 'mjutʃuəl ɪn'hænsmənt / 相使 xiāngshǐ

mutual inhibition / 'mjutʃuəl ˌɪnhɪ'bɪʃn / 相恶 xiāngwù

mutual promotion / 'mjutʃuəl prə'mouʃn / 相须 xiāng xū

natural crude drug / 'nætʃrəl krud drʌg / 天然药物 tiānrányàowù

natural medicine / 'nætʃrəl 'medɪsn / 天然药物 tiānrányàowù

nature and flavor / 'neɪtʃər ənd 'fleɪvər / 性味 xìngwèi

nineteen incompatibilities / ˌnaɪn'tin ˌɪnkəmˌpætə'bɪlətis / 十九畏 shíjiǔwèi

odor / 'oʊdər / 气 qì

peel / pil / 皮 pí

physical and chemical identification / 'fɪzɪkl ənd 'kemɪkl aɪˌdentɪfɪ'keɪʃn / 理化鉴定 lǐhuàjiàndìng

plain / pleɪn / 平 píng

processing in production place / 'prɑsesɪŋ ɪn prə'dʌkʃn pleɪs / 产地加工 chǎndìjiāgōng

pungent / 'pʌndʒənt / 辛 xīn

quality analysis / 'kwɑləti ə'næləsɪs / 质量分析 zhìliàngfēnxī

quality control / 'kwɑləti kən'troʊl / 质量控制 zhìliàngkòngzhì

quality standard / ˈkwɑləti ˈstændərd / 质量标准 zhìliàngbiāozhǔn

radial striation / ˈreɪdiəl straɪˈeɪʃn / 菊花心 júhuāxīn

rhizome / ˈraɪzoʊm / 根茎 gēnjīng

root / rut / 根 gēn

rotten due to insect bites / ˈrɑtn du tə ˈɪnsekt baɪts / 虫蛀 chóngzhù

salty / ˈsɔlti / 咸 xián

seed / sid / 种子 zhǒngzi

seven relations / ˈsevn rɪˈleʃənz / 七情 qīqíng

shape / ʃeɪp / 形状 xíngzhuàng

size / saɪz / 大小 dàxiǎo

smell / smel / 嗅 xiù

sour / ˈsaʊər / 酸 suān

spot of oil cavity / spɑt əv ɔɪl ˈkævəti / 朱砂点 zhūshādiǎn

storage / ˈstɔrɪdʒ / 贮藏 zhùcáng

surface character / ˈsɜrfɪs ˈkærəktər / 表面特征 biǎomiàntèzhēng

sweet / swit / 甘 gān

taste / teɪst / 味 wèi

tasteless / ˈteɪstləs / 淡 dàn

texture / ˈtekstʃər / 质地 zhìdì

warm / wɔrm / 温 wēn

whole herb / hoʊl hɜrb / 全草 quáncǎo

withering period / ˈwɪðərɪŋ ˈpɪriəd / 枯萎期 kūwěiqī

Section 2　Processing

第二节　炮　制

adjuvant material / ˈædʒəvənt məˈtɪriəl / 辅料 fǔliào

boiling / ˈbɔɪlɪŋ / 煮[制] zhǔ[zhì]

boiling with vinegar / ˈbɔɪlɪŋ wɪð ˈvɪnɪɡər / 醋煮 cù zhǔ

burn as charcoal with function preserved / bɜrn əz ˈtʃɑrkoʊl wɪð ˈfʌŋkʃn prɪˈzɜrvd / 制炭存性 zhì tàncúnxìng

calcining / kælˈsaɪnɪŋ / 煅[制] duàn[zhì]

calcining and quenching / kælˈsaɪnɪŋ ənd ˈkwentʃɪŋ / 煅淬 duàncuì

calcining openly / kælˈsaɪnɪŋ ˈoʊpənli / 明煅 míngduàn

carbonizing / ˈkɑbənaɪzɪŋ / 制炭 zhìtàn

carbonizing by calcining / ˈkɑbənaɪzɪŋ baɪ kælˈsaɪnɪŋ / 煅炭 duàntàn

carbonizing by stir-frying / ˈkɑbənaɪzɪŋ baɪ stɜr ˈfraiɪŋ / 炒炭 chǎotàn

chopping / ˈtʃɒpɪŋ / [切]块 [qiē]kuài

cleansing / ˈklɛnzɪŋ / 净制 jìngzhì

cutting / ˈkʌtɪŋ / 切[制] qiē[zhì]

fried with adjuvant material / fraɪd wɪð ˈædʒəvənt məˈtɪriəl / 加辅料炒 jiāfǔliàochǎo

frost-like powder / frɔst laɪk ˈpaʊdər / [制]霜 [zhì] shuāng

grinding in water / ˈɡraɪndɪŋ ɪn ˈwɔtər / 水飞 shuǐfēi

heated with sand / ˈhitɪd wɪð sænd / 砂烫 shātàng

immersion / ɪˈmɜrʒn / 浸润 jìnrùn

levigating / ˈlevɪgeɪtɪŋ / 水飞 shuǐfēi

moistening / ˈmɔɪsnɪŋ / 润 rùn

prepared drug in pieces / prɪˈpeɪd drʌg ɪn ˈpiːsɪz / 饮片 yǐnpiàn

processed with oil / ˈprɑsest wɪð ɔɪl / 油制 yóuzhì

processing / ˈprɑsesɪŋ / 炮制 páozhì

processing with salt-water / ˈprɑsesɪŋ ˈwɪð sɔlt ˈwɔtɚ / 盐制 yánzhì

processing with vinegar / ˈprɑsesɪŋ ˈwɪð ˈvɪnɪgər / 醋制 cùzhì

processing with wine / ˈprɑsesɪŋ ˈwɪð waɪn / 酒制 jiǔzhì

rinsing moistening / ˈrɪnsɪŋ ˈmɔɪsɪŋ / 洗润 xǐrùn

roasting / ˈroʊstɪŋ / 煨[制] wēi[zhì]

scalding / ˈskɔldɪŋ / 烫[制] tàng[zhì]

scalding / ˈskɔldɪŋ / 土炒 tǔchǎo

screening / ˈskrinɪŋ / 筛选 shāixuǎn

sectioning / ˈsɛkʃənɪŋ / [切]段 [qiē]duàn

selection in water / sɪˈlekʃn ɪn ˈwɔtər / 水选 shuǐxuǎn

selection in wind / sɪˈlekʃn ɪn wɪnd / 风选 fēngxuǎn

showering moistening / ˈʃaʊʃərɪŋ ˈmɔɪsnɪŋ / 淋润 línrùn

simple stir-frying / ˈsɪmpl stər ˈfraɪɪŋ / 清炒 qīngchǎo

slicing / ˈslaɪsɪŋ / [切]片 [qiē]piàn

sliver / ˈslɪvər / [切]丝 [qiē]sī

soaking moistening / ˈsoʊkɪŋ ˈmɔɪsnɪŋ / 泡润 pàorùn

sorting / ˈsɔrtɪŋ / 挑选 tiāoxuǎn

steaming / ˈstimɪŋ / 蒸[制] zhēng[zhì]

steaming with salt-water / ˈstimɪŋ wɪð sɔlt ˈwɔtɚ / 盐

蒸 yánzhēng

steaming with vinegar / ˈstimɪŋ wɪð ˈvɪnɪgər / 醋蒸 cùzhēng

steaming with wine / ˈstimɪŋ wɪð waɪn / 酒蒸 jiǔzhēng

stewing / stjuɪŋ / 炖[制] dùn[zhì]

stewing with wine / stjuɪŋ wɪð waɪn / 酒炖 jiǔdùn

stir-frying / stɜr ˈfraiiŋ / 炒[制] chǎo[zhì]

stir-frying with bran / stɜr ˈfraiiŋ wɪð bræn / 麸炒 fūchǎo

stir-frying with ginger juice / stɜr ˈfraiiŋ wɪð ˈdʒɪndʒər dʒus / 姜汁制 jiāngzhīzhì

stir-frying with honey / stɜr ˈfraiiŋ wɪð ˈhʌni / 蜜制 mìzhì

stir-frying with salt-water / stɜr ˈfraiiŋ wɪð sɔlt ˈwɔtər / 盐炙 yánzhì

stir-frying with vinegar / stɜr ˈfraiiŋ wɪð ˈvɪnɪgər / 醋炙 cùzhì

stir-frying with wine / stɜr ˈfraiiŋ wɪð waɪn / 酒炙 jiǔzhì

washing and rinsing / ˈwɑʃɪŋ ənd ˈrɪnsɪŋ / 洗漂 xǐpiǎo

Section 3   Chinese Medicinal Herbs
第三节   中   药

abalone shell / ˌæbəˈloʊni ʃel / 石决明 shíjuémíng

 # acanthopanax [**root bark**] 五加皮 wǔjiāpí

air potato / eə(r) pəˈteɪtəʊ / 黄药子 huángyàozǐ

 # akebia fruit 预知子 yùzhīzǐ

 # akebia stem 木通 mùtōng

albizia flower / ælˈbɪzɪə flaʊə / 合欢花 héhuānhuā

aloe / ˈæloʊ / 芦荟 lúhuì

alum / ˈæləm / 白矾 báifán

alum processed pinellia [tuber] 清半夏 qīngbànxià

American ginseng / əˈmerɪkən ˈdʒɪnseŋ / 西洋参 xī yángshēn

amur cork-tree / ɑˈmuə kɔk tri / 黄柏 huángbǎi

antelope horn / ˈæntɪləup hɔn / 羚羊角 língyángjiǎo

antler / ˈæntlə(r) / 鹿角 lùjiǎo

appendiculate cremastra pseudobulb 山慈菇 shāncígū

areca peel / əˈrikər pil / 大腹皮 dàfùpí

areca seed / əˈrikər sid / 槟榔 bīngláng

argy wormwood leaf / ɑdʒi ˈwɜrmwʊd lif / 艾叶 àiyè

armand clematis stem / ˈɑrmənd ˈklemətɪs stem / 川木 通 chuānmùtōng

arnebia root / ˈɑrnɪbiə rut / 紫草 zǐcǎo

ash bark / æʃ bɑk / 秦皮 qínpí

asiatic cornelian cherry fruit / ˌeɪʃiˈætɪk kɔrˈniliən ˈtʃeri frut / 山茱萸 shānzhūyú

asiatic moonseed rhizome / ˌeɪʃiˈætɪk ˈmunsid ˈraɪˌzoum / 北豆根 běidòugēn

asparagus / əˈspærəgəs / 芦笋 lúsǔn

ass hide glue / æs haɪd glu / 阿胶 ējiāo

atractylodes 苍术 cāngzhú

atrina glass 败酱草 bàijiàngcǎo

baical skullcap root 黄芩 huángqín

bamboo shavings / bæmˈbu ʃeɪvɪŋz / 竹茹 zhúrú

barbary wolfberry fruit / ˈbɑbəri ˈwʊlfbəri frut / 枸杞 子 gǒuqǐzǐ

barbated skullcup herb 半枝莲 bànzhīlián

bat's droppings / bæts ˈdrɒpɪŋz / 夜明砂 yèmíngshā

beautiful sweetgum fruit / ˈbjutəfəl ˈswitgʌm frut / 路路通 lùlùtōng

beautiful sweetgum resin / ˈbjutəfəl ˈswitgʌm ˈrezn / 枫香脂 fēngxiāngzhī

beeswax / ˈbizwæks / 蜂蜡 fēnglà

belvedere fruit / belvədɪr frut / 地肤子 dìfūzǐ

 # benzoin 安息香 ānxīxiāng

bezoar / bizor / 牛黄 niúhuáng

 # bile arisaema 胆南星 dǎnnánxīng

 # biond magnolia flower-bud 辛夷 xīnyí

bistort rhizome / ˈbɪstɔt ˈraɪzəʊm / 拳参 quánshēn

bitter apricot seed / ˈbɪtər ˈæprɪkɑt sid / 杏仁 xìngrén

black catechu / blæk ˈkætəˌtʃʊ / 儿茶 érchá

black sesame / blæk ˈsesəmi / 黑芝麻 hēizhīma

blackberry lily rhizome / ˈblækbəri ˈlɪli ˈraɪzəʊm / 射干 shègàn

 # blackend swallowwort root 白薇 báiwēi

black-tailsnake / blæk teɪlsneɪk / 乌梢蛇 wūshàoshé

blister beetle / ˈblɪstə(r) beetle / 斑蝥 bānmáo

boat-fruited sterculia seed / bəʊt frutɪd stɜˈkjulɪə sid / 胖大海 pàngdàhǎi

bone fossil of big mammals / bəʊn ˈfɑsl əv bɪg ˈmæmls / 龙骨 lónggǔ

 # borneol 冰片 bīngpiàn

buck-eye seed / ˈbʌk aɪ sid / 娑罗子 suōluózǐ

buffalo horn / ˈbʌfəloʊ hɔrn / 水牛角 shuǐniújiǎo

 # cablin patchouli herb 广藿香 guǎnghuòxiāng

calamine / ˈkæləmaɪn / 炉甘石 lúgānshí

calomel / ˈkæləmel / 轻粉 qīngfěn

canton love-pea vine / ˈkæntən lʌv pi vaɪn / 鸡骨草 jīgǔcǎo

cape jasmine fruit / keɪp ˈdʒæzmɪn frut / 栀子 zhīzi

carbonized hair 血余炭 xuèyútàn

cardamon fruit / ˈkadəmən frut / 白豆蔻 báidòukòu

cassia bark / ˈkæsɪə bɑrk / 肉桂 ròuguì

cassia seed 决明子 juémíngzǐ

cassia twig / ˈkæsɪə twɪg / 桂枝 guìzhī

castor seed / ˈkɑstə(r) sid / 蓖麻子 bìmázǐ

catclaw buttercup root / kætklɔ ˈbʌtəkʌp rut / 猫爪草 māozhuǎcǎo

cattail pollen / ˈkætteɪl ˈpɒlən / 蒲黄 púhuáng

centipede / ˈsentɪpid / 蜈蚣 wúgōng

cherokeerose fruit / ˈtʃerəkirəʊz frut / 金樱子 jīnyīngzǐ

Chinese angelica / ˌtʃaɪˈniz ænˈdʒelɪkə / 当归 dāngguī

Chinese arborvitae kernel / ˌtʃaɪˈniz ˌɑbəˈvaɪti ˈkɜnl / 柏子仁 bǎizǐrén

Chinese asafetida / tʃaɪˈniz æsəˈfɛtɪdə / 阿魏 āwèi

Chinese caterpillar fungus / ˌtʃaɪˈniz ˈkætərpɪlər fʌŋgəs / 冬虫夏草 dōngchóngxiàcǎo

Chinese cinquefoil / tʃaɪˈniz ˈsɪŋkˌfɔɪl / 委陵菜 wěilíngcài

Chinese clematis root / ˌtʃaɪˈniz ˈklemətɪs rut / 威灵仙 wēilíngxiān

Chinese date / ˌtʃaɪˈniz deɪt / 大枣 dàzǎo

Chinese dwarf cherry seed / tʃaɪˈniz dwɔrf ˈtʃeri sid /

郁李仁 yùlǐrén

Chinese eaglewood / ˌtʃaɪˈniz ˈiglwud / 沉香 chénxiāng

Chinese gall / ˌtʃaɪˈniz gɔl / 五倍子 wǔbèizǐ

Chinese gentian / ˌtʃaɪˈniz ˈdʒenʃn / 龙胆 lóngdǎn

Chinese honeylocust abnormal fruit / ˌtʃaɪˈniz ˈhʌniˈləʊkəst æbˈnɔml frut / 猪牙皂 zhūyázào

Chinese honeylocustspine / ˌtʃaɪˈniz hʌniˈloʊkəstspaɪn / 皂角刺 zàojiǎocì

Chinese lobelia herb / ˌtʃaɪˈniz loʊˈbiliə hɜb / 半边莲 bànbiānlián

Chinese lovage / ˌtʃaɪˈniz ˈlʌvɪdʒ / 藁本 gǎoběn

 # Chinese magnoliavine fruit 五味子 wǔwèizǐ

Chinese mahonia stem / ˌtʃaɪˈniz məˈhoniə stem / 功劳木 gōngláomù

 # Chinese mosla 香薷 xiāngrú

Chinese pulsatilla root / ˌtʃaɪˈniz pʌlsəˈtilə rut / 白头翁 báitóuwēng

Chinese rose flower / ˌtʃaɪˈniz roʊz ˈflaʊər / 月季花 yuèjìhuā

 # Chinese silkvine root-bark 香加皮 xiāngjiāpí

Chinese star anise / ˈtʃaɪˈniz stɑr ˈænɪs / 八角茴香 bājiǎohuíxiāng

Chinese starjasmine stem / ˌtʃaɪˈniz stɑ(r)ˈdʒæzmɪn stem / 络石藤 luòshíténg

Chinese tamarisk twig / ˌtʃaɪˈniz ˈtæməˌrɪsk twɪg / 西河柳 xīhéliǔ

 # Chinese taxillus herb 桑寄生 sāngjìshēng

 # Chinese thorowax root 柴胡 cháihú

 # Chinese viscum herb 槲寄生 hújìshēng

 # Chinese waxgourd peel 冬瓜皮 dōngguāpí

Chinese white olive / ˌtʃaɪ'niz waɪt 'ɑlɪv / 青果 qīng guǒ

Chinese wolfberry root-bark / ˌtʃaɪ'niz 'wʊlfˌbɛri rut bɑrk / 地骨皮 dìgǔpí

chlorite schist / 'klɔraɪt ʃɪst / 青礞石 qīngméngshí

christina loosestrife / krɪs'tinə 'lʊsˌstraɪf / 金钱草 jīn qiáncǎo

chrysanthemum flower / krɪ'zænθəməm 'flaʊə(r) / 菊花 júhuā

cibot / sɪbout / 狗脊 gǒujǐ

cicada slough / sɪ'kɑdə slaʊ / 蝉蜕 chántuì

cinnabar / 'sɪnəbɑr / 朱砂 zhūshā

citron fruit / 'sɪtrən frut / 香橼 xiāngyuán

clam shell / klæm ʃel / 蛤壳 géqiào

clam shell / klæm ʃel / 瓦楞子 wǎléngzǐ

climbing nightshade / 'klaɪmɪŋ 'naɪt'ʃed / 白英 báiyīng

clinopodium herb / ˌklinə'poudiəm hɜb / 断血流 duàn xuèliú

clove / kloʊv / 丁香 dīngxiāng

cluster mallow fruit / 'klʌstər 'mæloʊ frut / 冬葵子 dōngkuízǐ

 # coastal glehnia root 北沙参 běishāshēn

 # cochinchina momordica seed 木鳖子 mùbiēzǐ

 # cochinchinese asparagus root 天冬 tiāndōng

 # cockcomb inflorescence 鸡冠花 jīguānhuā

cogon grass rhizome / koˈɡon ɡræs ˈraɪzoʊm / 白茅根 báimáogēn

coin-like white-banded snake / kɔɪn laɪk waɪt bændɪd sneɪk / 金钱白花蛇 jīnqiánbáihuāshé

coix seed / kɔɪks sid / 薏苡仁 yìyǐrén

combined spicebush root / kəmˈbaɪnd ˈspaɪsbʊʃ rut / 乌药 wūyào

common andrographis herb 穿心莲 chuānxīnlián

common anemarrhena rhizome 知母 zhīmǔ

common aucklandia root 木香 mùxiāng

common bletilla rubber / ˈkɑmən blɪˈtɪlə rʌbər / 白及 báijí

common buried rubber / ˈkɑmən ˈbɛrɪd ˈrʌbər / 三棱 sānléng

common carpesium fruit / ˈkɑmən ˈkɑpˈsiəm frut / 鹤虱 hèshī

common clubmoss herb 伸筋草 shēnjīncǎo

common cnidium fruit / ˈkɑmən kˈnidiəm frut / 蛇床子 shéchuángzǐ

common coltsfoot flower / ˈkɒmən ˈkəʊltsfʊt ˈflaʊə(r) / 款冬花 kuǎndōnghuā

common curculigo rhizome 仙茅 xiānmáo

common ducksmeat herb 浮萍 fúpíng

common floweringqince fruit 木瓜 mùguā

common heron's bill herb 老鹳草 lǎoguàncǎo

common knotgrass herb / ˈkɒmən ˈnɒtɡrɑs hɜb / 萹蓄 biānxù

common monkshood mother root / ˈkɑmən ˈmʌŋkshʊd

ˈmʌðər rut / 川乌 chuānwū

common pleione pseudobulb 山慈菇 shāncígū

common ru 灯心草 dēngxīncǎo

common scouring rush herb / ˈkɑmən ˈskaʊrɪŋ rʌʃ hɜb / 木贼 mùzéi

common selfheal fruit-spike / ˈkɒmən ˈselfˌhil frut spaɪk / 夏枯草 xiàkūcǎo

common yam rhizome / ˈkɑmən jæm ˈraɪzoʊm / 山药 shānyào

cowherb seed / ˈkaʊˌhɜb sid / 王不留行 wángbùliúxíng

creeping euphorbia / ˈkripɪŋ juˈfɔbɪə / 地锦草 dìjǐn cǎo

croton fruit / ˈkrotən frut / 巴豆 bādòu

crystallized sodium sulfate / ˈkrɪstəlaɪzd ˈsoʊdiəm ˈsʌlˌfet / 芒硝 mángxiāo

cutch / kʌtʃ / 儿茶 érchá

cuttlebone / ˈkʌtlbəʊn / 海螵蛸 hǎipiāoxiāo

dahurian angelica root 白芷 báizhǐ

dahurian rhododendron leaf / ˌdəˈhjʊərɪən ˌroʊdəˈdɛndrən lif / 满山红 mǎnshānhóng

dandelion / ˈdændɪlaɪən / 蒲公英 púgōngyīng

danshen root 丹参 dānshēn

datura flower / dəˈtjʊərə ˈflaʊə(r) / 洋金花 yáng jīnhuā

dayflower herb / ˈdeɪˌflaʊə hɜb / 鸭跖草 yāzhícǎo

debark peony root / dɪˈbɑrk ˈpiəni rut / 白芍 báisháo

decumbent corydalis rhizome / dɪˈkʌmb(ə)nt kəˈrɪdəlɪs ˈraɪzəʊm / 夏天无 xiàtiānwú

deer horn / dɪə(r) hɔn / 鹿角 lùjiǎo

deer-horn glue / dɪə(r) hɔn glu / 鹿角胶 lùjiǎojiāo

 # degelatined deer-horn 鹿角霜 lùjiǎoshuāng

dendrobium / dɛn'drobiəm / 石斛 shíhú

 # densefruit pittany root-bark 白鲜皮 báixiǎnpí

 # desertliving cistanche 肉苁蓉 ròucōngróng

dichroa root / dɪk'rəʊə rut / 常山 chángshān

 # divaricate saposhnikovia root 防风 fángfēng

dodder seed / 'dɒdə sid / 菟丝子 tùsīzǐ

dogbane leaf / 'dɒgbeɪn lif / 罗布麻叶 luóbùmáyè

doubleteeth pubescent angelica root / 'dʌbltiθ pju'besnt æn'dʒelɪkə rut / 独活 dúhuó

 # draconis resin 血竭 xuèjié

dried fresh ginseng / draɪd freʃ 'dʒɪnseŋ / 生晒参 shēng shàishēn

dried ginger / draɪd dʒɪndʒər / 干姜 gānjiāng

dried lacquer / draɪd 'lækər / 干漆 gānqī

dried tangerine peel / draɪd 'tændʒərin pil / 陈皮 chénpí

 # dutchmanspipe vine 天仙藤 tiānxiānténg

 # dutohmanspipe fruit 马兜铃 mǎdōulíng

 # dwarf lilyturf tuber 麦冬 màidōng

 # dyers woad leaf 大青叶 dàqīngyè

earthworm / 'ɜrθwɜrm / 地龙 dìlóng

walnut seed / 'wɔlnʌt sid / 核桃仁 hétáorén

ephedra / i'fedrə / 麻黄 máhuáng

ephedra root / i'fedrə rut / 麻黄根 máhuánggēn

epimedium herb / ˌepəˈmidjəm hɜb / 淫羊藿 yínyáng huò

 # eucommia bark 杜仲 dùzhòng

European verbena herb / ˌjʊrəˈpiə vɜrˈbinə hɜb / 马鞭草 mǎbiāncǎo

feather cockscomb seed / ˈfɛðər ˈkɑksˌkom sid / 青葙子 qīngxiāngzǐ

 # fennel 小茴香 xiǎohuíxiāng

fenugreek seed / ˈfenjugrik sid / 胡芦巴 húlúbā

 # fermented pinellia 半夏曲 bànxiàqǔ

fermented soybean / fərˈmɛnted ˈsɒɪbin / 淡豆豉 dàn dòuchǐ

 # field thistle 小蓟 xiǎojì

figwort root / ˈfɪɡˌwərt rut / 玄参 xuánshēn

 # figwortflower picrorhiza rhizome 胡黄连 húhuáng lián

finger citron / ˈfɪŋɡər ˈsɪtrən / 佛手 fóshǒu

 # flatstem milkvetch seed 沙苑子 shāyuànzǐ

 # fleeceflower root 何首乌 héshǒuwū

fluorite / ˈfluəˌraɪt / 紫石英 zǐshíyīng

 # flying squirrel's droppings 五灵脂 wǔlíngzhī

fortune windmillpalm petiole / ˈfɔtʃun wɪndmɪlpɑm ˈpetɪəʊl / 棕榈 zōnglǘ

 # fortune's drynaria rhizome 骨碎补 gǔsuìbǔ

fourleaf ladybell root / fɔ(r)lif ˈleɪdibel rut / 南沙参 nánshāshēn

 # fragrant solomonseal rhizomehn / 玉竹 yùzhú

franchet groundcherry fruit / ˈfræntʃet ˈɡraʊndˈtʃɛrɪ

frut / 锦灯笼 jǐndēnglóng

frankincense / ˈfræŋkɪnsens / 乳香 rǔxiāng

fresh ginger / freʃ ˈdʒɪndʒər / 生姜 shēngjiāng

 # fresh rehmannia root 鲜地黄 xiāndìhuáng

fritillaria [**bulb**] / frɪtəˈlɛrɪə[bʌlb] / 贝母 bèimǔ

 # fruit of caoguo 草果 cǎoguǒ

 # galanga galangal fruit 红豆蔻 hóngdòukòu

 # galanga resurrectionlily rhizome 山奈 shānnài

gambir plant nod / ˈgæmbɪə plɑnt nɒd / 钩藤 gōu téng

gansui root / gænˈsui rut / 甘遂 gānsuí

garden balsam seed / ˈgɑrdn ˈbɔlsəm sid / 急性子 jí xìngzǐ

garden burnet root / ˈgɑrdn ˈbɜnɪt rut / 地榆 dìyú

germinated barley / ˈdʒɜmɪneɪtɪd ˈbɑlɪ / 麦芽 màiyá

germinated rice-grain / ˈdʒɜmɪneɪtɪd raɪs greɪn / 稻芽 dàoyá

giant knotweed rhizome / ˈdʒaɪənt ˈnɒtwid ˈraɪzoʊm / 虎杖 hǔzhàng

 # giant typhonium rhizome 白附子 báifùzǐ

 # ginger processed pinellia [**tuber**] 姜半夏 jiāngbàn xià

ginkgo leaf / ˈgɪŋkəʊ lif / 银杏叶 yínxìngyè

ginkgo seed / ˈgɪŋkoʊ sid / 白果 báiguǒ

ginseng / ˈdʒɪnseŋ / 人参 rénshēn

ginseng leaf / ˈdʒɪnseŋ lif / 人参叶 rénshēnyè

glabrous greenbrier rhizome / ˈglebrəs ˈgrinˌbraɪər ˈraɪzoʊm / 土茯苓 tǔfúlíng

glossy ganoderma / ˈglɑsi ganɔdərmə / 灵芝 língzhī

 # glossy privet fruit 女贞子 nǚzhēnzǐ

golden buckwheat rhizome / ˈgoldn ˈbʌkwit ˈraɪzoʊm / 金荞麦 jīnqiáomài

golden larch bark / ˈgouldən lɑrtʃ bɑrk / 土荆皮 tǔjīngpí

golden thread / ˈgəuldən θrɛd / 黄连 huánglián

 # gordon euryale seed 芡实 qiànshí

grand torreya seed / grænd ˈtɔriə sid / 榧子 fěizǐ

 # grassleaf sweetflag rhizome 石菖蒲 shíchāngpú

great burdock achene / greɪt ˈbɜrdɑk əˈkin / 牛蒡子 niúbàngzǐ

 # grosvenor momordica fruit 罗汉果 luóhànguǒ

ground beetle / graʊnd ˈbitl / 土鳖虫 tǔbiēchóng

gypsum / ˈdʒɪpsəm / 石膏 shígāo

 # hairyvein agrimonia herb 仙鹤草 xiānhècǎo

halloysite / ˈhælɔisait / 赤石脂 chìshízhī

hawthorn fruit / ˈhɔθɔrn frut / 山楂 shānzhā

 # heartleaf houttuynia herb 鱼腥草 yúxīngcǎo

hedge prinsepia nut / hɛdʒ prɪnˈsɪpiə nʌt / 蕤仁 ruírén

 # hedyotis 白花蛇舌草 báihuāshéshécǎo

hemp seed / hemp sid / 火麻仁 huǒmárén

 # hempleaf negundo chastetree leaf 牡荆叶 mǔjīngyè

henbane seed / ˈhenbeɪn sid / 天仙子 tiānxiānzǐ

 # heterophylly falsestarwort root 太子参 tàizǐshēn

himalayan teasel root / ˌhiməˈleiən ˈtizl rut / 续断 xùduàn

hirsute shiny bugleweed herb / irsyt ˈʃaɪni ˈbjugəlˌwid hɜb / 泽兰 zélán

hogfennel root 前胡 qiánhú

honey / ˈhʌni / 蜂蜜 fēngmì

honeycomb / ˈhʌnikəʊm / 蜂房 fēngfáng

honeysuckle stem / ˈhʌnisʌkl stem / 忍冬藤 rěndōng téng

honeysucklebud and flower / ˈhʌnisʌklbʌd ənd ˈflaʊə(r) / 金银花 jīnyínhuā

human placenta / ˈhjumən pləˈsentə / 紫河车 zǐhéchē

hyacinth bean / ˈhaɪəsɪnθ bin / 白扁豆 báibiǎndòu

immature orange fruit / ˌɪməˈtjʊr ɒrɪndʒ frut / 枳实 zhǐshí

immature tangerine peel / ˌɪməˈtʃʊr ˈtændʒərin pil / 青皮 qīngpí

immature wheat / ˌɪməˈtjʊr wit / 浮小麦 fúxiǎo mài

incised notopterygium rhizome and root 羌活 qiāng huó

India madder root / ˈɪndɪə ˈmædə rut / 茜草 qiàncǎo

Indian bread / ˈɪndiən bred / 茯苓 fúlíng

Indian mock strawberry / ˈɪndiən mɒk ˈstrɔbəri / 蛇莓 shéméi

Indian trumpetflower seed 木蝴蝶 mùhúdié

ineleaf schizonepeta herb 荆芥 jīngjiè

inner membrane of chicken gizzard / ˈɪnər membreɪn əv ˈtʃɪkɪn ˈgɪzərd / 鸡内金 jīnèijīn

inula flower / iˈnjulə ˈflaʊə(r) / 旋覆花 xuánfùhuā

inula herb / iˈnjulə hɜb / 金沸草 jīnfèicǎo

inula root / iˈnjulə rut / 土木香 tǔmùxiāng

\# isatis root 板蓝根 bǎnlángēn

lychee seed / ˈlaɪtʃi sid / 荔枝核 lìzhīhé

jack bean / dʒæk bin / 刀豆 dāodòu

\# jackinthepulpit tuber 天南星 tiānnánxīng

Japanese ampelopsis root / ˌdʒæpəˈniz æmpəˈlɑpsɪs rut / 白蔹 báiliǎn

Japanese climbing fern spore / ˌdʒæpəˈniz ˈklaɪmɪŋ fɜn spɔ(r) / 海金沙 hǎijīnshā

Japanese ginseng / ˌdʒæpəˈniz ˈdʒɪnseŋ / 竹节参 zhújiéshēn

Japanese pagodatree pod / ˌdʒæpəˈniz pəˈgəʊdətri pɑd / 槐角 huáijiǎo

Japanese thistle root / ˌdʒæpəˈniz ˈθɪsl rut / 大蓟 dàjì

\# java brucea fruit 鸦胆子 yādǎnzǐ

\# kadsura pepper stem 海风藤 hǎifēngténg

\# katsumada galangal seed 草豆蔻 cǎodòukòu

kelp / kelp / 昆布 kūnbù

\# knoxia root 红大戟 hóngdàjǐ

kudzuvine root / ˈkudzuvaɪn rut / 葛根 gěgēn

\# kusnezoff monkshood root 草乌 cǎowū

\# largehead atractylodes rhizome 白术 báizhú

largeleaf gentian root / lɑdʒlif ˈdʒenʃn rut / 秦艽 qínjiāo

largeleaf Japanese ginseng rhizome / lɑdʒlif ˌdʒæpəˈniz ˈdʒɪnseŋ ˈraɪzəum / 珠子参 zhūzǐshēn

\# largetrifoliolious bugbane rhizome 升麻 shēngmá

leech / litʃ / 水蛭 shuǐzhì

lesser galangal rhizome / ˈlesə(r) ˈgæl(ə)ŋgæl ˈraɪzəʊm / 高良姜 gāoliángjiāng

 # lightyellow sophora root 苦参 kǔshēn

lilac daphne flower bud / ˈlaɪlək ˈdæfnɪ ˈflaʊər bʌd / 芫花 yuánhuā

lilac pink herb / ˈlaɪlək pɪŋk hɜb / 瞿麦 qúmài

lily bulb / ˈlɪli bʌlb / 百合 bǎihé

limonite / ˈlaɪmənaɪt / 禹余粮 yǔyúliáng

linseed / ˈlɪnˌsid / 亚麻子 yàmázǐ

liquorice root / ˈlɪkərɪʃ rut / 甘草 gāncǎo

liriope root tuber / ləˈraiəpi rut ˈtubər / 山麦冬 shān màidōng

long pepper / lɒŋ ˈpepə(r) / 荜茇 bìbá

longan aril / ˈlɒŋgən ˈærɪl / 龙眼肉 lóngyǎnròu

long-nosed pit viper / lɒŋ nəʊzd pɪt vaɪpɜr / 蕲蛇 qíshé

longstamen onion bulb / lɒŋˈsteɪmən ˈʌnjən bʌlb / 薤白 xièbái

 # longtube ground ivy herb 连钱草 liánqiáncǎo

lophatherum herb / ləˈfæθrəm hɜb / 淡竹叶 dàn zhúyè

loquat leaf / ˈloʊkwɑt lif / 枇杷叶 pípáyè

lotus leaf / ˈləʊtəs lif / 荷叶 héyè

lotus plumule / ˈləʊtəs ˈplumjul / 莲子心 liánzǐxīn

lotus receptacle / ˈləʊtəs rɪˈseptəkl / 莲房 liánfáng

lotus rhizome node / ˈləʊtəs ˈraɪzəʊm nəʊd / 藕节 ǒujié

lotus seed / ˈləʊtəs sid / 莲子 liánzǐ

lotus stamen / ˈləʊtəs ˈsteɪmən / 莲须 liánxū

luffa vegetable sponge / ˈlʌfə ˈvedʒtəbl spʌndʒ / 丝瓜络 sīguāluò

magnetite / ˈmægnItaIt / 磁石 císhí

mahonia [**leaf**] / məˈhoniə [lif] / 功劳叶 gōngláoyè

malaytea scurfpea fruit 补骨脂 bǔgǔzhī

male fern rhizome / meIl fɜn ˈraIzəʊm / 绵马贯众 mián mǎguànzhòng

manchurian dutchmanspipe stem 关木通 guānmùtōng

manchurian wild ginger / mænˈtʃuəriən waIld ˈdʒIndʒə(r) / 细辛 xìxīn

mantis egg-case / ˈmæntIs eg keIs / 桑螵蛸 sāngpiāo xiāo

manyinflorescenced sweetvetch root 红芪 hóngqí

mealyfangji [**root**] 防己 fángjǐ

medicated leaven / ˈmedIkeItId ˈlevn / 神曲 shénqǔ

medicinal changium root 明党参 míngdǎngshēn

medicinal cyathula root 川牛膝 chuānniúxī

medicinal evodia fruit 吴茱萸 wúzhūyú

medicine terminalia fruit 诃子 hēzǐ

micaschist / ˈmaIkəʃIst / 金礞石 jīnméngshí

mile swertia herb 青叶胆 qīngyèdǎn

milkvetch root / mIlkvetʃ rut / 黄芪 huángqí

milkwort root / ˈmIlkwɜt rut / 远志 yuǎnzhì

millet sprout / ˈmIlIt spraʊt / 谷芽 gǔyá

morinda root 巴戟天 bājǐtiān

motherwort fruit / ˈmʌðəwɜt frut / 茺蔚子 chōngwèizǐ

motherwort herb / ˈmʌðəwɜt hɜb / 益母草 yìmǔcǎo

mountain spicy fruit / ˈmaʊntən ˈspaIsi frut / 荜澄茄

bìchéngqié

mulberry fruit / ˈmʌlbəri frut / 桑椹 sāngshèn

mulberry leaf / ˈmʌlbəri lif / 桑叶 sāngyè

mulberry twig / ˈmʌlbəri twɪg / 桑枝 sāngzhī

 # murraya jasminorage 九里香 jiǔlǐxiāng

musk / mʌsk / 麝香 shèxiāng

 # muskroot-like semiaquilegia root 天葵子 tiānkuízǐ

mustard seed / ˈmʌstərd sid / 芥子 jièzǐ

myrrh / mɜ(r) / 没药 mòyào

nacre / ˈneɪkə / 珍珠母 zhēnzhūmǔ

 # nardostachys root 甘松 gānsōng

native achyranthes [**root**] / ˈneɪtɪv ækəˈrænθiz [rut] / 土牛膝 tǔniúxī

natural indigo / ˈnætʃrəl ɪndɪgoʊ / 青黛 qīngdài

 # nutgrass galingale rhizome 香附 xiāngfù

nutmeg / ˈnʌtmeg / 肉豆蔻 ròudòukòu

 # obscured homalomena rhizome 千年健 qiānniánjiàn

 # obtuseleaf erycibe 丁公藤 dīnggōngténg

ocher / ˈəʊkə / 赭石 zhěshí

officinal magnolia bark / əˈfɪsɪn(ə)l mægˈnəʊliə bɑk / 厚朴 hòupò

officinal magnolia flower / əˈfɪsɪn(ə)l mægˈnəʊliə ˈflaʊə(r) / 厚朴花 hòupòhuā

ophicalcite / ɔfiˈkælsait / 花蕊石 huāruǐshí

orange fruit / ˈɒrɪndʒ frut / 枳壳 zhǐqiào

oriental waterplantain rhizome / ˌɒriˈentl ˈwɔtə(r) ˈplæntɪn ˈraɪzəʊm / 泽泻 zéxiè

 # orientvine vine 青风藤 qīngfēngténg

oyster shel / ˈɔɪstər ʃel / 牡蛎 mǔlì

pagodatree flower / pəˈɡəʊdətri ˈflaʊə(r) / 槐花 huáihuā

pale butterflybush flower / peɪl ˈbʌtəflaɪbʊʃ ˈflaʊə(r) / 密蒙花 mìménghuā

palmleaf raspberry fruit / pɑmlif ˈrɑzbəri frut / 覆盆子 fùpénzǐ

pangolin scales / ˈpæŋɡəlɪn skeɪlz / 穿山甲 chuānshānjiǎ

paniculate bolbostemma rhizome / pəˈnɪkjʊˌleɪt bɑlbəʊˈstɛmə ˈraɪzoʊm / 土贝母 tǔbèimǔ

paniculate swallowwort root / pəˈnɪkjʊˌleɪt ˈswɒləɪwɜt rut / 徐长卿 xúchángqīng

papermulberry fruit / ˈpeɪpə(r) ˈmʌlbəri frut / 楮实子 chǔshízǐ

paris root / ˈpærɪs rut / 重楼 chónglóu

peach seed / pitʃ sid / 桃仁 táorén

pearl / pɜl / 珍珠 zhēnzhū

peking euphorbia root / ˈpiˈkiŋ juˈfɔbɪə rut / [京]大戟 [jīng]dàjǐ

peony root / ˈpiəni rut / 赤芍 chìsháo

pepper fruit / ˈpepə(r) frut / 胡椒 hújiāo

peppermint / ˈpepəmɪnt / 薄荷 bòhe

pepperweed seed / ˈpepə(r) wid sid / 葶苈子 tínglìzǐ

perilla fruit / pəˈrɪlə frut / 紫苏子 zǐsūzǐ

perilla leaf / pəˈrɪlə lif / 紫苏叶 zǐsūyè

perilla stem / pəˈrɪlə stem / 紫苏梗 zǐsūgěng

persimmon calyx / pəˈsɪmən ˈkeɪlɪks / 柿蒂 shìdì

 # pharbitis seed 牵牛子 qiānniúzǐ

pilose antler / ˈpaɪləʊz ˈæntlə(r) / 鹿茸 lùróng

pine pollen / paɪn ˈpɑlən / 松花粉 sōnghuāfěn

 # pinellia tuber 半夏 bànxià

pipefish / ˈpaɪpfɪʃ / 海龙 hǎilóng

 # pipewort flower 谷精草 gǔjīngcǎo

plantain herb / ˈplæntɪn hɜb / 车前草 chēqiáncǎo

plantain seed / ˈplæntɪn sid / 车前子 chēqiánzǐ

 # platycodon root 桔梗 jiégěng

plum flower / plʌm ˈflaʊə(r) / 梅花 méihuā

poison yam / ˈpɔɪzn jæm / 萆薢 bìxiè

pokeberry root / ˈpəʊkˌberɪ rut / 商陆 shānglù

pomegranate rind / ˈpɑmɪgrænɪt raɪnd / 石榴皮 shíliúpí

poppy capsule / ˈpɒpi ˈkæpsjul / 罂粟壳 yīngsùqiào

prepared common monkshood branched root / prɪˈperd ˈkɑmən ˈmʌŋkshʊd ˈbræntʃed rut / 附子 fùzǐ

prepared common monkshood mother root / prɪˈperd ˈkɑmən ˈmʌŋkshʊd ˈmʌðər rut / 制川乌 zhìchuānwū

 # prepared fleeceflower root 制何首乌 zhìhéshǒuwū

 # prepared kusnezoff monkshood root 制草乌 zhìcǎowū

 # prepared rehmannia root 熟地黄 shúdìhuáng

 # pricklyash peel 花椒 huājiāo

 # prince's-feather fruit 水红花子 shuǐhónghuāzǐ

 # processed pinellia tuber 法半夏 fǎbànxià

puff-ball / pʌfbɔl / 马勃 mǎbó

puff-ball / pʌfbɔl / 马钱子 mǎqiánzǐ

pummelo peel / ˈpʌmələʊ pil / 化橘红 huàjúhóng

puncturevine caltrop fruit / ˈpʌŋktʃə(r)vaɪn ˈkæltrəp

frut / 蒺藜 jílí

purslane 马齿苋 mǎchǐxiàn

pyrite / ˈpaɪraɪt / 自然铜 zìrántóng

pyrola herb / ˌpaɪəˈrəʊlə hɜb / 鹿衔草 lùxiáncǎo

qianjinzi / tʃʃændʒɪntsɪ / 千金子 qiānjīnzǐ

radish seed / ˈrædɪʃ sid / 莱菔子 láifúzǐ

rana oviduct 哈蟆油 hāmayóu

rangooncreeper fruit 使君子 shǐjūnzǐ

realgar / rɪˈælgə / 雄黄 xiónghuáng

red ginseng / red ˈdʒɪnseŋ / 红参 hóngshēn

red tangerine peel / red ˌtændʒəˈrin pil / 橘红 júhóng

reed rhizome / rid ˈraɪzoʊm / 芦根 lúgēn

rhubarb root and rhizome / ˈrubɑrb rut ənd ˈraɪzoʊm /
大黄 dàhuáng

rice bean / raɪs bin / 赤小豆 chìxiǎodòu

ricepaperplant pith / raɪsˈpeɪpə(r) plɑnt pɪθ / 通草
tōngcǎo

root and vine of manyprickle acanthopanax 刺五加
cìwǔjiā

rose flower / roʊz ˈflaʊər / 玫瑰花 méiguīhuā

rose-boot 红景天 hóngjǐngtiān

rosewood / ˈrəʊzwʊd / 降香 jiàngxiāng

safflower 红花 hónghuā

saffron / ˈsæfrən / 西红花 xīhónghuā

sandalwood / ˈsændlwʊd / 檀香 tánxiāng

sanqi / santʃi / 三七 sānqī

sappan wood 苏木 sūmù

sarcandra 肿节风 zhǒngjiéfēng

sargentgloryvine stem / ˈsɑrdʒəntˈglɔrivaɪn stem / 大血藤 dàxuèténg

scorpion 全蝎 quánxiē

sea horse / si hɔs / 海马 hǎimǎ

seabuckthorn fruit 沙棘 shājí

seaweed / ˈsiwid / 海藻 hǎizǎo

senna leaf / ˈsenə lif / 番泻叶 fānxièyè

sesame oil / ˈsesəmi ɔɪl / 麻油 máyóu

sharp-leaf glangal fruit 益智 yìzhì

shearer's pyrrosia leaf 石韦 shíwéi

shinyleaf pricklyash root 两面针 liǎngmiànzhēn

shrub chastetree fruit / ʃrʌb tʃeɪstrɪ frut / 蔓荆子 mànjīngzǐ

siberian cocklebur fruit 苍耳子 cāngěrzǐ

Sichuan chinaberry bark 苦楝皮 kǔliànpí

Sichuan lovage rhizome 川芎 chuānxiōng

siegesbeckia herb / ˈsidʒɪzˈbɛkɪə hɜb / 豨莶草 xīxiāncǎo

silktree albizia bark 合欢皮 héhuānpí

silk-worm droppings / sɪlk wɜm ˈdrɒpɪŋz / 蚕沙 cánshā

slender dutchmanspipe root 青木香 qīngmùxiāng

small centipeda herb / smɔl sɛntəˌpidə hɜb / 鹅不食草 ébùshícǎo

smoked plum / smokt plʌm / 乌梅 wūméi

snake slough / sneɪk slaʊ / 蛇蜕 shétuì

snakegourd fruit 瓜蒌 guālóu

snakegourd fruit 瓜蒌子 guālóuzǐ

snakegourd peel 瓜蒌皮 guālóupí

snakegourd root 天花粉 tiānhuāfěn

snowbell-leaf tickclover herb / ˈsnəʊbel lif tɪkkloʊvər hɜb / 广金钱草 guǎngjīnqiáncǎo

sodium sulfate powder / ˈsoʊdiəm ˈsʌlˌfet ˈpaʊdər / 玄明粉 xuánmíngfěn

solomon's seal rhizome / ˈsɑləmənz ˌsil ˈraɪˌzoʊm / 黄精 huángjīng

songaria cynomorium herb / sənˈgeriə ˌsɪnəˈmɔriəm hɜb / 锁阳 suǒyáng

southern fangchi root 广防己 guǎngfángjǐ

spikemoss 卷柏 juànbǎi

spine date seed / spaɪn deɪt sid / 酸枣仁 suānzǎorén

stalactite / ˈstæləktaɪt / 钟乳石 zhōngrǔshí

star-wort root / stɑ(r) wɜt rut / 银柴胡 yíncháihú

stemona root 百部 bǎibù

stiff silkworm / stɪf sɪlkwɜm / 僵蚕 jiāngcán

stink-bug / stɪŋk bʌg / 九香虫 jiǔxiāngchóng

storax / ˈstɔræks / 苏合香 sūhéxiāng

stringy stonecrop herb / ˈstrɪŋi ˈstoʊnkrɒp ɜb / 垂盆草 chuípéncǎo

suberect spatholobus stem 鸡血藤 jīxuèténg

sulfur / ˈsʌlfər / 硫黄 liúhuáng

sweet wormwood herb / ˈswit wɜmwʊd hɜb / 青蒿 qīnghāo

szechwan chinaberry fruit 川楝子 chuānliànzǐ

tabasheer / tæbəˈʃiə / 天竹黄 tiānzhúhuáng

talc / tælk / ·滑石 huáshí

tall gastrodia tuber 天麻 tiānmá

tangerine seed / ˌtændʒəˈrin sid / 橘核 júhé

tangle / ˈtæŋgl / 昆布 kūnbù

tangshen 党参 dǎngshēn

tatarian aster root / tɑˈtɛəriən ˈæstə(r) rut / 紫菀 zǐwǎn

tendrilleaf fritillary bulb 川贝母 chuānbèimǔ

thunberbg fritillary bulb 浙贝母 zhèbèimǔ

thunder ball / ˈθʌndə(r) bɔl / 雷丸 léiwán

toad venom / təʊd ˈvenəm / 蟾酥 chánsū

tokay gecko / təʊˈkeɪ ˈgekəʊ / 蛤蚧 géjiè

Tokyo violet herb / ˈtəʊkjəʊ ˈvaɪələt hɜb / 紫花地丁 zǐhuādìdīng

tortoise carapace and plastron 龟甲 guījiǎ

tree peony root bar / tri ˈpiəni rut bɑr / 牡丹皮 mǔdānpí

tree-of-heaven bark / tri əv ˈhevn bɑk / 椿皮 chūnpí

trumpet-creeper flower / ˈtrʌmpɪt kripə(r) ˈflaʊə(r) / 凌霄花 língxiāohuā

tuber fleeceflower stem 首乌藤 shǒuwūténg

tuber onion seed / ˈtjubə(r) ˈʌnjən sid / 韭菜子 jiǔcàizǐ

turmeric / ˈtɜmərɪk / 姜黄 jiānghuáng

turmeric root tuber / ˈtɜrmərɪk rut ˈtubər / 郁金 yùjīn

turtle carapace / ˈtɜtl ˈkærəpeɪs / 鳖甲 biējiǎ

twotoothed achyranthes root 牛膝 niúxī

uniflower swisscentaury root / ˌjunɪˈflaʊər swɪsˈsɛnˌtɔri rut / 漏芦 lòulú

\# **unprocessed rehmannia root** 生地黄 shēngdìhuáng

vietnamese sophora root / ˌviɛtnəˈmiz sɔfɔrɑ rut / 山豆根 shāndòugēn

\# **villous amomum fruit** 砂仁 shārén

virgate wormwood herb / ˈvɜgət ˈwɜmwʊd hɜb / 茵陈 yīnchén

\# **waxgourd seed** 冬瓜子 dōngguāzǐ

weeping forsythia capsule / ˈwipɪŋ fərˈsɪθiə ˈkæpsl / 连翘 liánqiáo

white mulberry root-bark / waɪt ˈmʌlbəri rut bɑk / 桑白皮 sāngbáipí

wild chrysanthemum flower / waɪld krɪˈzænθəməm ˈflaʊə(r) / 野菊花 yějúhuā

wild ginseng / waɪld ˈdʒɪnseŋ / 野山参 yěshānshēn

\# **wilford granesbill herb** 老鹳草 lǎoguàncǎo

\# **willowleaf rhizome** 白前 báiqián

\# **yanhusuo** 延胡索 yánhúsuǒ

\# **yerbadetajo herb** 墨旱莲 mòhànlián

\# **zedoray rhizome** 莪术 ézhú

zhuling / ˈdʒulɪŋ / 猪苓 zhūlíng

zingiber / ˈzindʒibə / 干姜 gānjiāng

Chapter 5   Prescriptions of Chinese Materia Medica

第五章　方　剂　学

Section 1   General Introduction

第一节　概　　论

assistant drug / ə'sɪstənt drʌg / 佐药 zuǒyào

channel ushering drug / 'tʃænl 'ʌʃərɪŋ drʌg / 引经药 yǐnjīngyào

classical prescriptions / 'klæsɪkl prɪ'skrɪpʃnz / 经方 jīngfāng

compound prescription / 'kɑmpaʊnd prɪ'skrɪpʃn / 复方 fùfāng

contrary drug / 'kɒntrəri drʌg / 反佐药 fǎnzuǒyào

couplet medicines / 'kʌplət 'medɪsnz / 药对 yàoduì

discourse on prescription / 'dɪskɔrs ɑn prɪ'skrɪpʃn / 方论 fānglùn

envoy drug / 'envɔɪ drʌg / 使药 shǐyào

experiential effective recipe / ɪkspɪri'enʃl ɪ'fektɪv 'resəpi / 验方 yànfāng

harmonizing drug / 'hɑmənaɪzɪŋ drʌg / 调和药 tiáohéyào

minister drug / 'mɪnɪstə(r) drʌg / 臣药 chényào

non-classical prescriptions / nɑn 'klæsɪkl prɪ'skrɪpʃnz / 时方 shífāng

prescribing method / prɪ'skraɪbɪŋ 'meθəd / 处方法 chùfāngfǎ

prescription / prɪˈskrɪpʃn / 方剂 fāngjì

secret recipe / ˈsikrət ˈresəpi / 秘方 mìfāng

simple recipe / ˈsɪmpl ˈresəpi / 单方 dānfāng

sovereign drug / ˈsɒvrɪn drʌg / 君药 jūnyào

supplementary drug / ˌsʌplɪˈmentri drʌg / 佐助药 zuǒzhùyào

supplementary inhibitory medicines / ˌsʌplɪˈmentri ɪnˈhɪbɪtərɪ ˈmedɪsnz / 佐制药 zuǒzhìyào

synergy / ˈsɪnərdʒi / 配伍 pèiwǔ

Section 2　Preparations/Decoctions

第二节　剂型、煎服法

a. c. / eɪ ˈsi / 饭前服 fànqiánfú

administered after dissolved / ədˈministərd ˈæftər dɪˈzɑlvd / 冲服 chōngfú

administered after meal / ədˈministərd ˈæftər mil / 饭后服 fànhòufú

administered at draught / ədˈministərd ət dræft / 顿服 dùnfú

administered at empty stomach / ədˈministərd ət ˈempti ˈstʌmək / 空腹服 kōngfùfú

administered before bed time / ədˈministərd bɪˈfɔr bed taɪm / 临睡服 línshuìfú

administered before meal / ədˈministərd bɪˈfɔr mil / 饭前服 fànqiánfú

administered cold / ədˈministərd koʊld / 冷服 lěngfú

administered hot / ədˈministə hɑt / 热服 rèfú

administered under tongue / ədˈministərd ˈʌndər tʌŋ /

嚓化 qínhuà

administered warm / əd'ministərd wɔrm / 温服 wēnfú

aerosol / 'eərəsɒl / 气雾剂 qìwùjì

ante cibum / 'ænti 'sibəm / 饭前服 fànqiánfú

cake / keɪk / 糕剂 gāojì

capsule / 'kæpsjul / 胶囊剂 jiāonángjì

compression formula / kəm'preʃn 'fɔmjələ / 熨剂 yùnjì

concentrated decoction / 'kɑnsntreɪtɪd dɪ'kɑkʃn / 浓缩煎剂 nóngsuōjiānjì

concentrated pill / 'kɑnsntreɪtɪd pɪl / 浓缩丸 nóngsuōwán

decoct with water / 'dɪ'kɑkt wɪð 'wɔtər / 水煎 shuǐjiān

decoct with wine / 'dɪ'kɑkt wɪð waɪn / 酒煎 jiǔjiān

decocted earlier / 'dɪ'kɑktɪd 'ərlɪr / 先煎 xiānjiān

decocted later / 'dɪ'kɑktɪd 'leɪtər / 后下 hòuxià

decocted separately / 'dɪ'kɑktɪd 'seprətli / 另煎 lìngjiān

decoction / dɪ'kɑkʃn / 汤剂 tāngjì

dissolve / dɪ'zɑlv / 溶化 rónghuà

distillate formula / 'dɪstɪleɪt 'fɔrmjələ / 露剂 lùjì

dripping pill / 'drɪpɪŋ pɪl / 滴丸剂 dīwánjì

ear drop / ɪr drɑp / 滴耳剂 dī'ěrjì

effervescent tablet / ˌefər'vesnt 'tæblət / 泡腾片 pàoténgpiàn

emulsion / ɪ'mʌlʃn / 乳剂 rǔjì

enema / 'enəmə / 灌肠剂 guànchángjì

extract / 'ekstrækt / 浸膏剂 jìngāojì

eye drop / aɪ drɑp / 滴眼剂 dīyǎnjì

fermented medicine / fər'mentɪd 'medɪsn / 曲剂 qǔjì

flour and water paste pill / ˈflaʊər ənd ˈwɔtə peɪst pɪl / 糊丸 húwán

gel / dʒel / 胶剂 jiāojì

granules / ˈgrænjuls / 颗粒剂 kēlìjì

hard capsule / hɑrd ˈkæpsjul / 硬胶囊剂 yìngjiāonángjì

honeyed pill / ˈhʌnid pɪl / 蜜丸 mìwán

injection / ɪnˈdʒekʃn / 注射剂 zhùshèjì

liniment / ˈlɪnəmənt / 搽剂 chájì

liquid extract / ˈlɪkwɪd ˈekstrækt / 流浸膏剂 liújìngāojì

lozenge / ˈlɒzɪndʒ / 锭剂 dìngjì

medicinal tea / məˈdɪsɪnl ti / 茶剂 chájì

medicinal usher / məˈdɪsɪnl ˈʌʃər / 药引 yàoyǐn

melt / melt / 烊化 yánghuà

micro-capsule / ˈmaɪkrəʊ ˈkæpsjul / 微囊剂 wēinángjì

mild fire / maɪld ˈfaɪər / 文火 wénhuǒ

mini-pill / ˈmɪni pɪl / 微丸 wēiwán

mix / mɪks / 兑入 duìrù

mix with fresh juice / mɪks wɪð freʃ dʒus / 生汁兑入 shēngzhīduìrù

mixture / ˈmɪkstʃə(r) / 合剂 héjì

moxibustion formula / ˌmɒksɪˈbʌstʃ(ə)n ˈfɔmjələ / 灸剂 jiǔjì

nasal drop / ˈneɪzl drɑp / 滴鼻剂 dībíjì

ointment / ˈɔɪntmənt / 软膏剂 ruǎngāojì

optimal fire / ˈɑptɪməl ˈfaɪər / 火候 huǒhou

oral liquid / ˈɔrəl ˈlɪkwɪd / 口服液 kǒufúyè

oral thick paste / ˈɔrəl θɪk peɪst / 膏滋 gāozī

p. c. / pi ˈsi / 饭后服 fànhòufú

pill / pɪl / 丸剂 wánjì

plaster / ˈplæstər / 膏药 gāoyào

post cibum / poʊst ˈsibəm / 饭后服 fànhòufú

powder / ˈpaʊdər / 散剂 sǎnjì

preparation / ˌprepəˈreɪʃn / 剂型 jìxíng

smoke fumigant / sməʊk ˈfjumɪgənt / 烟熏剂 yānxūnjì

soft capsule / sɒft ˈkæpsjul / 软胶囊剂 ruǎnjiāonángjì

spray / spreɪ / 喷雾剂 pēnwùjì

stripe formula / straɪp ˈfɔrmjələ / 条剂 tiáojì

strong fire / strɔŋ ˈfaɪər / 武火 wǔhuǒ

suppository / səˈpɒzətri / 栓剂 shuānjì

syrup / ˈsɪrəp / 糖浆剂 tángjiāngjì

tablet / ˈtæblət / 片剂 piànjì

taken frequently / ˈtekən ˈfrikwəntli / 频服 pínfú

taken separately / ˈtekən ˈseprətli / 分服 fēnfú

thread formula / θred ˈfɔrmjələ / 线剂 xiànjì

tincture / ˈtɪŋktʃə(r) / 酊剂 dīngjì

watered pill / ˈwɔtəd pɪl / 水丸 shuǐwán

water-honeyed pill / ˈwɔtə hʌnid pɪl / 水蜜丸 shuǐmì wán

wax pill / wæks pɪl / 蜡丸 làwán

wine / waɪn / 酒剂 jiǔjì

wrap-boiling / ræp ˈbɔɪlɪŋ / 包煎 bāojiān

Section 3 Classification of Prescriptions

第三节 方剂分类

anti-helminthic formula / ˈænti hɛlˈmɪnθɪk ˈfɔrmjələ / 驱虫剂 qūchóngjì

astringent formula / əˈstrɪndʒənt ˈfɔrmjələ / 固涩剂 gùsèjì

blood-activating formula / blʌd ˈæktəˌvetɪŋ ˈfɔrmjələ / 活血剂 huóxuèjì

blood-regulating formula / blʌd ˈrɛgjəˌleɪtɪŋ ˈfɔrmjələ / 理血剂 lǐxuèjì

blood-stanching formula / blʌd stɑntʃɪŋ ˈfɔrmjələ / 止血剂 zhǐxuèjì

blood-supplementing formula / blʌd ˈsʌplɪməntɪŋ ˈfɔrmjələ / 补血剂 bǔxuèjì

carminative formula / kɑrˈmɪnətɪv ˈfɔrmjələ / 理气剂 lǐqìjì

cold cathartic formula / koʊld kəˈθɑrtɪk ˈfɔrmjələ / 寒下剂 hánxiàjì

cold formula for resuscitation / koʊld ˈfɔrmjələ fər rɪsʌsɪˈteɪʃn / 凉开剂 liángkāijì

desiccating formula / ˈdɛsɪˌkeɪtɪŋ ˈfɔrmjələ / 祛湿剂 qūshījì

digestive formula / daɪˈdʒestɪv ˈfɔrmjələ / 消食剂 xiāoshíjì

drastic diuretics formula / ˈdræstɪk daɪjuˈrɛtɪks ˈfɔrmjələ / 逐水剂 zhúshuǐjì

emetic formula / ɪˈmetɪk ˈfɔrmjələ / 涌吐剂 yǒngtǔjì

formula for activating qi flowing / ˈfɔrmjələ fər ˈæktəˌvetɪŋ tʃi ˈfloɪŋ / 行气剂 xíngqìjì

formula for arresting leucorrhea and metrorrhagia / ˈfɔrmjələ fər əˈrestɪŋ ˌljukəˈriə ənd ˌmitrəˈredʒɪə / 固崩止带剂 gùbēngzhǐdàijì

formula for astringing intestine and arresting proptosis / ˈfɔrmjələ fər əˈstrɪŋɪŋ ɪnˈtestɪn ənd əˈrestɪŋ proˈtosɪs / 涩肠固脱剂 sèchánggùtuōjì

formula for astringing lung for relieving cough / ˈfɔrmjələ fər əˈstrɪŋɪŋ lʌŋ fər rɪˈlivɪŋ kɔf / 敛肺止咳剂 liǎnfèizhǐkéjì

formula for astringing spermatorrhea / ˈfɔrmjələ fər əˈstrɪŋɪŋ spərˌmætoˈrɪr / 涩精止遗剂 sèjīngzhǐyíjì

formula for benefiting both qi and blood / ˈfɔrmjələ fər ˈbenɪfɪtɪŋ boʊθ tʃi ənd blʌd / 气血双补剂 qìxuèshuāngbǔjì

formula for benefiting both yin and yang / ˈfɔrmjələ fər ˈbenɪfɪtɪŋ boʊθ jɪn ənd jæŋ / 阴阳并补剂 yīnyángbìngbǔjì

formula for calming down internal wind / ˈfɔrmjələ fər ˈkamɪŋ daʊn ɪnˈtɜrnl wɪnd / 平熄内风剂 píngxī nèifēngjì

formula for clearing asthenic fever / ˈfɔrmjələ fər ˈklɪrɪŋ æsˈθenɪk ˈfivər / 清虚热剂 qīngxūrèjì

formula for clearing heat and eliminating dampness / ˈfɔrmjələ fər ˈklɪrɪŋ hit ɪˈlɪmənetɪŋ ˈdæmpnəs / 清热祛湿剂 qīngrèqūshījì

formula for clearing heat and removing toxicity / ˈfɔrmjələ fər ˈklɪrɪŋ hit ənd riˈmuvɪŋ tɑkˈsɪsəti / 清热解毒剂 qīngrèjiědújì

formula for clearing heat at qi level / ˈfɔrmjələ fər ˈklɪrɪŋ hit ət tʃi ˈlevl / 清气分热剂 qīngqìfēnrèjì

formula for clearing heat in viscerae / ˈfɔrmjələ fər ˈklɪrɪŋ hit ɪn ˈvɪsərə / 清脏腑热剂 qīngzàngfǔrèjì

formula for clearing nutrient level and cooling blood / ˈfɔrmjələ fər ˈklɪrɪŋ ˈnutriənt ˈlevl ənd ˈkʊlɪŋ blʌd / 清营凉血剂 qīngyíngliángxuèjì

formula for clearing summerheat / ˈfɔrmjələ fər ˈklɪrɪŋ ˈsʌmərhit / 清热解暑剂 qīngrèjiěshǔjì

formula for consolidating superficies for arresting sweating / ˈfɔrmjələ fər kənˈsɒlɪdeɪtɪŋ ˌsupərˈfɪʃiz fər əˈrestɪŋ ˈswetɪŋ / 固表止汗剂 gùbiǎozhǐhànjì

formula for descending qi / ˈfɔrmjələ fər dɪˈsɛndɪŋ tʃi / 降气剂 jiàngqìjì

formula for dispersing external wind / ˈfɔrmjələ fər dɪˈspərsɪŋ ɪkˈstɜrnl wɪnd / 疏散外风剂 shūsànwàifēngjì

formula for diuresis and diffusing dampness / ˈfɔrmjələ fər ˌdaɪjʊ(ə)ˈrisɪs ənd dɪˈfjuzɪŋ ˈdæmpnəs / 利水渗湿剂 lìshuǐshènshījì

formula for harmonizing stomach and drying dampness / ˈfɔrmjələ fər ˈhɑmənaɪzɪŋ ˈstʌmək ənd ˈdraɪɪŋ ˈdæmpnəs / 和胃燥湿剂 héwèizàoshījì

formula for purgation / ˈfɔrmjələ fər pərˈgeʃən / 泻下剂 xièxiàjì

formula for relieving both superficial and internal disorders / ˈfɔrmjələ fər rɪˈlivɪŋ boʊθ ˌsupərˈfɪʃl ənd ɪnˈtɜrnl dɪsˈɔrdərz / 表里双解剂 biǎolǐshuāngjiějì

formula for relieving superficies and catharsis / ˈfɔrmjələ fər rɪˈlivɪŋ ˌsupərˈfɪʃiz ənd kəˈθɑrsɪs / 解表通里剂 jiěbiǎotōnglǐjì

formula for relieving superficies and clearing interior / ˈfɔrmjələ fər rɪˈlivɪŋ ˌsupərˈfɪʃiz ənd ˈklɪrɪŋ ɪnˈtɪriər / 解表清里剂 jiěbiǎoqīnglǐjì

formula for relieving superficies and warming interior / ˈfɔrmjələ fər rɪˈlivɪŋ ˌsupərˈfɪʃiz ənd ˈwɔrmɪŋ ɪnˈtɪriər / 解表温里剂 jiěbiǎowēnlǐjì

formula for relieving superficies syndrome with pungent and cool natured drugs / ˈfɔrmjələ fər rɪˈlivɪŋ ˌsupərˈfɪʃiz ˈsɪndroʊm wɪð ˈpʌndʒənt ənd kul neɪtʃərd drʌgz / 辛凉解表剂 xīnliángjiěbiǎojì

formula for relieving superficies syndrome with pungent and warm natured drugs / ˈfɔrmjələ fər rɪˈlivɪŋ ˌsupərˈfɪʃiz ˈsɪndroʊm wɪð ˈpʌndʒənt ənd wɔrm neɪtʃərd drʌgz / 辛温解表剂 xīnwēnjiěbiǎojì

formula for resolving phlegm with arresting wind / ˈfɔrmjələ fər rɪˈzɑlvɪŋ flem wɪð əˈrestɪŋ wɪnd / 治风化痰剂 zhìfēnghuàtánjì

formula for resolving phlegm with clear-moistening drugs / ˈfɔrmjələ fər rɪˈzɑlvɪŋ flem wɪð klɪr ˈmɔɪsnɪŋ drʌgz / 清润化痰剂 qīngrùnhuàtánjì

formula for resolving phlegm with warm drugs / ˈfɔrmjələ fər rɪˈzɑlvɪŋ flem wɪð wɔrm drʌgz / 温燥化痰剂 wēnzàohuàtánjì

formula for restoring yang and rescuing patient from collapse / ˈfɔrmjələ fər rɪˈstorɪŋ jæŋ ənd ˈreskjuɪŋ ˈpeɪʃnt frəm kəˈlæps / 回阳救逆剂 huíyángjiùnìjì

formula for resuscitation / ˈfɔrmjələ fər rɪsʌsɪˈteɪʃn / 开窍剂 kāiqiàojì

formula for strengthening body resistance for relieving superficies / ˈfɔrmjələ fər ˈstreŋθənɪŋ ˈbɑdi rɪˈzɪstəns fər rɪˈlivɪŋ ˌsupərˈfɪʃiz / 扶正解表剂 fúzhèng jiěbiǎojì

formula for warming channel for dispersing cold / ˈfɔrmjələ fər ˈwɔrmɪŋ ˈtʃænl fər dɪˈspərsɪŋ koʊld / 温经散寒剂 wēnjīngsànhánjì

formula for warming interior for dispersing cold / ˈfɔrmjələ fər ˈwɔrmɪŋ ɪnˈtɪriər fər dɪˈspərsɪŋ koʊld / 温中散寒剂 wēnzhōngsànhánjì

formula for warmly resolving watery dampness / ˈfɔrmjələ fər ˈwɔrmli rɪˈzɑlvɪŋ ˈwɔtəri ˈdæmpnəs / 温化水湿剂 wēnhuàshuǐshījì

formula for wind disorder / ˈfɔrmjələ fər wɪnd dɪsˈɔrdər / 治风剂 zhìfēngjì

heat-clearing formula / hit ˈklɪrɪŋ ˈfɔrmjələ / 清热剂 qīngrèjì

moistened cathartic formula / ˈmɔɪsnd kəˈθɑrtɪk ˈfɔrmjələ / 润下剂 rùnxiàjì

phlegm-expelling formula / flem ɪkˈspɛlɪŋ ˈfɔrmjələ / 祛痰剂 qūtánjì

qi regulated formula / tʃi ˈrɛgjəˌleɪtɪd ˈfɔrmjələ / 理气剂 lǐqìjì

qi supplementing formula / tʃi ˈsʌplɪməntɪŋ ˈfɔrmjələ / 补气剂 bǔqìjì

reconciling shaoyang formula / ˈrɛkənsaɪlɪŋ ˈʃaujæŋ ˈfɔrmjələ / 和解少阳剂 héjiěshàoyángjì

sedative / ˈsedətɪv / 安神剂 ānshénjì

superficies-relieving formula / sʊpərˈfɪʃiz rɪˈlivɪŋ ˈfɔrmjələ / 解表剂 jiěbiǎojì

supplementing formula / ˈsʌplɪməntɪŋ ˈfɔrmjələ / 补益剂 bǔyìjì

tranquillizing formula / ˈtræŋkwəlaɪzɪŋ ˈfɔrmjələ / 安神剂 ānshénjì

warm cathartic formula / wɔrm kəˈθɑrtɪk ˈfɔrmjələ / 温下剂 wēnxiàjì

warm formula for resuscitation / wɔrm ˈfɔrmjələ fər rɪsʌsɪˈteɪʃn / 温开剂 wēnkāijì

warming interior formula / ˈwɔrmɪŋ ɪnˈtɪriər ˈfɔrmjələ / 温里剂 wēnlǐjì

yang-supplementing formula / jæŋˈsʌplɪməntɪŋ ˈfɔrmjələ / 补阳剂 bǔyángjì

yin-supplementing formula / jɪn ˈsʌplɪməntɪŋ ˈfɔrmjələ / 补阴剂 bǔyīnjì

Section 4 Classic formulas
第四节 方　剂

an'gong niuhuang pills / ˈankʊŋ ˈnjuhwɑŋ pɪlz / 安宫牛黄丸 āngōngniúhuángwán

an'gong niuhuang wan / ˈankʊŋ ˈnjuhwɑŋ wæn / 安宫牛黄丸 āngōngniúhuángwán

baidu powder / baiˌdu ˈpaʊdər / 败毒散 bàidúsǎn

baihe gujin decoction / baɪhɛ kudʒɪn dɪˈkɑkʃn / 百合固金汤 bǎihégùjīntāng

baihu decoction / baihu dɪˈkɑkʃn / 白虎汤 báihǔtāng

baitouweng decoction / baitouˈwɛn dɪˈkɑkʃn / 白头翁汤 báitóuwēngtāng

banxia baizhu tianma decoction / bænʃjɑ paɪdʒu tjænmɑ dɪˈkɑkʃn / 半夏白术天麻汤 bànxiàbáizhútiānmátāng

banxia houpo decoction / bænʃjɑ ˈhɑʊpoʊ dɪˈkɑkʃn / 半夏厚朴汤 bànxiàhòupòtāng

banxia xiexin decoction / bænʃjɑ ˈʃjɛʃɪn dɪˈkɑkʃn / 半夏泻心汤 bànxiàxièxīntāng

baohe pills / bɑʊhɛ pɪlz / 保和丸 bǎohéwán

baohe wan / bɑʊhɛ wan / 保和丸 bǎohéwán

bazhen decoction / bʌʤen dɪˈkɑkʃn / 八珍汤 bāzhēn tāng

bazheng powder / bʌʤeŋ ˈpɑʊdər / 八正散 bāzhèng sǎn

beimu gualou powder / beɪmu kuɑlu ˈpɑʊdər / 贝母瓜蒌散 bèimǔguālóusǎn

biejiajian pills / pjɛdʒiadʒjæn pɪlz / 鳖甲煎丸 biējiǎ jiānwán

bixie fenqing drink / baɪˈʃɪ feŋˈtʃɪŋ drɪŋk / 萆薢分清饮 bìxièfēnqīngyǐn

budai pills / buˈtaɪ pɪlz / 布袋丸 bùdàiwán

bufei e'jiao decoction / bufeɪ eˈdʒjɑʊ dɪˈkɑkʃn / 补肺阿胶汤 bǔfèi'ējiāotāng

buyang huanwu decoction / bujæŋ haɪwu dɪˈkɑkʃn / 补阳还五汤 bǔyánghuánwǔtāng

buzhong yiqi decoction / buʤʊŋ jitʃi dɪˈkɑkʃn / 补中益气汤 bǔzhōngyìqìtāng

cang'er powder / ˈtsɑŋər ˈpɑʊdər / 苍耳散 cāng'ersǎn

chaige jieji decoction / tʃaɪkɜ dʒjɛdʒi dɪˈkɑkʃn / 柴葛解肌汤 cháigějiějītāng

chaihu shugan powder / tʃaɪhu ʃukan ˈpɑʊdər / 柴胡疏肝散 cháihúshūgānsǎn

chuanxiong chatiao powder / tʃwanʃɒŋ tʃatjaʊ ˈpaʊdər / 川芎茶调散 chuānxiōngchátiáosǎn

chuanxiong chatiao san / tʃwanʃɒŋ tʃa tjaʊ san / 川芎茶调散 chuānxiōngchátiáosǎn

cizhu pills / tsiˈdʒu pɪlz / 磁朱丸 cízhūwán

congchi decoction / tsaŋtʃi dɪkakʃn / 葱豉汤 cōngchǐtāng

dabuyin pills / daˈbujɪn pɪlz / 大补阴丸 dàbǔyīnwán

dabuyin wan / daˈbujɪn wæn / 大补阴丸 dàbǔyīnwán

dachaihu decoction / datʃaɪhu dɪˈkakʃn / 大柴胡汤 dàcháihútāng

dachengqi decoction / daˈdʒɛntʃi dɪˈkakʃn / 大承气汤 dàchéngqìtāng

dading fengzhu pills / dadɪŋ ˈfʌŋdʒu pɪlz / 大定风珠 dàdìngfēngzhū

dahuang fuzi decoction / dahwaŋ futsɪ dɪˈkakʃn / 大黄附子汤 dàhuángfùzǐtāng

dahuang mudan decoction / dahwaŋ mudæn dɪˈkakʃn / 大黄牡丹汤 dàhuángmǔdāntāng

dajianzhong decoction / dadʒjændʒʊŋ dɪˈkakʃn / 大建中汤 dàjiànzhōngtāng

danggui buxue decoction / tæŋˈkweɪ buʃuɛ dɪˈkakʃn / 当归补血汤 dāngguībǔxuètāng

danggui liuhuang decoction / tæŋˈkweɪ ljuhwaŋ dɪˈkakʃn / 当归六黄汤 dāngguīliùhuángtāng

danggui sini decoction / tæŋˈkweɪ sini dɪˈkakʃn / 当归四逆汤 dāngguīsìnìtāng

daochi powder / dəʊtʃi ˈpaʊdər / 导赤散 dǎochìsǎn

daqinjiao decoction / datʃɪndʒɑʊ dɪˈkɑkʃn / 大秦艽汤 dàqínjiāotāng

dihuang drink / dihwɑŋ drɪŋk / 地黄饮子 dìhuáng yǐnzǐ

dingchuan decoction / dɪŋtʃwɑn dɪˈkɑkʃn / 定喘汤 dìngchuǎntāng

dingxian pills / dɪŋʃjan pɪlz / 定痫丸 dìngxiánwán

dingxiang shidi decoction / tɪŋʃjaŋ ˈʃɪdi dɪˈkɑkʃn / 丁香柿蒂汤 dīngxiāngshìdìtāng

dingzhi pills / dɪŋʤi pɪlz / 定志丸 dìngzhìwán

duhuo jisheng decoction / duhwo dʒiˈʃeŋ dɪˈkɑkʃn / 独活寄生汤 dúhuójìshēngtāng

er'chen decoction / ˈərtʃən dɪˈkɑkʃn / 二陈汤 èrchéntāng

er'miao powder / ˈərmjɑʊ ˈpɑʊdər / 二妙散 èrmiàosǎn

er'zhi pills / ˈərʤi pɪlz / 二至丸 èrzhìwán

fangfeng tongsheng powder / faŋˈfʌŋ tɒŋʃeŋ ˈpɑʊdər / 防风通圣散 fángfēngtōngshèngsǎn

fangji huangqi decoction / faŋˈdʒi hwɑŋtʃi dɪˈkɑkʃn / 防己黄芪汤 fángjǐhuángqítāng

fei'er pills / feɪˈər pɪlz / 肥儿丸 féi'érwán

fei'er wan / feɪˈər wæn / 肥儿丸 féi'érwán

fengsui micropills / ˈfeŋsweɪ ˈmaɪkroʊpɪlz / 封髓丹 fēngsuǐdān

fuling pills / fulɪŋ pɪlz / 茯苓丸 fúlíngwán

fuyuan huoxue decoction / ˈfujuan hwoˈʃuɛ dɪˈkɑkʃn / 复元活血汤 fùyuánhuóxuètāng

fuyuan huoxue tang / ˈfujuɑn hwoˈʃuɛ tɑŋ / 复元活血汤 fùyuánhuóxuètāng

ganlu xiaodu pills / kanlu ʃaʊdu pɪlz / 甘露消毒丹 gānlùxiāodúdān

ganmai dazao decoction / kanmaɪ datsɑʊ dɪˈkɑkʃn / 甘麦大枣汤 gānmàidàzǎotāng

gegen decoction / kɜkən dɪˈkɑkʃn / 葛根汤 gěgēntāng

gegen qinlian decoction / kɜkən tʃɪnlian dɪˈkɑkʃn / 葛根芩连汤 gěgēnqínliántāng

guadi powder / kuɑˈdi ˈpaʊdər / 瓜蒂散 guādìsǎn

guchong decoction / kuˈtʃʊŋ dɪˈkɑkʃn / 固冲汤 gùchōngtāng

guifu dihuang pills / ˈkweɪfu dihwɑŋ pɪlz / 桂附地黄丸 guìfùdìhuángwán

guifu dihuang wan / ˈkweɪfu dihwɑŋ wæn / 桂附地黄丸 guìfùdìhuángwán

guilu er'xian glue / ˈkweɪlu ərˈʃjæn glu / 龟鹿二仙胶 guīlùèrxiānjiāo

guipi decoction / ˈguipi dɪˈkɑkʃn / 归脾汤 guīpítāng

guizhi decoction / ˈkwedʒi dɪˈkɑkʃn / 桂枝汤 guìzhītāng

guizhi fuling pills / ˈkwedʒi fulɪŋ pɪlz / 桂枝茯苓丸 guìzhīfúlíngwán

guizhi fuling wan / ˈkwedʒi fulɪŋ wæn / 桂枝茯苓丸 guìzhīfúlíngwán

gujing pills / ˈkudʒɪŋ pɪlz / 固经丸 gùjīngwán

gujing wan / ˈkudʒɪŋ wæn / 固经丸 gùjīngwán

haoqin qingdan decoction / hɑʊtʃɪn 'tʃɪŋdan dɪ'kɑkʃn / 蒿芩清胆汤 hāoqínqīngdǎntāng

houpo wenzhong decoction / 'haʊpoʊ wenʤʊŋ dɪ'kɑkʃn / 厚朴温中汤 hòupòwēnzhōngtāng

huachong pills / huatʃʊŋ pɪlz / 化虫丸 huàchóngwán

huaihua powder / hwaɪhua paʊdər / 槐花散 huáihuāsǎn

huanglian jiedu decoction / hwɑŋljæn dʒjɛdu dɪ'kɑkʃn / 黄连解毒汤 huángliánjiědútāng

huangtu decoction / hwɑŋtu dɪ'kɑkʃn / 黄土汤 huáng tǔtāng

huoxiang zhengqi powder / hwoʃjæŋ ʤɛŋtʃi paʊdər / 藿香正气散 huòxiāngzhèngqìsǎn

jiajian weirui decoction / dʒjɑdʒæn weɪrweɪ dɪ'kɑkʃn / 加减葳蕤汤 jiājiǎnwēiruítāng

jichuan decoction / 'dʒitʃwɑn dɪ'kɑkʃn / 济川煎 jìchuānjiān

jinfeicao powder / dʒɪnfeɪtsau 'paʊdər / 金沸草散 jīnfèicǎosǎn

jinlingzi powder / dʒɪnlɪŋtsɪ 'paʊdər / 金铃子散 jīnlíngzǐsǎn

jinsuo gujing pills / dʒɪn'suoʊ kudʒɪn pɪlz / 金锁固精丸 jīnsuǒgùjīngwán

jiuji xixian powder / dʒjudzi ʃiʃjɑn 'paʊdər / 救急稀涎散 jiùjíxīxiánsǎn

jiuwei qianghuo decoction / dʒɪuweɪ tʃjɑŋhwo dɪ'kɑkʃn / 九味羌活汤 jiǔwèiqiānghuótāng

jiuxian powder / dʒɪuʃjæn 'paʊdər / 九仙散 jiǔxiānsǎn

juanbi decoction / dʒwanpi dɪkakʃn / 蠲痹汤 juānbì tāng

juhe pills / dʒuhɛ pɪlz / 橘核丸 júhéwán

jupi zhuru decoction / dʒupi dʒuru dɪkakʃn / 橘皮竹茹汤 júpízhúrútāng

kexue formula / kɛʃuɛ ˈfɔrmjələ / 咳血方 kéxuèfāng

liangge powder / ljɑŋkə ˈpaʊdər / 凉膈散 liánggésǎn

lianpu drink / ljænpu drɪŋk / 连朴饮 liánpǔyǐn

linggui zhugan decoction / lɪŋˈkweɪ ʃukan dɪˈkakʃn / 苓桂术甘汤 língguìzhúgāntāng

lingjiao gouteng decoction / lɪŋdʒjɑʊ kəʊtəŋ dɪˈkakʃn / 羚角钩藤汤 língjiǎogōuténgtāng

liuwei dihuang pills / ljuweɪ dihwɑŋ pɪlz / 六味地黄丸 liùwèidìhuángwán

liuwei dihuang wan / ljuweɪ dihwɑŋ wæn / 六味地黄丸 liùwèidìhuángwán

liuyi powder / ljuji ˈpaʊdər / 六一散 liùyìsǎn

liuyi san / ljuji san / 六一散 liùyìsǎn

lizhong decoction / lidʒʊŋ dɪˈkakʃn / 理中汤 lǐzhōng tāng

mahuang decoction / mɑhwɑŋ dɪˈkakʃn / 麻黄汤 má huángtāng

mahuang xingren gancao shigao decoction / mɑhwɑŋ hɪŋrən kantsaʊ ʃikaʊ dɪˈkakʃn / 麻黄杏仁甘草石膏汤 máhuángxìngréngāncǎoshígāotāng

maimendong decoction / maɪmɛndɔŋ dɪˈkakʃn / 麦门冬汤 màiméndōngtāng

maziren pills / mɑtsɪrən pɪlz / 麻子仁丸 mázǐrén

wán

mengshi guntan pills / meŋʃɪ kuəntæn pɪlz / 礞石滚痰丸 méngshígǔntánwán

muli powder / muli ˈpaʊdər / 牡蛎散 mǔlìsǎn

muxiang binglang pills / muʃjɑŋ bɪŋlæŋ pɪlz / 木香槟榔丸 mùxiāngbīnglángwán

muxiang binglang wan / muʃjɑŋ bɪŋlæŋ wæn / 木香槟榔丸 mùxiāngbīnglángwán

neibu huangqi decoction / neɪbu hwɑŋtʃi dɪˈkɑkʃn / 内补黄芪汤 nèibǔhuángqítāng

nuangan decoction / nwankan dɪkɑkʃn / 暖肝煎 nuǎngānjiān

pingwei powder / pɪŋweɪ ˈpaʊdər / 平胃散 píngwèisǎn

puji xiaodu drink / pudʒi ʃaʊdu drɪŋk / 普济消毒饮 pǔjìxiāodúyǐn

qianghuo shengshi decoction / tʃiɑŋhwo ʃɛŋʃi dɪˈkɑkʃn / 羌活胜湿汤 qiānghuóshèngshītāng

qianzheng powder / ˈtʃɪˈændʒɛŋ ˈpaʊdər / 牵正散 qiānzhèngsǎn

qibao meiran mini-pills / tʃibaʊ meɪrən ˈmɪni pɪlz / 七宝美髯丹 qībǎoměirándān

qili powder / tʃili ˈpaʊdər / 七厘散 qīlísǎn

qili san / tʃi li san / 七厘散 qīlísǎn

qinggu powder / ˈtʃɪŋku ˈpaʊdər / 清骨散 qīnggǔsǎn

qinghao biejia decoction / ˈtʃɪŋhɑʊ pjɛdʒia dɪˈkɑkʃn / 青蒿鳖甲汤 qīnghāobiējiǎtāng

qingluo drink / ˈtʃɪŋlwo drɪŋk / 清络饮 qīngluòyǐn

qingqi huatan pills / ˈtʃɪŋtʃi huɑtæn pɪlz / 清气化痰丸

qīngqìhuàtánwán

qingshu yiqi decoction / ˈtʃɪŋʃu ɪtʃi dɪˈkɑkʃn / 清暑益气汤 qīngshǔyìqìtāng

qingwei powder / ˈtʃɪŋweɪ ˈpaʊdər / 清胃散 qīngwèisǎn

qingwen baidu powder / ˈtʃɪŋwen baidu ˈpaʊdər / 清瘟败毒散 qīngwēnbàidúsǎn

qingying decoction / ˈtʃɪŋjɪn dɪˈkɑkʃn / 清营汤 qīngyíngtāng

qingzao jiufei decoction / ˈtʃɪŋtsɑʊ dʒɪufeɪ dɪˈkɑkʃn / 清燥救肺汤 qīngzàojiùfèitāng

sangju drink / sæŋdʒu drɪŋk / 桑菊饮 sāngjúyǐn

sangpiaoxiao powder / sæŋˈpjaʊʃaʊ ˈpaʊdər / 桑螵蛸散 sāngpiāoxiāosǎn

sangxing decoction / sæŋˈʃɪŋ dɪˈkɑkʃn / 桑杏汤 sāngxìngtāng

sanjia fumai decoction / sanˈdʒia fuˈmaɪ dɪˈkɑkʃn / 三甲复脉汤 sānjiǎfùmàitāng

sanren decoction / sanrən dɪˈkɑkʃn / 三仁汤 sānréntāng

sanwu beiji pills / sanwʊ beɪdʒi pɪlz / 三物备急丸 sān wùbèijíwán

sanzi yangqin decoction / santsɪ jæŋtʃɪn dɪˈkɑkʃn / 三子养亲汤 sānzǐyǎngqīntāng

shaoyao decoction / ʃaʊjaʊ dɪˈkɑkʃn / 芍药汤 sháoyàotāng

shenfu decoction / ʃənsu dɪˈkɑkʃn / 参附汤 shēnfùtāng

shenghua decoction / ˈʃʌŋhua dɪˈkɑkʃn / 生化汤 shēnghuàtāng

shengma gegen decoction / ˈʃʌŋma kɜkən dɪˈkɑkʃn / 升麻葛根汤 shēngmágěgēntāng

shengmai powder / ˈʃʌŋmaɪ ˈpaʊdər / 生脉散 shēngmàisǎn

shengmai san / ˈʃʌŋmaɪ san / 生脉散 shēngmàisǎn

shenling baizhu powder / ʃənlɪŋ paɪdʒu ˈpaʊdər / 参苓白术散 shēnlíngbáizhúsǎn

shenling baizhu san / ʃənlɪŋ paɪdʒu san / 参苓白术散 shēnlíngbáizhúsǎn

shenqi pills / ʃəntʃi pɪlz / 肾气丸 shènqìwán

shensu drink / ʃənsu drɪŋk / 参苏饮 shēnsūyǐn

shihu yeguang pills / ʃɪhu jɛˈkwæŋ pɪlz / 石斛夜光丸 shíhúyèguāngwán

shihu yeguang wan / ʃɪhu jɛˈkwæŋ wæn / 石斛夜光丸 shíhúyèguāngwán

shihui powder / ʃɪˈhuɪ ˈpaʊdər / 十灰散 shíhuīsǎn

shipi powder / ʃɪpi ˈpaʊdər / 实脾散 shípísǎn

shixiao powder / ʃiˈʃjaʊ ˈpaʊdər / 失笑散 shīxiàosǎn

shizao decoction / ʃɪtsaʊ dɪˈkɑkʃn / 十枣汤 shízǎotāng

shuzuo drink / ʃutsaʊ drɪŋk / 疏凿饮子 shūzáoyǐnzi

sijunzi decoction / ˈsidʒuəntsɪ dɪˈkɑkʃn / 四君子汤 sìjūnzǐtāng

simiao yong'an decoction / ˈsimjɑʊ ˈjɒŋan dɪˈkɑkʃn / 四妙勇安汤 sìmiàoyǒng'āntāng

sini decoction / siˈni dɪˈkɑkʃn / 四逆汤 sìnìtāng

sini powder / si'ni 'paʊdər / 四逆散 sìnìsǎn

sini tang / si'ni tɑŋ / 四逆汤 sìnìtāng

sishen pills / si'ʃən pɪlz / 四神丸 sìshénwán

sishen wan / si'ʃən wæn / 四神丸 sìshénwán

siwu decoction / si'wʊ dɪ'kɑkʃn / 四物汤 sìwùtāng

suanzaoren decoction / swɑn'tsɑʊrən dɪkɑkʃn / 酸枣仁汤 suānzǎoréntāng

suhexiang pills / su'heʃjɑŋ pɪlz / 苏合香丸 sūhéxiāng wán

suhexiang wan / su'heʃjɑŋ wæn / 苏合香丸 sūhéxiāng wán

suzi jiangqi decoction / su'tsɪ 'dʒjæŋtʃi dɪ'kɑkʃn / 苏子降气汤 sūzǐjiàngqìtāng

tiantai wuyao powder / 'tjæntaɪ wʊjaʊ 'paʊdər / 天台乌药散 tiāntāiwūyàosǎn

tianma gouteng drink / 'tjænmɑ koʊtəŋ drɪŋk / 天麻钩藤饮 tiānmágōuténgyǐn

tianwang buxin mini-pills / 'tjænwæŋ buʃɪn 'mɪni pɪlz / 天王补心丹 tiānwángbǔxīndān

tongxieyao formula / 'tʊŋʃjejaʊ fɔrmjələ / 痛泻要方 tòngxièyàofāng

tounong powder / 'toʊnɒŋ 'paʊdər / 透脓散 tòunóngsǎn

wandai decoction / wæn'taɪ dɪ'kɑkʃn / 完带汤 wándàitāng

weijing decoction / weɪ'dʒɪŋ dɪ'kɑkʃn / 苇茎汤 wěijīngtāng

wendan decoction / wen'dan dɪ'kɑkʃn / 温胆汤 wēn

dǎntāng

wenjing decoction / wenˈdʒɪŋ dɪˈkɑkʃn / 温经汤 wēn jīngtāng

wenpi decoction / wenˈpi dɪˈkɑkʃn / 温脾汤 wēnpí tāng

wuji powder / wʊdʒi ˈpaʊdər / 五积散 wǔjīsǎn

wuling powder / wʊlɪŋ ˈpaʊdər / 五苓散 wǔlíngsǎn

wuling san / wʊlɪŋ san / 五苓散 wǔlíngsǎn

wumei pills / wʊmeɪ pɪlz / 乌梅丸 wūméiwán

wupi drink / wʊpi drɪŋk / 五皮饮 wǔpíyǐn

wuren pills / wʊrən pɪlz / 五仁丸 wǔrénwán

wuwei xiaodu drink / wʊweɪ ʃaʊdu drɪŋk / 五味消毒饮 wǔwèixiāodúyǐn

wuzhuyu decoction / wudʒuju dɪˈkɑkʃn / 吴茱萸汤 wúzhūyútāng

xianglian pills / ʃjɑŋljæn pɪlz / 香连丸 xiāngliánwán

xianglian wan / ʃjɑŋljæn wæn / 香连丸

xiangru powder / ʃjɑŋru ˈpaʊdər / 香薷散 xiāngrúsǎn

xiangsu powder / ʃjɑŋsu ˈpaʊdər / 香苏散 xiāngsūsǎn

xiaochaihu decoction / ʃaʊʃaɪdʒu dɪˈkɑkʃn / 小柴胡汤 xiǎocháihútāng

xiao'er huichun mini-pills / ʃaʊˈər ˈhuɪˈtʃʌn ˈmɪni pɪlz / 小儿回春丹 xiǎoˈérhuíchūndān

xiaofeng powder / ʃjaʊˈfəŋ ˈpaʊdər / 消风散 xiāofēngsǎn

xiaohuoluo mini-pills / ʃaʊhwolwo ˈmɪni pɪlz / 小活络丹 xiǎohuóluòdān

xiaoji drink / ʃaʊdʒi drɪŋk / 小蓟饮子 xiǎojìyǐnzi

xiaojianzhong decoction / ʃaʊˈdʒjænˈdʒʊŋ dɪˈkakʃn / 小建中汤 xiǎojiànzhōngtāng

xiaojin mini-pills / ʃaʊˈdʒɪn ˈmɪni pɪlz / 小金丹 xiǎo jīndān

xiaoqinglong decoction / ʃaʊˈtʃɪŋlʊŋ dɪˈkakʃn / 小青龙汤 xiǎoqīnglóngtāng

xiaoxuming decoction / ʃaʊˈsumɪŋ dɪˈkakʃn / 小续命汤 xiǎoxùmìngtāng

xiaoyao powder / ʃaʊjau ˈpaʊdər / 逍遥散 xiāoyáosǎn

xiebai powder / ʃjɛpaɪ ˈpaʊdər / 泻白散 xièbáisǎn

xijiao dihuang decoction / ʃidʒjaʊ dihwaŋ dɪˈkakʃn / 犀角地黄汤 xījiǎodìhuángtāng

xingsu powder / ˈhɪŋsu ˈpaʊdər / 杏苏散 xìngsūsǎn

xuanfu daizheshi decoction / ˈʃwanfu taɪdʒeʃɪ dɪˈkakʃn / 旋覆代赭石汤 xuánfùdàizhěshítāng

xuefu zhuyu decoction / ʃuɛfu dʒuju dɪˈkakʃn / 血府逐瘀汤 xuèfǔzhúyūtāng

yanghe decoction / jæŋhe dɪˈkakʃn / 阳和汤 yánghé tāng

yangyin qingfei decoction / jæŋjɪn ˈtʃɪŋfeɪ dɪˈkakʃn / 养阴清肺汤 yǎngyīnqīngfèitāng

yiguan decoction / jiˈkwan dɪˈkakʃn / 一贯煎 yíguàn jiān

yihuang decoction / ˈjihwaŋ dɪˈkakʃn / 易黄汤 yìhuáng tāng

yinchen wuling powder / jɪnˈtʃən wulɪŋ ˈpaʊdər / 茵陈五苓散 yīnchénwǔlíngsǎn

yinchenhao decoction / jɪnˈtʃənhaʊ dɪˈkakʃn / 茵陈蒿

汤 yīnchénhāotāng

yinqiao powder / ɪɪn'tʃjaʊ 'paʊdər / 银翘散 yínqiáo sǎn

yiwei decoction / ji'weɪ dɪ'kɑkʃn / 益胃汤 yìwèitāng

yougui drink / ju'kweɪ drɪŋk / 右归饮 yòuguīyǐn

yougui pills / ju'kweɪ pɪlz / 右归丸 yòuguīwán

yueju pills / 'juedʒu pɪlz / 越鞠丸 yuèjūwán

yunü decoction / 'juənnu dɪ'kɑkʃn / 玉女煎 yùnǚ jiān

yupingfeng powder / 'jupɪŋˌfʌŋ 'paʊdər / 玉屏风散 yùpíngfēngsǎn

yuzhen powder / 'judʒen 'paʊdər / 玉真散 yùzhēnsǎn

yuzhen san / 'judʒen san / 玉真散 yùzhēnsǎn

zaizao powder / 'tsaɪtsɑʊ 'paʊdər / 再造散 zàizàosǎn

zaizao san / 'tsaɪtsɑʊ san / 再造散 zàizàosǎn

zhengan xifeng decoction / 'dʒeŋkæn ʃi'feŋ dɪkɑkʃn / 镇肝熄风汤 zhèngānxīfēngtāng

zhenren yangzang decoction / dʒenrən jæŋ'zæŋ dɪ'kɑkʃn / 真人养脏汤 zhēnrényǎngzàngtāng

zhenwu decoction / dʒenwu dɪ'kɑkʃn / 真武汤 zhēn wǔtāng

zhibao mini-pills / 'dʒibaʊ 'mɪni pɪlz / 至宝丹 zhì bǎodān

zhigancao decoction / 'dʒikankau dɪ'kɑkʃn / 炙甘草汤 zhìgāncǎotāng

zhijing powder / dʒi'dʒɪŋ 'paʊ'dər / 止痉散 zhǐjìngsǎn

zhishi daozhi pills / dʒi'ʃɪ dɑʊ'dʒi pɪlz / 枳实导滞丸 zhǐshídǎozhìwán

zhishi daozhi wan / dʒi'ʃɪ dɑʊ'dʒi wæn / 枳实导滞丸 zhǐshídǎozhìwán

zhishi xiaopi pills / dʒi'ʃɪ ʃjɑʊpi pɪlz / 枳实消痞丸 zhǐshíxiāopǐwán

zhishi xiebai guizhi decoction / dʒi'ʃɪ 'ʃjɛbai 'kweɪdʒi dɪ'kakʃn / 枳实薤白桂枝汤 zhǐshíxièbáiguìzhī tāng

zhisou powder / dʒisoʊ 'paʊdər / 止嗽散 zhǐsòusǎn

zhizhu pills / dʒiʃu pɪlz / 枳术丸 zhǐzhúwán

zhizhu wan / dʒiʃu wæn / 枳术丸 zhǐzhúwán

zhizichi decoction / dʒitsɪ'tʃi dɪ'kakʃn / 栀子豉汤 zhīzichǐtāng

zhouche pills / tʃəʊtʃɛ pɪlz / 舟车丸 zhōuchēwán

zhuling decoction / dʒulɪŋ dɪ'kakʃn / 猪苓汤 zhūlíng tāng

zhusha an'shen pills / dʒuʃa anʃən pɪlz / 朱砂安神丸 zhūshā'ānshénwán

zhuye shigao decoction / dʒujɛ ʃɪkɑʊ dɪ'kakʃn / 竹叶石膏汤 zhúyèshígāo tāng

zixue powder / tsɪʃuə paʊdər / 紫雪 zǐxuě

zuogui drink / tswo'kweɪ drɪŋk / 左归饮 zuǒguīyǐn

zuogui pills / tswo'kweɪ pɪlz / 左归丸 zuǒguīwán

zuojin pills / tswo'dʒɪn pɪlz / 左金丸 zuǒjīnwán

zuojin wan / tswo'dʒɪn wæn / 左金丸 zuǒjīnwán

Section 5　Chinese Patent Medicine
第五节　中　成　药

aifu nuangong pills / 'aɪfu nwankʊŋ pɪlz / 艾附暖宫丸

àifùnuǎngōngwán

an'kun zanyu pills / ɑnkuən ˈtsɑnju pɪlz / 安坤赞育丸 ānkūnzànyùwán

an'shen buxin pills / ɑnʃən buʃɪn pɪlz / 安神补心丸 ānshénbǔxīnwán

awei huapi plaster / aˈweɪ ˈhuɑpi plæstər / 阿魏化痞膏 āwèihuàpǐgāo

badu shengji powder / badu ʃɛŋdʒi paʊdər / 拔毒生肌散 bádúshēngjīsǎn

baidai pills / paɪtaɪ pɪlz / 白带丸 báidàiwán

baizi yangxin pills / baɪtsɪ jæŋʃɪn pɪlz / 柏子养心丸 bǎizǐyǎngxīnwán

banlangen granules / bænlankən grænjuls / 板蓝根颗粒 bǎnlángēnkēlì

banliu pills / bænlju pɪlz / 半硫丸 bànliúwán

bazhen yimu pills / bʌdʒen jimu pɪlz / 八珍益母丸 bāzhēnyìmǔwán

bazheng mixture / bʌdʒeŋ mɪkstʃər / 八正合剂 bāzhènghéjì

bidouyan mixture / biˈdoʊjən mɪkstʃər / 鼻窦炎口服液 bídòuyánkǒufúyè

bingpeng powder / bɪŋ pəŋpaʊdər / 冰硼散 bīngpéngsǎn

biyan qingdu granules / biˈjən tʃɪŋdu grænjuls / 鼻咽清毒颗粒 bíyānqīngdúkēlì

biyan tablets / biˈjən tæblɪts / 鼻炎片 bíyánpiàn

boyun tuiyi pills / bojuən tweɪi pɪlz / 拨云退翳丸 bōyúntuìyìwán

bushen guchi pills / buˈʃən ˈkutʃi pɪlz / 补肾固齿丸 bǔshèngùchǐwán

chaihu oral liquid / ˈtʃaɪhu ɔrəl lɪkwɪd / 柴胡口服液 cháihúkǒufúyè

chuanbei pipa syrup / tʃwanˈbeɪ pipɑ sɪrəp / 川贝枇杷糖浆 chuānbèipípatángjiāng

chuanxinlian tablets / ˈtʃwanʃɪnljæn tæblɪts / 穿心莲片 chuānxīnliánpiàn

ciwujia tablets / ˈtsiwudʒia tæblɪts / 刺五加片 cìwǔjiāpiàn

compound caoshanhu tablets / kɑmpaʊnd kauʃanhu tæblɪts / 复方草珊瑚含片 fùfāngcǎoshānhú hánpiàn

compound danshen dripping pills / kɑmpaʊnd dænʃən drɪpɪŋ pɪlz / 复方丹参滴丸 fùfāngdānshēndīwán

compound danshen injections / kɑmpaʊnd dænʃən ɪnˈdʒɛkʃən / 复方丹参注射液 fùfāngdānshēnzhùshèyè

compound danshen tablets / kɑmpaʊnd dænʃən tæblɪts / 复方丹参片 fùfāngdānshēnpiàn

compound dantong tablets / kɑmpaʊnd dæntɒŋ tæblɪts / 复方胆通片 fùfāngdǎntōngpiàn

dahuang zhechong pills / ˈdahwɑŋ dʒətʃʊŋ pɪlz / 大黄蟅虫丸 dàhuángzhèchóngwán

dahuoluo pills / ˈdɑhwolwo pɪlz / 大活络丹 dàhuóluòdān

daige powder / taɪkə paʊdər / 黛蛤散 dàigésǎn

danggui extract / dɑŋkui ˈekstrækt / 当归流浸膏 dāngguīliújìngāo

danggui longhui pills / tæŋkui luŋhui pɪlz / 当归龙荟丸 dāngguīlónghuìwán

danshen injections / dænʃən ɪn'dʒɛkʃəns / 丹参注射液 dānshēnzhùshèyè

danshitong capsules / danʃɪ'tɒŋ 'kæpsəlz / 胆石通胶囊 dǎnshítōngjiāonáng

danzhi xiaoyao pills / dændʒi ʃjaʊjaʊ pɪlz / 丹栀逍遥丸 dānzhīxiāoyáowán

dashanzha bolus / daʃandʒa boʊləs / 大山楂丸 dà shānzhāwán

di'ao xinxuekang capsules / diaʊ ʃɪnʃuekaŋ 'kæpsəlz / 地奥心血康胶囊 dì'àoxīnxuèkāngjiāonáng

dieda pills / djɛda pɪlz / 跌打丸 diēdǎwán

dieda wanhua oil / djɛda wænhua ɔɪl / 跌打万花油 diēdǎwànhuāyóu

diyu huaijiao pills / diju huadʒjaʊ pɪlz / 地榆槐角丸 dìyúhuáijiǎowán

er'long zuoci pills / ər'lʊŋ tswotsi pɪlz / 耳聋左慈丸 ěr'lóngzuǒcíwán

fangfeng tongsheng pills / 'faŋfəŋ tɒŋʃɛŋ pɪlz / 防风通圣丸 fángfēngtōngshèngwán

fresh bamboo sap / freʃ bæm'bu sæp / 鲜竹沥 xiānzhúlì

fule granules / fulə 'grænjuls / 妇乐颗粒 fùlèkēlì

fuyanping capsules / fu'jənpɪŋ 'kæpsəlz / 妇炎平胶囊 fùyánpíngjiāonáng

fuzi lizhong pills / fu'tsɪ lidʒʊŋ pɪlz / 附子理中丸 fùzǐlǐzhōngwán

gejie dingchuan pills / 'kədʒjɛ 'dɪŋtʃwan pɪlz / 蛤蚧

定喘丸 géjièdìngchuǎnwán

gengnian'an pills / kəŋnjan an pɪlz / 更年安片 gēng nián'ānpiàn

goupi plaster / koʊpi plæstər / 狗皮膏 gǒupígāo

guanxin suhe pills / ˈkwanʃɪn suhɛ pɪlz / 冠心苏合丸 guānxīnsūhéwán

guci pills / kuˈtsi pɪlz / 骨刺丸 gǔcìwán

guifu lizhong pills / ˈkweɪfu liʤʊŋ pɪlz / 桂附理中丸 guìfùlǐzhōngwán

guilingji capsules / ˈkweɪlɪŋji ˈkæpsəlz / 龟龄集胶囊 guīlíngjíjiāonáng

guogong wine / kuoˈkʊŋ waɪn / 国公酒 guógōngjiǔ

heche dazao pills / hɛtʃɛ ˈdatsɑʊ pɪlz / 河车大造丸 héchēdàzàowán

huaijiao pills / hwaɪˈdʒjɑʊ pɪlz / 槐角丸 huáijiǎowán

huatuo zaizao pills / hwɑtwo ˈtsaɪtsɑʊ pɪlz / 华佗再造丸 huátuózàizàowán

huixiang juhe pills / hweɪʃjɑŋ dʒuhɛ pɪlz / 茴香橘核丸 huíxiāngjúhéwán

huodan pills / ˈhoudan pɪlz / 藿胆丸 huòdǎnwán

huoxue zhitong powder / hwoˈʃuɛ dʒiˈtʊŋ paʊdər / 活血止痛散 huóxuèzhǐtòngsǎn

jiaogulan total glucoside tablets / ˈdʒjɑʊkulan toʊtl glʊkəˌsaɪd ˈtæblɪts / 绞股兰总苷片 jiǎogǔlánzǒnggānpiàn

jidesheng sheyao tablets / dʒideʃɛŋ ʃɛjɑʊ ˈtæblɪts / 季德胜蛇药片 jìdéshèngshéyàopiàn

jingwanhong soft plaster / dʒɪŋˈwænhʊŋ sɔft plæstər /

京万红软膏 jīngwànhóngruǎngāo

jinyinhua distillate / dʒɪn'jɪnhuɑ dɪstɪleɪt / 金银花露 jīnyínhuālù

jisheng shenqi pills / dʒiʃeŋ 'ʃəntʃi pɪlz / 济生肾气丸 jìshēngshènqìwán

jiuhua plaster / dʒɪuhuɑ plæstər / 九华膏 jiǔhuágāo

jizhi syrup / 'dʒidʒi sɪrəp / 急支糖浆 jízhītángjiāng

juhong pills / 'dʒuhʊŋ pɪlz / 橘红丸 júhóngwán

kaixiong shunqi pills / kaɪʃʊŋ shun'tʃi pɪlz / 开胸顺气丸 kāixiōngshùnqìwán

kanggu zengsheng pills / 'kɑŋku 'zəŋʃəŋ pɪlz / 抗骨增生丸 kànggǔzēngshēngwán

kanlisha coarse sand granules / 'kɑnliʃɑ kɔrs sænd grænjuls / 坎离砂 kǎnlíshā

kouyanqing granules / koʊ'jəntʃɪŋ grænjuls / 口炎清颗粒 kǒuyánqīngkēlì

leigongteng tablets / 'leɪkʊŋtəŋ tæblɪts / 雷公藤片 léigōngténgpiàn

liangfu pills / ljɑŋ'fu pɪlz / 良附丸 liángfùwán

lidan paishi tablets / 'lidan paɪʃɪ tæblɪts / 利胆排石片 lìdǎnpáishípiàn

liuhe dingzhong pills / 'ljuhɛ 'dɪŋdʒʊŋ pɪlz / 六合定中丸 liùhédìngzhōngwán

liujunzi pills / 'ljudʒuntsɪ pɪlz / 六君子丸 liùjūnzǐ wán

liushen pills / 'ljuʃən pɪlz / 六神丸 liùshénwán

mayinglong shexiang zhichuang ointments / mɑ'jɪŋlʊŋ 'ʃɛʃjɑŋ dʒitʃwɑŋ ɔɪntmənts / 马应龙麝香痔疮膏 mǎyìnglóngshèxiāngzhìchuānggāo

mingmu dihuang pills / mɪŋˈmu dihwɑŋ pɪlz / 明目地黄丸 míngmùdìhuángwán

mingmu shangqing pills / mɪŋˈmu ˈʃɑŋtʃɪŋ pɪlz / 明目上清丸 míngmùshàngqīngwán

mugua pills / ˈmukuɑ pɪlz / 木瓜丸 mùguāwán

muxiang shunqi pills / ˈmuʃjɑŋ shunˈtʃi pɪlz / 木香顺气丸 mùxiāngshùnqìwán

naoliqing pills / nɑʊˈlitʃɪŋ pɪlz / 脑立清丸 nǎolìqīngwán

neixiao luoli pills / ˈneiʃjɑʊ lwoˈli pɪlz / 内消瘰疬丸 nèixiāoluǒlìwán

niaosaitong tablets / ˈnjɑʊsaɪtɒŋ tæblɪts / 尿塞通片 niàosāitōngpiàn

niuhuang baolong pills / ˈnjuhwɑŋ ˈbaʊlʊŋ pɪlz / 牛黄抱龙丸 niúhuángbàolóngwán

niuhuang jiangya capsules / ˈnjuhwɑŋ ˈʤjɑŋjɑ kæpsls / 牛黄降压胶囊 niúhuángjiàngyājiāonáng

niuhuang jiedu tablets / ˈnjuhwɑŋ ˈdʒjɛdu tæblɪts / 牛黄解毒片 niúhuángjiědúpiàn

niuhuang qingxin pills / ˈnjuhwɑŋ tʃɪŋʃɪn pɪlz / 牛黄清心丸 niúhuángqīngxīnwán

niuhuang shangqing pills / ˈnjuhwɑŋ ˈʃɑŋtʃɪŋ pɪlz / 牛黄上清丸 niúhuángshàngqīngwán

niuhuang shedan chuanbei mixture / ˈnjuhwɑŋ ʃəˈdan tʃwanˈbeɪ mɪkstʃər / 牛黄蛇胆川贝液 niúhuáng shédǎnchuānbèiyè

niuhuang zhibao pills / ˈnjuhwɑŋ ˈʤibaʊ pɪlz / 牛黄至宝丸 niúhuángzhìbǎowán

paishi granules / paɪʃɪ grænjuls / 排石颗粒 páishíkēlì

qianbai biyan tablets / tʃjɑnbaɪ bijən tæblɪts / 千柏鼻炎片 qiānbǎibíyánpiàn

qianlietong tablets / tʃʃænljetʊŋ tæblɪts / 前列通片 qiánliètōngpiàn

qiju dihuang pills / 'tʃidʒu dihwɑŋ pɪlz / 杞菊地黄丸 qǐjúdìhuángwán

qingdai powder / tʃɪŋ'taɪ paʊdər / 青黛散 qīngdàisǎn

qingkailing injections / tʃɪŋkaɪ'lɪŋ ɪn'dʒɛkʃəns / 清开灵注射液 qīngkāilíngzhùshèyè

qingkailing oral liquid / tʃɪŋkaɪ'lɪŋ ɔrəl lɪkwɪd / 清开灵口服液 qīngkāilíngkǒufúyè

qingliang oil / tʃɪŋ'ljɑŋ ɔɪl / 清凉油 qīngliángyóu

qingyan pills / tʃɪŋ'jan pɪlz / 清咽丸 qīngyānwán

qizhi weitong granules / tʃi'dʒi weɪtʊŋ grænjuls / 气滞胃痛颗粒 qìzhìwèitòngkēlì

qizhi xiangfu pills / tʃi'dʒi ʃjɑŋfu pɪlz / 七制香附丸 qīzhìxiāngfùwán

qufu shengji powder / 'tʃufu ʃəŋdʒi paʊdər / 去腐生肌散 qùfǔshēngjīsǎn

rendan mini-pills / rəndæn mɪni pɪlz / 人丹 réndān

renshen jianpi pills / rənʃən 'dʒjænpi pɪlz / 人参健脾丸 rénshēnjiànpíwán

renshen yangrong pills / rənʃən jæŋrʊŋ pɪlz / 人参养荣丸 rénshēnyǎngróngwán

renshen zaizao pills / rənʃən 'tsaɪtsɑʊ pɪlz / 人参再造丸 rénshēnzàizàowán

rupixiao tablets / ru'piʃjɑʊ tæblɪts / 乳癖消片 rǔpǐ

xiāopiàn

ruyi jinhuang powder / ru'ji dʒɪnhwɑŋ paʊdər / 如意金黄散 rúyìjīnhuángsǎn

sanhuang plaster / 'sɑnhwɑŋ plæstər / 三黄膏 sānhuánggāo

sanhuang tablets / 'sɑnhwɑŋ tæblɪts / 三黄片 sānhuángpiàn

sanjiu weitai capsules / sɑn'dʒɪu weɪtaɪ kæpsls / 三九胃泰 sānjiǔwèitài

sanqi shangyao tablets / sɑntʃi ʃɑŋjaʊ tæblɪts / 三七伤药片 sānqīshāngyàopiàn

sanqi tablets / sɑntʃi tæblɪts / 三七片 sānqīpiàn

shangqing pills / 'ʃɑŋtʃɪŋ pɪlz / 上清丸 shàngqīngwán

shangshi zhitong plaster / ʃɑnʃi dʒitʊŋ plæstər / 伤湿止痛膏 shāngshīzhǐtònggāo

shengji yuhong plaster / ʃəŋdʒi juhʊŋ plæstər / 生肌玉红膏 shēngjīyùhónggāo

shengmai injections / ʃəŋ'maɪ ɪn'dʒɛkʃənz / 生脉注射液 shēngmàizhùshèyè

shexiang baoxin pills / 'ʃɛʃjɑŋ baʊʃɪn pɪlz / 麝香保心丸 shèxiāngbǎoxīnwán

shexiang qutong aerosol / 'ʃɛʃjɑŋ tʃutʊŋ erəsal / 麝香祛痛气雾剂 shèxiāngqūtòngqìwùjì

shexiang zhuifeng plaster / ʃɛʃjɑŋ dʒweɪfəŋ plæstər / 麝香追风膏 shèxiāngzhuīfēnggāo

shidishui tincture / ʃɪdi'ʃweɪ tɪŋktʃər / 十滴水 shídīshuǐ

shiguogong wine / ʃiˈkwəʊkʊŋ waɪn / 史国公药酒 shǐguógōngyàojiǔ

shihu mingmu pills / ʃɪhu mɪŋˈmu pɪlz / 石斛明目丸 shíhúmíngmùwán

shiquan dabu pills / ʃɪtʃwæn dabu pɪlz / 十全大补丸 shíquándàbǔwán

shixiang fansheng pills / ʃɪʃjaŋ fɑnʃəŋ pɪlz / 十香返生丸 shíxiāngfǎnshēngwán

shouwu pills / ˈʃoʊwʊ pɪlz / 首乌丸 shǒuwūwán

shuanghuanglian mixture / ʃwaŋhwaŋljæn mɪkstʃər / 双黄连口服液 shuānghuángliánkǒufúyè

suoyang gujing pills / swoˈjæŋ kudʒɪŋ pɪlz / 锁阳固精丸 suǒyánggùjīngwán

suxiao jiuxin pills / ˈsuʃjɑʊ dʒɪuʃɪn pɪlz / 速效救心丸 sùxiàojiùxīnwán

tianma pills / tjænmɑ pɪlz / 天麻丸 tiānmáwán

tiedi pills / tjɛdi pɪlz / 铁笛丸 tiědíwán

tongguan powder / tɒŋkwan paʊdər / 通关散 tōngguānsǎn

tongxuan lifei pills / tɒŋʃwan liˈfeɪ pɪlz / 通宣理肺丸 tōngxuānlǐfèiwán

wangbi granules / wɑŋˈbi grænjuls / 尪痹颗粒 wāngbìkēlì

wanshi niuhuang qingxin pills / ˈwɑnʃɪ njuhwɑŋ tʃɪŋʃɪn pɪlz / 万氏牛黄清心丸 wànshìniúhuángqīngxīnwán

wanying troches / ˈwɑnjɪŋ troks / 万应锭 wànyìngdìng

weisu granules / ˈweɪsu grænjuls / 胃苏颗粒 wèisūkēlì

wind medicated oil / wɪnd medɪkeɪtɪd ɔɪl / 风油精 fēngyóujīng

wufu huadu pills / wufu ˈhuɑdu pɪlz / 五福化毒丸 wǔfúhuàdúwán

wuji baifeng pills / wʊdʒi paɪˈfəŋ pɪlz / 乌鸡白凤丸 wūjībáifèngwán

wuren runchang pills / wurən ˈruntʃɑŋ pɪlz / 五仁润肠丸 wǔrénrùnchángwán

wushicha granules / wuʃɪtʃɑ grænjuls / 午时茶颗粒 wǔshíchákēlì

wuzi yanzong pills / wutsɪ ˈjənzʊŋ pɪlz / 五子衍宗丸 wǔzǐyǎnzōngwán

xianglian tablets / ʃjɑŋljæn tæblɪts / 香连片 xiāngliánpiàn

xiangsha liujun pills / ʃjɑŋʃɑ ljudʒuən pɪlz / 香砂六君丸 xiāngshāliùjūnwán

xiangsha yangwei pills / ʃjɑŋʃɑ jæŋˈweɪ pɪlz / 香砂养胃丸 xiāngshāyǎngwèiwán

xiangsha zhizhu pills / ʃjɑŋʃɑ dʒiʃu pɪlz / 香砂枳术丸 xiāngshāzhǐzhúwán

xiao'er ganmao granules / ʃjaʊər kanmɑʊ grænjuls / 小儿感冒颗粒 xiǎo'érgǎnmàokēlì

xiao'er ganyan granules / ˈʃjaʊər kanjən grænjuls / 小儿肝炎颗粒 xiǎo'érgānyánkēlì

xiao'er zhibao pills / ˈʃjaʊər dʒibaʊ pɪlz / 小儿至宝丸 xiǎo'érzhìbǎowán

xiaojin pills / ˈʃjaʊdʒɪn pɪlz / 小金丸 xiǎojīnwán

xiaokechuan syrup / ʃjaʊkɛtʃwɑn sɪrəp / 消咳喘糖浆 xiāokéchuǎntángjiāng

xiaoshuan tongluo tablets / ʃjaʊʃwan tɒŋˈlwo tæblɪts / 消栓通络片 xiāoshuāntōngluòpiàn

xiaoshuan zaizao pills / ʃjaʊʃwan tsaɪˈtsɑʊ pɪlz / 消栓再造丸 xiāoshuānzàizàowán

xiaozhiling injections / ʃjaʊʤilɪŋ ɪnˈdʒɛkʃəns / 消痔灵 xiāozhìlíng

xiguashuang runhou tablets / ʃikuɑʃwɑŋ ˈruənhəʊ tæblɪts / 西瓜霜润喉片 xīguāshuāngrùnhóupiàn

xingren zhike syrup / ʃɪŋrən dʒikə sɪrəp / 杏仁止咳糖浆 xìngrénzhǐkétángjiāng

xinmaitong tablets / ʃɪnmaɪtɒŋ tæblɪts / 心脉通片 xīnmàitōngpiàn

xinqingning tablets / ʃɪntʃɪŋnɪŋ tæblɪts / 新清宁片 xīnqīngníngpiàn

xiongju shangqing pills / ʃɒŋdʒu ʃɑŋtʃɪŋ pɪlz / 芎菊上清丸 xiōngjúshàngqīngwán

xuanshi solution / ʃwanʃi səˈluʃn / 癣湿药水 xuǎnshīyàoshuǐ

yangweishu capsules / jæŋˈweɪʃu kæpsls / 养胃舒胶囊 yǎngwèishūjiāonáng

yangxue an'shen pills / jæŋˈʃuɛ anʃən pɪlz / 养血安神丸 yǎngxuè'ānshénwán

yiganning granules / jikannɪŋ grænjuls / 乙肝宁颗粒 yǐgānníngkēlì

yimucao paste / jimukau peɪst / 益母草膏 yìmǔcǎogāo

yiyuan powder / jijuɑn paʊdər / 益元散 yìyuánsǎn

yuanhu zhitong tablets / jwɑnhu dʒitʊŋ tæblɪts / 元胡止痛片 yuánhúzhǐtòngpiàn

yueju baohe pills / juedʒu baʊhɛ pɪlz / 越鞠保和丸 yuèjūbǎohéwán

yufeng ningxin tablets / jufɛŋ nɪŋʃɪn tæblɪts / 愈风宁心片 yùfēngníngxīnpiàn

yunnan baiyao powder / juənnɑn paɪjaʊ paʊdər / 云南白药 yúnnánbáiyào

zanglian pills / tsæŋljæn pɪlz / 脏连丸 zàngliánwán

zangqingguo tablets / ˈzæŋtʃɪŋkou tæblɪts / 藏青果喉片 zàngqīngguǒhóupiàn

zhenggu mixture / ˈʤeŋku mɪkstʃər / 正骨水 zhènggǔshuǐ

zhenqi fuzheng granules / ʤentʃi fuˈʤeŋ grænjuls / 贞芪扶正颗粒 zhēnqífúzhèngkēlì

zhenzhuming eye drops / ʤendʒumɪŋ aɪ drɑps / 珍珠明滴眼液 zhēnzhūmíngdīyǎnyè

zhibai dihuang pills / ʤibaɪ dihwɑŋ pɪlz / 知柏地黄丸 zhībǎidìhuángwán

zhongganling tablets / ˈʤʊŋkanlɪŋ tæblɪts / 重感灵片 zhònggǎnlíngpiàn

zhuanggu guanjie pills / ˈʤwɑŋku kwandʒj pɪlz / 壮骨关节丸 zhuànggǔguānjiéwán

zhuche pills / ˈdʒutʃɛ pɪlz / 驻车丸 zhùchēwán

zicao soft plaster / ˈtsɪkau sɔft plæstər / 紫草膏 zǐcǎogāo

zijin troches / ˈtsɪdʒɪn troks / 紫金锭 zǐjīndìng

Chapter 6 Health Preservation and Rehabilitation

第六章 养生康复学

adjusting ways to cultivating health / əˈdʒʌstɪŋ wez tə kʌltɪveɪtɪŋ helθ / 和于术数 héyúshùshù

antenatal training / ˌænti'neɪtl 'treɪnɪŋ / 胎教 tāijiào

baduanjin / badwandʒɪn / 八段锦 bāduànjǐn

changing tendon exercise / tʃendʒɪŋ 'tendən 'eksərsaɪz / 易筋经 yìjīnjīng

choice and creation of healthy environment / tʃɔɪs ənd kriˈeɪʃn əv helθi ɪnˈvaɪrənmənt / 环境养生 huánjìngyǎngshēng

dietetic contraindication / daɪə'tɛtɪk ˌkɑntrəɪndɪ'keɪʃn / 饮食禁忌 yǐnshíjìnjì

dietetic regulation / daɪə'tɛtɪk ˌrɛgjə'leʃən / 饮食调理 yǐnshítiáolǐ

eight-sectioned exercise / eɪt 'sekʃnd 'eksərsaɪz / 八段锦 bāduànjǐn

exhalation and inhalation / ˌekshə'leɪʃn ənd ˌɪnhə'leɪʃn / 吐纳 tǔnà

five mimic-animal exercise / faɪv mɪmɪk 'ænɪml 'eksərsaɪz / 五禽戏 wǔqínxì

following rule of yin and yang / 'fɑloʊɪŋ rul əv jɪn ənd jæŋ / 法于阴阳 fǎyúyīnyáng

harmony of body and spirit / 'hɑrməni əv 'bɑdi ənd 'spɪrɪt / 形与神俱 xíngyǔshénjù

health maintenance / helθ 'meɪntənəns / 养生 yǎng

shēng

health maintenance in four seasons / helθ ˈmeɪntənəns ɪn fɔr siznz / 四时调摄 sìshítiáoshè

health preserving with drugs / helθ prɪˈzɝvɪŋ wɪð drʌgz / 药养 yàoyǎng

health preserving with food / helθ prɪˈzɝvɪŋ wɪð fud / 食养 shíyǎng

hiding and storing / ˈhaɪdɪŋ ənd storŋ / 闭藏 bìcáng

inhaling pure air / ɪnˈheɪlɪŋ pjʊr ɛr / 呼吸精气 hū xījīngqì

keeping essence and spirit in interior / ˈkipɪŋ ˈesns ənd ˈspɪrɪt ɪn ɪnˈtɪriər / 精神内守 jīngshénnèishǒu

mouth cleaning for newborn / maʊθ ˈklinɪŋ fə(r) ˈnubɔrn / 拭口 shìkǒu

natural life span / ˈnætʃrəl laɪf spæn / 天年 tiānnián

nourishing fetus / ˈnɜrɪʃɪŋ ˈfitəs / 胎养 tāiyǎng

nourishing yang in spring and summer while nourishing yin in autumn and winter / ˈnɜrɪʃɪŋ jæŋ ɪn sprɪŋ ənd ˈsʌmər hwaɪl ˈnɜrɪʃɪŋ jɪn ɪn ˈatəm ənd ˈwɪntər / 春夏养阳，秋冬养阴 chūnxiàyǎngyáng qiūdōngyǎngyīn

physical and breathing exercise / ˈfɪzɪkl ənd ˈbriðɪŋ ˈeksərsaɪz / 导引 dǎoyǐn

prosperity and blossom / prɑˈspɛrətɪ ənd ˈblɑsəm / 蕃秀 fānxiù

puerperium / pjuəˈperɪəm / 产褥 chǎnrù

quality of food / ˈkwɑləti əv fud / 食性 shíxìng

rehabilitation / ˌriəbɪlɪˈteʃn / 康复 kāngfù

ripening and moderating / ˈraɪpənɪŋ ənd ˈmɔdəreitɪŋ / 容平 róngpíng

self controlling mentality / self kənˈtrolŋ menˈtæləti / 独立守神 dúlìshǒushén

seven impairments and eight benefits / ˈsevn ɪmˈpeɪrmənts ənd eɪt ˈbɛnəfɪts / 七损八益 qīsǔnbāyì

shi'er'duanjin / ʃɪɚˈdwandʒɪn / 十二段锦 shí'èrduànjǐn

special monthly care during pregnancy / ˈspɛʃəl ˈmʌnθli ker ˈdʊrɪŋ ˈpregnənsi / 逐月养胎法 zhúyuèyǎngtāifǎ

spiritual health care / ˈspɪrɪtʃuəl helθ ker / 精神修养 jīngshénxiūyǎng

sprouting and growing / sprɑʊtɪŋ ənd ˈgrouɪŋ / 发陈 fāchén

taijiquan / taɪdʒɪtʃwan / 太极拳 tàijíquán

taking medicine / ˈtekɪŋ ˈmedɪsn / 服食 fúshí

tranquilized mind and empty thinking / ˈtræŋkwɪˌlaɪzd maɪnd ənd ˈɛmptɪ ˈθɪŋkɪŋ / 恬淡虚无 tiándànxūwú

twelve-sectioned exercise / twelv ˈsekʃnd ˈeksərsaɪz / 十二段锦 shí'èrduànjǐn

wuqinxi / wutʃɪŋʃi / 五禽戏 wǔqínxì

yijinjing / jidʒɪndʒɪŋ / 易筋经 yìjīnjīng

Chapter 7　Internal Medicine of Traditional Chinese Medicine

第七章　中医内科学

Section 1　Febrile Diseases

第一节　热　病

autumn-dryness disease / ˈɔtəm ˈdraɪnəs dɪˈziz / 秋燥 qiūzào

cold pathogenic disease / koʊld pæθəˈdʒenɪk dɪˈziz / 伤寒 shānghán

common cold / ˈkɑmən koʊld / 感冒 gǎnmào

damp warm / dæmp wɔrm / 湿温 shīwēn

dysentery / ˈdɪsənteri / 痢疾 lìjí

epidemic infectious disease / ˌepɪˈdemɪk ɪnˈfekʃəs dɪˈziz / 瘟疫 wēnyì

fever with swollen head / ˈfivər wɪð ˈswoʊlən hed / 大头瘟 dàtóuwēn

fulminant dysentery / ˈfʊlmɪnənt ˈdɪsənteri / 疫毒痢 yìdúlì

heat stroke and sunstroke / hit stroʊk ənd ˈsʌnstroʊk / 中暑 zhòngshǔ

influenza / ˌɪnfluˈenzə / 时行感冒 shíxínggǎnmào

malaria / məˈleriə / 疟疾 nüèjí

malignant malaria / məˈlɪgnənt məˈleriə / 瘴疟 zhàngnuè

recurrent dysentery / rɪˈkɜrənt ˈdɪsənteri / 休息痢 xiū

xīlì

scarlet fever / ˈskɑrlɪt ˈfivər / 烂喉丹痧 lànhóudānshā

spring warm disorder / sprɪŋ wɔrm dɪsˈɔrdər / 春温 chūnwēn

syncope due to summer-heat / ˈsɪŋkəpi du tə ˈsʌmər hit / 暑厥 shǔjué

＊ **warm disease** / wɔrm dɪˈziz / 温病 wēnbìng

＊ **warm disease caused by incubating pathogens** / wɔrm dɪˈziz kɔzd baɪ ɪŋkjubeɪtɪŋ ˈpæθədʒəns / 伏邪温病 fúxiéwēnbìng

warm disease in summer / wɔrm dɪˈziz ɪn ˈsʌmər / 暑温 shǔwēn

warm disease in winter / wɔrm dɪˈziz ɪn ˈwɪntər / 冬温 dōngwēn

wind warm disorder / wɪnd wɔrm dɪsˈɔrdər / 风温 fēngwēn

Section 2　Lung System Diseases
第二节　肺系疾病

abscess of lung / ˈæbses əv lʌŋ / 肺痈 fèiyōng

asthma / ˈæzmə / 哮病 xiàobìng

atrophic lung disease / əˈtrɑfɪk lʌŋ dɪˈziz / 肺痿 fèiwěi

＊ **cough** / kɔf / 咳嗽 késou

dyspnea / dɪspˈniə / 喘病 chuǎnbìng

dyspnea of deficiency type / dɪspˈniə əv dɪˈfɪʃnsi taɪp / 虚喘 xūchuǎn

dyspnea of excess type / dɪspˈniə əv ɪkˈses taɪp / 实喘

shíchuǎn

endogenous cough / enˈdɑdʒənəs kɔf / 内伤咳嗽 nèi shāngkésou

exogenous cough / ekˈsɑdʒənəs kɔf / 外感咳嗽 wài gǎnkésou

lung cancer / lʌŋ kænsə / 肺癌 fèiˈái

lung-distention / lʌŋ dɪsˈtenʃən / 肺胀 fèizhàng

pulmonary tuberculosis / ˈpʌlməneri tubɜrkjəˈloʊsɪs / 肺痨 fèiláo

suspending fluid / səˈspɛndɪŋ ˈfluɪd / 悬饮 xuányǐn

Section 3   Heart System Diseases

第三节　心系疾病

angina pectoris / ænˈdʒaɪnə ˈpektərɪs / 真心痛 zhēn xīntòng

chest discomfort / tʃest dɪsˈkʌmfərt / 胸痹 xiōngbì

＊ **palpitation** / ˌpælpəˈteʃən / 心悸 xīnjì

palpitation due to alarm / ˌpælpəˈteʃən du tə əˈlɑrm / 惊悸 jīngjì

precordial pain with cold limbs / priˈkɔdjəl peɪn wɪð koʊld lɪmz / 厥心痛 juéxīntòng

real heart pain / riəl hɑrt peɪn / 真心痛 zhēnxīntòng

severe palpitation / səˈvɪr ˌpælpəˈteʃən / 怔忡 zhēng chōng

sudden precordial pain / sʌdn priˈkɔdjəl peɪn / 卒心痛 cùxīntòng

Section 4 Brain System Diseases

第四节　脑系疾病

amnesia / æmˈniʒə / 健忘 jiànwàng

apoplexy / ˈæpəpleksi / 中风 zhòngfēng

cerebroma / sɪrbromə / 脑瘤 nǎoliú

＊**dementia** / dɪˈmenʃə / 痴呆 chīdāi

depressive psychosis / dɪˈpresɪv saɪˈkoʊsɪs / 癫病 diān bìng

dwarfism / ˈdwɔrfɪzəm / 侏儒 zhūrú

insomnia / ɪnˈsɑmniə / 不寐 bùmèi

lily disease / ˈlɪli dɪˈziz / 百合病 bǎihébìng

manic psychosis / ˈmænɪk saɪˈkoʊsɪs / 狂病 kuáng bìng

somnolence / ˈsɑmnələns / 多寐 duōmèi

vertigo / vɜrtɪɡoʊ / 眩晕 xuànyūn

wry mouth / raɪ maʊθ / 口僻 kǒupì

Section 5 Spleen and Stomach System Diseases

第五节　脾胃疾病

abdominal pain / æbˈdɑmɪnl peɪn / 腹痛 fùtòng

acid regurgitation / ˈæsɪd rɪɡɜrdʒɪˈteɪʃn / 吐酸 tǔsuān

chronic diarrhea / ˈkrɑnɪk ˌdaɪəˈriə / 久泻 jiǔxiè

constipation / ˌkɑnstɪˈpeɪʃn / 便秘 biànmì

diarrhea / ˌdaɪəˈriə / 泄泻 xièxiè

distention and fullness / dɪsˈtenʃən ənd ˈfʊlnəs / 痞满 pǐmǎn

dysphagia / dɪsˈfedʒɪə / 噎膈 yēgé

fulminant diarrhea / ˈfʊlmɪnənt daɪəˈriə / 暴泻 bàoxiè

fulminant vomiting / ˈfʊlmɪnənt ˈvɑmɪtɪŋ / 暴吐 bàotǔ

hiccough / ˈhɪkəp / 呃逆 ènì

intestinal cancer / ɪnˈtestɪnl ˈkænsər / 肠癌 cháng'ái

pancreas cancer / ˈpæŋkriəs ˈkænsər / 胰癌 yí'ái

regurgitation / rɪgɜrdʒɪˈteɪʃn / 反胃 fǎnwèi

stomach cancer / ˈstʌmək ˈkænsər / 胃癌 wèi'ái

Section 6　Hepatobiliary System Diseases

第六节　肝胆疾病

fulminant jaundice / ˈfʊlmɪnənt ˈdʒɔndɪs / 急黄 jíhuáng

gallstones / ˈgɔlstoʊns / 胆石 dǎnshí

hypochondriac pain / ˌhaɪpəˈkɑndriæk peɪn / 胁痛 xiétòng

jaundice / ˈdʒɔndɪs / 黄疸 huángdǎn

liver abscess / ˈlɪvər ˈæbses / 肝痈 gānyōng

liver cancer / ˈlɪvər ˈkænsər / 肝癌 gān'ái

liver syncope / ˈlɪvər ˈsɪŋkəpi / 肝厥 gānjué

stagnancy of liver-Qi and blood / ˈstægnənsi əv ˈlɪvər tʃi ənd blʌd / 肝著 gānzhuó

syncope due to ascariasis / ˈsɪŋkəpi du tə æskəˈraɪəsɪs / 蛔厥 huíjué

tympanites / ˌtɪmpəˈnaɪtiz / 臌胀 gǔzhàng

yang jaundice / jæŋ ˈdʒɔndɪs / 阳黄 yánghuáng

yin jaundice / jɪn ˈdʒɔndɪs / 阴黄 yīnhuáng

Section 7　Kidney and Bladder System Diseases

第七节　肾膀胱疾病

affection of kidney by cold-dampness / əˈfɛkʃən əv ˈkɪdni baɪ koʊld ˈdæmpnɪs / 肾著 shènzhuó

anuria and vomiting / ənˈjʊərɪr ənd ˈvɑmɪtɪŋ / 关格 guāngé

carcinoma of bladder / ˌkɑrsɪˈnoʊmə əv ˈblædə / 膀胱癌 pángguāng'ái

carcinoma of kidney / ˌkɑrsɪˈnoʊmə əv ˈkɪdni / 肾癌 shèn'ái

edema / iˈdimə / 水肿 shuǐzhǒng

heat stranguria / hit stˈræŋgjʊrɪr / 热淋 rèlín

impotence / ˈɪmpətəns / 阳痿 yángwěi

nocturnal emission / nɑkˈtɜrnl ɪˈmɪʃn / 梦遗 mèngyí

persistent erection of penis / pərˈsɪstənt ɪˈrekʃn əv ˈpinɪs / 阳强 yángqiáng

prospermia / prəˈspəmiə / 早泄 zǎoxiè

retention of urine / rɪˈtɛnʃən əv ˈjʊrən / 癃闭 lóngbì

skin edema / skɪn iˈdimə / 皮水 píshuǐ

spermatorrhea / spɝˌmætoˈrɪr / 遗精 yíjīng

spermatorrhea / spɝˌmætoˈrɪr / 滑精 huájīng

sterility / stəˈrɪləti / 不育 bùyù

stony edema / ˈstoʊni iˈdimə / 石水 shíshuǐ

stranguria due to chyluria / stˈræŋgjʊrɪr du tə kaɪljʊərɪr / 膏淋 gāolín

stranguria due to disturbance of qi / stˈræŋgjʊrɪr du tə dɪˈstɜrbəns əv tʃi / 气淋 qìlín

stranguria due to hematuria / stˈræŋɡjʊrɪr du tə ˌhiməˈtjurɪr / 血淋 xuèlín

stranguria due to overstrain / stˈræŋɡjʊrɪr du tə ˈovəstren / 劳淋 láolín

stranguria / stˈræŋɡjʊrɪr / 淋证 línzhèng

urolithic stranguria / ˈʊərəlɪθɪk stˈræŋɡjʊrɪr / 石淋 shílín

wind edema / wɪnd iˈdimə / 风水 fēngshuǐ

yang edema / jæŋ iˈdimə / 阳水 yángshuǐ

yin edema / jɪn iˈdimə / 阴水 yīnshuǐ

Section 8   The Diseases of Qi Blood and Boby Fluid

第八节　气血津液疾病

blood disease / blʌd dɪˈziz / 血证 xuèzhèng

cold syncope / koʊld ˈsɪŋkəpi / 寒厥 hánjué

consumptive disease / kənˈsʌmptɪv dɪˈziz / 虚劳 xūláo

consumptive thirst / kənˈsʌmptɪv θɜrst / 消渴 xiāokě

crapulent syncope / ˈkræpjulənt ˈsɪŋkəpi / 食厥 shíjué

depression disease / dɪˈpreʃn dɪˈziz / 郁病 yùbìng

desertion disease / dɪˈzɜrʃn dɪˈziz / 脱证 tuōzhèng

fever due to internal injury / ˈfivər du tə ɪnˈtɜrnl ˈɪndʒəri / 内伤发热 nèishāngfārè

heat syncope / hit ˈsɪŋkəpi / 热厥 rèjué

hematemesis / ˌhɛməˈtɛmɪsɪs / 吐血 tùxiě

hematochezia / ˈhimətokɪzɪr / 便血 biànxiě

hematuria / himəˈtjurɪə / 尿血 niàoxiě

night sweating / naɪt ˈswetɪŋ / 盗汗 dàohàn

phlegm syncope / flem ˈsɪŋkəpi / 痰厥 tánjué

purpura / ˈpɜˑpjʊrə / 紫癜 zǐdiàn

spontaneous sweating / spanˈteɪniəs ˈswetɪŋ / 自汗 zìhàn

sweating disease / ˈswetɪŋ dɪˈziz / 汗证 hànzhèng

syncope due to disorder of qi / ˈsɪŋkəpi du tə dɪsˈɔrdər əv tʃi / 气厥 qìjué

syncope due to disorder of bleeding / ˈsɪŋkəpi du tə dɪsˈɔrdər əv ˈblidɪŋ / 血厥 xuèjué

syncope / ˈsɪŋkəpi / 厥证 juézhèng

weak foot / wik fʊt / 脚气病 jiǎoqìbìng

yellowish sweating / ˈjelouɪʃ ˈswetɪŋ / 黄汗 huánghàn

Section 9   Meridian and Limb Diseases
第九节　经络肢体疾病

arthralgia / ɑrˈθræld3ə / 痹病 bìbìng

arthralgia aggravated by cold / ɑrˈθræld3ə ˈægrəveɪtɪd baɪ koʊld / 痛痹 tòngbì

arthralgia due to dampness / ɑrˈθræld3ə du tə ˈdæmpnəs / 著痹 zhuóbì

arthralgia due to heat-toxicity / ɑrˈθræld3ə du tə ˌhit tɑkˈsɪsəti / 热痹 rèbì

bi disease / pɪ dɪˈziz / 痹病 bìbìng

convulsive disease / kənˈvʌlsɪv dɪˈziz / 痉病 jìngbìng

fixed arthralgia / fɪkst ɑrˈθræld3ə / 著痹 zhuóbì

flaccidity disease / flækˈsɪdɪti dɪˈziz / 痿病 wěibìng

gout / gaʊt / 痛风 tòngfēng

lumbago / lʌmˈbeɪgou / 腰痛 yāotòng

migratory arthralgia / maɪɡrətɔri ɑrˈθrældʒə / 行痹 xíngbì

tremor / ˈtremər / 颤振 chànzhèn

wind-cold-dampness arthralgia / wɪnd koʊld ˈdæmpnəs ɑrˈθrældʒə / 风寒湿痹 fēnghánshībì

Section 10　Other Internal Medical Diseases

第十节　内科其他疾病

ancylostomiasis / ˌænsɪˌlɑstəˈmaɪəsɪs / 钩虫病 gōuchóngbìng

ascariasis / æskəˈraɪəsɪs / 蛔虫病 huíchóngbìng

enterobiasis / ˌentərəʊˈbaɪəsɪs / 蛲虫病 náochóngbìng

oxyuriasis / ɒksɪjʊəˈraɪəsɪs / 蛲虫病 náochóngbìng

Chapter 8　Surgery of Traditional Chinese Medicine

第八章　中医外科学

Section 1　Sores and Ulcers

第一节　疮疡疾病

abscess / ˈæbses / 脓肿 nóngzhǒng

acute suppurative parotitis / əˈkjut ˈsʌpjʊəretɪv ˌpærəˈtaɪtɪs / 发颐 fāyí

amassment and accumulation / əˈmæsmənt ənd əkjumjəˈleɪʃn / 积聚 jījù

bump / bʌmp / 瘤 liú

carbuncle / ˈkɑrbʌŋkl / 有头疽 yǒutóujū

carbuncle / ˈkɑrbʌŋkl / 痈 yōng

carbuncle complicated by septicemia / ˈkɑrbʌŋkl ˈkɑmplɪkeɪtɪd baɪ ˌsɛptəˈsimɪə / 走黄 zǒuhuáng

carbuncle of Huantiao point / ˈkɑrbʌŋkl əv hwantjɑʊ pɔɪnt / 环跳疽 huántiàojū

cat's eye sore / kæts aɪ sor / 猫眼疮 māoyǎnchuāng

chilblain / ˈtʃɪlbleɪn / 冻疮 dòngchuāng

chronic suppurative abscess of bones and joints / ˈkrɑnɪk ˈsʌpjʊəretɪv ˈæbses əv bonz ənd dʒɔɪnts / 流痰 liútán

comedo / kəˈmidəʊ / 粉刺 fěncì

condyloma acuminatum / kɑndəˈlomə əˈkjumənɪtəm / 尖锐湿疣 jiānruìshīyóu

congestion / kənˈdʒestʃən / 淤血 yūxuè

contact dermatitis / ˈkɑntækt ˌdɜrməˈtaɪtɪs / 接触性皮炎 jiēchùxìngpíyán

deep carbuncle / dip ˈkɑrbʌŋkl / 无头疽 wútóujū

deep-rooted carbuncle / dip ˈrutɪd ˈkɑrbʌŋkl / 疽 jū

ecthyma / ˈɛkθɪmə / 臁疮 liánchuāng

eczema / ɪgˈzimə / 湿疮 shīchuāng

erysipelas / ˌerɪˈsɪpələs / 丹毒 dāndú

external treatment / ɪkˈstɜrnl ˈtritmənt / 外治法 wàizhìfǎ

facial wandering wind / ˈfeɪʃl ˈwɑndərɪŋ wɪnd / 面游风 miànyóufēng

furuncle / ˈfjʊərʌŋk(ə)l / 疖 jiē

gangrene of digit / ˈgæŋgrin əv ˈdɪdʒɪt / 脱疽 tuōjū

gonorrhea / ɡɑnəˈriə / 花柳毒淋 huāliǔdúlín

gravitational abscess / ˌgrævɪˈteɪʃənl ˈæbses / 流注 liúzhù

hard furuncle / hɑrd ˈfjʊərʌŋk(ə)l / 疔疮 dīngchuāng

herpes simplex / ˈhɜrpiz ˈsɪmpleks / 热疮 rèchuāng

herpes / ˈhɜrpiz / 疱疹 pàozhěn

herpes zoster / ˈhɜrpiz ˈzɑstə / 蛇串疮 shéchuànchuāng

huanglian jiedu decoction / hwɑŋljæn dʒjɛdu dɪˈkɑkʃn / 黄连解毒汤 huángliánjiědútāng

incentive ogenesis / ɪnˈsentɪv ʊəˈdʒɛnɪsɪs / 诱因 yòuyīn

invagination / ɪnvædʒəˈneʃən / 内陷 nèixiàn

longdan xiegan decoction / lʊŋdan ʃjɛkan dɪˈkɑkʃn /

龙胆泻肝汤 lóngdǎnxiègāntāng

medicinal poison rash / məˈdɪsɪnl ˈpɔɪzn ræʃ / 药毒疹 yàodúzhěn

miliaria / ˌmɪlɪˈɛrɪə / 痱子 fèizi

pathogenesis / ˌpæθəˈdʒenɪsɪs / 病机 bìngjī

pemphigus / ˈpɛmfɪgəs / 天疱疮 tiānpàochuāng

pruritus due to wind pathogen / prʊˈraɪtəs du tə wɪnd ˈpæθədʒən / 风瘙痒 fēngsàoyǎng

red butterfly sore / red ˈbʌtərflaɪ sor / 红蝴蝶疮 hóng húdiéchuāng

rheumatic arthritis / ruˈmætɪk ɑrˈθraɪtɪs / 风湿性关节炎 fēngshīxìngguānjiéyán

rosacea / rəʊˈzeɪʃɪə / 酒渣鼻 jiǔzhābí

scabies / ˈskeɪbiz / 疥疮 jièchuāng

scrofula / ˈskrɔfjʊlə / 瘰疬 luǒlì

seborrheic alopecia / sɪˈbɒrhaɪk ˌæləˈpiʃə / 油风脱发 yóufēng tuōfà

six climatic exopathogens / sɪks klaɪˈmætɪk eksəˈpæθ əʊdʒəns / 六淫 liùyín

snake-like sores / sneɪk laɪk sɔrz / 蛇串疮 shéchuànchuāng

sore and ulcer / sɔr ənd ˈʌlsər / 疮疡 chuāngyáng

ulcer / ˈʌlsər / 溃疡 kuìyáng

verqruca / vəˈrukə / 疣 yóu

vine tangling / vaɪn ˈtæŋglɪn / 瓜藤缠 guāténgchán

wind-heat sores / wɪnd hit sorz / 风热疮 fēngrèchuāng

wuwei xiaodu drink / wuweɪ ʃaʊdu drɪŋk / 五味消毒

饮 wǔwèixiāodúyǐn

xianfang huoming drink / ʃjænfɑŋ hwomɪŋ drɪŋk / 仙方活命饮 xiānfānghuómìngyǐn

yanghe decoction / jæŋhɛ dɪˈkɑkʃn / 阳和汤 yánghé tāng

yellow fluid ulcers / ˈjeloʊ ˈfluɪd ˈʌlsərz / 黄水疮 huáng shuǐchuāng

Section 2　Breast Diseases
第二节　乳房疾病

acute mastitis / əˈkjut mæˈstaɪtɪs / 乳痈 rǔyōng

adenoma of thyroid / ˌædəˈnomə əv ˈθaɪrɔɪd / 肉瘿 ròuyǐng

angioma / ændʒɪˈomə / 血瘤 xuèliú

lump in breast / lʌmp ɪn brest / 乳癖 rǔpǐ

mammary fistula / ˈmæməri ˈfɪstʃələ / 乳漏 rǔlòu

nodular varicosity / ˈnɑdʒələ ˌværɪˈkɑsəti / 筋瘤 jīnliú

nodule in breast / ˈnɑdʒul ɪn brest / 乳核 rǔhé

qi goiter / tʃi ˈgɔɪtə / 气瘿 qìyǐng

qufu shengji powder / tʃufu ʃeŋqdʒi ˈpaʊdər / 去腐生肌散 qùfǔshēngjīsǎn

sarcoma / sɑrˈkoʊmə / 肉瘤 ròuliú

sebaceous cyst / sɪˈbeɪʃəs sɪst / 脂瘤 zhīliú

stony goiter / ˈstoʊni ˈgɔɪtə / 石瘿 shíyǐng

suppurative mastitis / ˈsʌpjʊəretɪv mæˈstaɪtɪs / 乳发 rǔfā

tuberculosis of breast / tubɜrkjəˈloʊsɪs əv brest / 乳痨 rǔláo

tumor due to disorder of qi / ˈtjʊmə du tə dɪsˈɔrdər əv tʃi / 气瘤 qìliú

Section 3　Anorectal Diseases
第三节　肛肠科疾病

anal fissure / ˈeɪnl ˈfɪʃər / 肛裂 gāngliè

anal fistula / ˈeɪnl ˈfɪstʃələ / 肛漏 gānglòu

anal prolapse / ˈeɪnl ˈproʊlæps / 脱肛 tuōgāng

epididymitis and orchitis / ˈepiˌdidiˈmaitis ənd ɔrˈkaɪtɪs / 子痈 zǐyōng

hemorrhoid / hɛməˈrɔɪd / 痔 zhì

hypertrophy of prostate / haɪˈpɜrtrəfi əv ˈprɑsteɪt / 精癃 jīnglóng

locked anus pile / lɔkt ˈeɪnəs paɪl / 锁肛痔 suǒgāng zhì

perianal or perirectal abscess / periˈeinəl ɔr peraɪˈrektl ˈæbses / 肛痈 gāngyōng

rectal polyp / ˈrektəl ˈpɑlɪp / 息肉痔 xīròuzhì

scrotal abscess / ˈskrəutəl ˈæbses / 囊痈 nángyōng

turbid semen / ˈtɜrbɪd ˈsimən / 精浊 jīngzhuó

Section 4　Dermatological Diseases
第四节　皮肤科疾病

drug eruption / drʌg ɪˈrʌpʃn / 药物性皮炎 yàowù xìngpíyán

ecchymosis / ɛkəˈmosɪs / 瘀斑 yūbān

hidden rashes / ˈhɪdn ræʃɪz / 瘾疹 yǐnzhěn

leprosy / ˈleprəsi / 麻风 máfēng

pruritus / prʊˈraɪtəs / 瘙痒症 sàoyǎngzhèng

urticaria / ˌɜrtɪˈkeriə / 瘾疹 yǐnzhěn

venomous snake bite / ˈvenəməs sneɪk baɪt / 毒蛇咬伤 dúshéyǎoshāng

vitiligo / ˌvɪtəˈlaɪgo / 白癜风 báidiànfēng

Chapter 9　Orthopedics and Traumatology of Traditional Chinese Medicine

第九章　中医骨伤科学

achilles tendinitis / ə'kiliz ˌtendi'naitis / 跟腱炎 gēn jiànyán

acromioclavicular dislocation / əˌkrəumiəuklə'vikjulə ˌdislou'keiʃn / 肩锁关节脱位 jiānsuǒguānjié tuōwèi

acute lumbar muscle sprain / ə'kjut 'lʌmbər 'mʌsl sprein / 急性腰扭伤 jíxìngyāoniǔshāng

ankylosing spondylitis / 'æŋkiˌləusiŋ spɑndi'laitis / 强直性脊柱炎 qiángzhíxìngjǐzhùyán

atlantoaxial dislocation / ætlæn'təuksiəl ˌdislou'keiʃn / 寰枢关节脱位 huánshūguānjiétuōwèi

bifid sacrum / 'baifid 'seikrəm / 骶椎裂 dǐzhuīliè

bone disease / boun di'ziz / 骨病 gǔbìng

carpal tunnel syndrome / 'kɑrpl 'tʌnl 'sindroum / 腕管综合征 wànguǎnzōnghézhēng

cauda equina injury / 'kaudə 'ikwinə 'indʒəri / 马尾神经损伤 mǎwěishénjīngsǔnshāng

cerebral palsy / sə'ribrəl 'pɔlzi / 大脑性瘫痪 dànǎo xìngtānhuàn

cerebral paralysis / sə'ribrəl pə'ræləsis / 大脑性瘫痪 dànǎoxìngtānhuàn

cervical spondylosis / 's3rvikl spɔndi'ləusis / 颈椎病 jǐngzhuībìng

coccygeal fracture / kɑk'sidʒiəl 'fræktʃər / 尾骨骨折

wěigǔgǔzhé

congenital dislocation of hip joint / kənˈdʒenɪtl ˌdɪsloʊˈkeɪʃn əv hɪp dʒɔɪnt / 先天性髋关节脱位 xiāntiānxìngkuānguānjiétuōwèi

congenital pseudoarthrosis of tibia / kənˈdʒenɪtl ˌsjudɑˈθrəʊsɪs əv ˈtɪbiə / 先天性胫骨假关节 xiāntiānxìngjìnggǔjiǎguānjié

congenital talipes equinovarus / kənˈdʒenɪtl ˈtælɪpiz ekwɪnəˈveərəs / 先天性马蹄内翻足 xiāntiānxìng mǎtínèifānzú

contusion / kənˈtuʒn / 挫伤 cuòshāng

costal fracture / ˈkɑstl ˈfræktʃər / 肋骨骨折 lèigǔgǔzhé

crush syndrome / krʌʃ ˈsɪndroʊm / 挤压综合征 jǐyā zōnghézhēng

cubital tunnel syndrome / ˈkjubitəl ˈtʌnl ˈsɪndroʊm / 腕管综合征 wànguǎnzōnghézhēng

delayed union / dɪˈled ˈjuniən / 骨折延迟愈合 gǔzhé yánchíyùhé

dislocation / ˌdɪsloʊˈkeɪʃn / 脱位 tuōwèi

dislocation of bone / ˌdɪsloʊˈkeɪʃn əv bone / 骨错缝 gǔcuòfèng

dislocation of elbow joint / ˌdɪsloʊˈkeɪʃn əv ˈelboʊ dʒɔɪnt / 肘关节脱位 zhǒuguānjiétuōwèi

dislocation of hip joint / ˌdɪsloʊˈkeɪʃn əv hɪp dʒɔɪnt / 髋关节脱位 kuānguānjiétuōwèi

dislocation of inter-phalangeal joint / ˌdɪsloʊˈkeɪʃn əv ɪnˈtɜr ˌfelənˈdʒiəl dʒɔɪnt / 趾间关节脱位 zhǐjiān guānjiétuōwèi

dislocation of knee joint / ˌdɪsloʊˈkeɪʃn əv ni dʒɔɪnt / 膝关节脱位 xīguānjiétuōwèi

dislocation of metacarpal-phalangeal joint / ˌdɪsloʊˈkeɪʃn əv ˌmetəˈkɑrpl felənˈdʒiəl dʒɔɪnt / 掌指关节脱位 zhǎngzhǐguānjiétuōwèi

dislocation of metatarsal-phalangeal joint / ˌdɪsloʊˈkeɪʃn əv ˌmetəˈkɑrpl ˌfelənˈdʒiəl dʒɔɪnt / 跖趾关节脱位 zhízhǐguānjiétuōwèi

dislocation of sacroiliac joint / ˌdɪsloʊˈkeɪʃn əv ˌsækroˈɪliæk dʒɔɪnt / 骶髂关节错缝 dǐqiàguānjiécuòfèng

dislocation of small joint of cervical vertebrae / ˌdɪsloʊˈkeɪʃn əv smɔl dʒɔɪnt əv ˈsɜrvɪkl ˈvətɪbrə / 颈椎小关节错缝 jǐngzhuīxiǎoguānjiécuòfèng

dislocation of small joint of thoracic vertebrae / ˌdɪsloʊˈkeɪʃn əv smɔl dʒɔɪnt əv θɔˈræsɪk ˈvətɪbrə / 胸椎小关节错缝 xiōngzhuīxiǎoguānjiécuòfèng

dislocation of talus / ˌdɪsloʊˈkeɪʃn əv ˈteləs / 距骨脱位 jùgǔtuōwèi

dislocation of tarsometatarsal joint / ˌdɪsloʊˈkeɪʃn əv ˈtɑsəʊˌmetəˈtɑsəl dʒɔɪnt / 跗跖关节脱位 fūzhíguānjiétuōwèi

dislocation of temporomandibular joint / ˌdɪsloʊˈkeɪʃn əv ˌtempəromænˈdɪbjələ dʒɔɪnt / 颞颌关节脱位 nièhéguānjiétuōwèi

disorder of temporomandibular joint / dɪsˈɔrdər əv ˌtempəromænˈdɪbjələ dʒɔɪnt / 颞颌关节紊乱症 nièhéguānjiéwěnluànzhèng

distal fracture of radius / ˈdɪstl ˈfræktʃər əv ˈreɪdiəs / 桡骨远端骨折 ráogǔyuǎnduāngǔzhé

disturbance of postlumbar joint / dɪˈstɜrbəns əv poʊstlʌmbər dʒɔɪnt / 腰椎后关节紊乱症 yāozhuī hòuguānjiéwěnluànzhèng

double fracture of shafts of ulna and radius / ˈdʌbl ˈfræktʃər əv ʃæfts əv ˈʌlnə ənd ˈreɪdiəs / 尺桡骨干双骨折 chǐráogǔgànshuānggǔzhé

epiphysitis / ɪˌpɪfɪˈsaɪtɪs / 骨骺炎 gǔhóuyán

external humeral epicondylitis / ekˈstɜrnəl ˈhjʊmərəl ˈepiˌkɔndiˈlaitis / 肱骨外上髁炎 gōnggǔwàishàng kēyán

fasciitis of nape muscle / fəˈsaitis əv neɪp ˈmʌsl / 项背筋膜炎 xiàngbèijīnmóyán

fasciitis of waist and gluteal region / fəˈsaitis əv weɪst ənd glʊˈtiəl ˈridʒən / 腰臀部筋膜炎 yāotúnbù jīnmóyán

fissured fracture / ˈfɪʃərd ˈfræktʃər / 裂缝骨折 lièfèng gǔzhé

fluorosis of bone / flʊəˈrosɪs əv boʊn / 氟骨病 fúgǔ bìng

fracture / ˈfræktʃər / 骨折 gǔzhé

fracture of calcaneus / ˈfræktʃər əv kælˈkenɪəs / 跟骨骨折 gēngǔgǔzhé

fracture of cervical vertebrae / ˈfræktʃər əv ˈsɜrvɪkl ˈvətɪbrə / 颈椎骨折 jǐngzhuīgǔzhé

fracture of clavicle / ˈfræktʃər əv ˈklævɪkl / 锁骨骨折 suǒgǔgǔzhé

fracture of femoral condyle / ˈfræktʃər əv ˈfiːmər ˈkɑndəl / 股骨髁骨折 gǔgǔkēgǔzhé

fracture of fibular shaft / ˈfræktʃər əv ˈfɪbjələ ʃæft / 腓骨干骨折 féigǔgàngǔzhé

fracture of greater tuberosity of humerus / ˈfræktʃər əv ˈɡreɪtər ˌtʊbəˈrɑsɪti əv ˈhjuːmərəs / 肱骨大结节骨折 gōnggǔdàjiéjiégǔzhé

fracture of head of radius / ˈfræktʃər əv hed əv ˈreɪdiəs / 桡骨头骨折 ráogǔtóugǔzhé

fracture of lateral epicondyle of humerus / ˈfræktʃər əv ˈlætərəl ˌɛpɪˈkɑndaɪl əv ˈhjuːmərəs / 肱骨外上髁骨折 gōnggǔwàishàngkēgǔzhé

fracture of lower 1/3 of radius combined with dislocation of lower ulna radius joint / ˈfræktʃər əv ˈloə 1/3 əv reɪdiəs kəmˈbaɪnd wɪð ˌdɪsloʊˈkeɪʃn əv ˈloə ˈʌlnə reɪdiəs dʒɔɪnt / 桡骨下 1/3 骨折合并下桡尺骨关节脱位 ráogǔxià 1/3 gǔzhéhébìngxiàráochǐgǔguānjiétuōwèi

fracture of lumbar vertebrae / ˈfræktʃər əv ˈlʌmbə ˈvətɪbrə / 腰椎骨折 yāozhuīgǔzhé

fracture of malleolus / ˈfræktʃər əv məˈliələs / 踝部骨折 huáibùgǔzhé

fracture of medial epicondyle of humerus / ˈfræktʃər əv ˈmidiəl ˌɛpɪˈkɑndaɪl əv ˈhjuːmərəs / 肱骨内上髁骨折 gōnggǔnèishàngkēgǔzhé

fracture of metacarpal bones / ˈfræktʃər əv metəˈkɑrpl bonz / 掌骨骨折 zhǎnggǔgǔzhé

fracture of metatarsus / ˈfræktʃər əv ˌmɛtəˈtɑrsəs / 跖

骨骨折 zhígǔgǔzhé

fracture of neck of femur / ˈfræktʃər əv nek əv ˈfimər / 股骨颈骨折 gǔgǔjǐnggǔzhé

fracture of olecranon / ˈfræktʃər əv oˈlɛkrənɑn / 尺骨鹰嘴骨折 chǐgǔyīngzuǐgǔzhé

fracture of phalanges of fingers / ˈfræktʃər əv fəˈlændʒiz əv ˈfiŋgəs / 指骨骨折 zhǐgǔgǔzhé

fracture of scaphoid bone of wrist / ˈfræktʃər əv ˈskæfɔid əv rist / 腕舟骨骨折 wànzhōugǔgǔzhé

fracture of scaphoid of foot / ˈfræktʃər əv ˈskæfɔid əv fut / 足舟骨骨折 zúzhōugǔgǔzhé

fracture of scapula / ˈfræktʃər əv ˈskæpjulə / 肩胛骨骨折 jiānjiǎgǔgǔzhé

fracture of shaft of femur / ˈfræktʃər əv ʃæft əv ˈfimər / 股骨干骨折 gǔgǔgàngǔzhé

fracture of shaft of humerus / ˈfræktʃər əv ˈʃæft əv ˈhjumərəs / 肱骨干骨折 gōnggǔgàngǔzhé

fracture of shaft of radius / ˈfræktʃər əv ʃæft əv ˈreidiəs / 桡骨干骨折 ráogǔgàngǔzhé

fracture of shaft of tibia and fibula / ˈfræktʃər əv ʃæft əv ˈtibiəl ənd ˈfibjələ / 胫腓骨干双骨折 jìngféigǔgànshuānggǔzhé

fracture of shaft of ulna / ˈfræktʃər əv ʃæft əv ˈʌlnə / 尺骨干骨折 chǐgǔgàngǔzhé

fracture of surgical neck of humerus / ˈfræktʃər əv ˈsɜrdʒikl nek əv ˈhjumərəs / 肱骨外髁颈骨折 gōng gǔwàikējǐnggǔzhé

fracture of talus / ˈfræktʃər əv ˈteləs / 距骨骨折 jùgǔ

gǔzhé

fracture of thoracic vertebrae / ˈfræktʃər əv θəˈræsɪk ˈvətɪbrə / 胸椎骨折 xiōngzhuīgǔzhé

fracture of tibial malleolus / ˈfræktʃər əv ˈtɪbɪəl məˈliələs / 胫骨髁骨折 jìnggǔkēgǔzhé

fracture of upper 1/3 of ulna combined with dislocation of head of radius / ˈfræktʃər əv ˈʌpər 1/3 əv ˈʌlnə kəmˈbaɪnd wɪð ˌdɪslouˈkeɪʃn əv hed əv ˈreɪdiəs / 尺骨上 1/3 骨折合并桡骨头脱位 chǐgǔshàng 1/3 gǔzhéhébìngráogǔtoutuōwèi

fresh fracture / freʃ ˈfræktʃər / 新鲜骨折 xīnxiāngǔzhé

genu valgum / ˈdʒɛnju ˈvælgəm / 膝外翻 xīwàifān

genu varum / ˈdʒɛnju ˈveərəm / 膝内翻 xīnèifān

gouty arthritis / ˈgauti ɑrˈθraɪtɪs / 痛风性关节炎 tòngfēngxìngguānjiéyán

greenstick fracture / grinstɪk ˈfræktʃər / 青枝骨折 qīngzhīgǔzhé

grinding contusion / ˈgraɪndɪŋ kənˈtuʒn / 碾挫伤 niǎncuòshāng

heel pain / hil peɪn / 跖痛症 zhítòngzhèng

herniation of cervical disc / ˌhəniˈeiʃən əv ˈsɜrvɪkl dɪsk / 颈椎间盘突出症 jǐngzhuījiānpántūchūzhèng

injury / ˈɪndʒəri / 损伤 sǔnshāng

injury of cruciate ligament of knee joint / ˈɪndʒəri əv ˈkruʃiit ˈlɪgəmənt əv ni dʒɔɪnt / 膝关节交叉韧带损伤 xīguānjiéjiāochārèndàisǔnshāng

injury of elbow fascia / ˈɪndʒəri əv ˈelbou ˈfeɪʃə / 肘

部筋伤 zhǒubùjīnshāng

injury of infrapatellar fat pad / ˈɪndʒəri əv ˈɪnfrəpəˈtelə fæt pæd / 髌下脂肪垫损伤 bìnxiàzhīfáng diànsǔnshāng

injury of medial and lateral ligaments of knee joint / ˈɪndʒəri əv ˈmidiəl ənd ˈlætərəl ˈlɪgəmənts əv ni dʒɔɪnt / 膝关节内外侧副韧带损伤 xīguānjiénèi wàicèfùrèndàisǔnshāng

injury of meniscus of knee joint / ˈɪndʒəri əv məˈnɪskəs əv ni dʒɔɪnt / 膝关节半月板损伤 xīguānjié bànyuèbǎnsǔnshāng

injury of shoulder fascia / ˈɪndʒəri əv ˈʃouldər ˈfeɪʃə / 肩部筋伤 jiānbùjīnshāng

injury of tendons / ˈɪndʒəri əv ˈtendənz / 筋伤 jīnshāng

injury of adductor of femur / ˈɪndʒəri əv əˈdʌktər əv fimər / 股内收肌群损伤 gǔnèishōujīqúnsǔnshāng

inner disorder due to injury / ˈɪnər dɪsˈɔrdər du tə ˈɪndʒəri / 损伤内证 sǔnshāngnèizhèng

intercondylar fracture of humerus / intzrkənˈdɪla ˈfræktʃər əv ˈhjumərəs / 肱骨髁间骨折 gōnggǔ kējiāngǔzhé

internal humeral epicondylitis / ɪnˈtɜrnl ˈhjumərəl ˈepiˌkɔndiˈlaitis / 肱骨内上髁炎 gōnggǔnèishàng kēyán

internal injury of abdomen / ɪnˈtɜrnl ˈɪndʒəri əv ˈæbdəmən / 腹部内伤 fùbùnèishāng

internal injury of chest / ɪnˈtɜrnl ˈɪndʒəri əv tʃest / 胸部内伤 xiōngbùnèishāng

internal injury of head / ɪnˈtɜrnl ˈɪndʒəri əv hed / 头部内伤 tóubùnèishāng

interphalangeal dislocation / ˌɪntəfəˈlændʒiəl ˌdɪsloʊˈkeɪʃn / 指间关节脱位 zhǐjiānguānjiétuōwèi

intertrochanteric fracture of femur / intətrəkənˈterik ˈfræktʃər əv ˈfimər / 股骨粗隆间骨折 gǔgǔcūlóngjiāngǔzhé

ischemic necrosis of head of femur / ɪsˈkimɪk neˈkroʊsɪs əv hed əv ˈfimər / 股骨头缺血性坏死 gǔgǔtouquēxuèxìnghuàisǐ

 # Kaschin-Beck disease 大骨节病 dàgǔjiébìng

laceration / ˌlæsəˈreɪʃn / 撕裂伤 sīlièshāng

laceration of muscle and tendon / ˌlæsə ˈreɪʃn əv ˈmʌsl ənd ˈtendən / 筋断 jīnduàn

lumbar muscle strain / ˈlʌmbər ˈmʌsl streɪn / 腰肌劳损 yāojīláosǔn

lumbar spondylolisthesis / ˈlʌmbər ˌspɒndiləulisˈθisis / 腰椎滑脱症 yāozhuīhuátuōzhèng

lunate dislocation / ˈlʊnet ˌdɪsloʊˈkeɪʃn / 月骨脱位 yuègǔtuōwèi

malunion / mæˈljunjən / 骨折畸形愈合 gǔzhéjīxíngyùhé

metatarsal tunnel syndrome / ˌmetəˈtɑrsl ˈtʌnl ˈsɪndroʊm / 跖管综合征 zhíguǎnzōnghézhēng

myositis ossificans / maɪəˈsaɪtɪs ˈossificans / 骨化性肌炎 gǔhuàxìngjīyán

myotenositis of long head of biceps brachii / maɪəˈtenəsaɪtɪs əv ˈlɒŋ ˈhɛd əv ˈbaɪseps bˈreɪtʃɪi / 肱二头肌长头肌腱炎 gōng'èrtóujīchángtóujī jiànyán

neuropathic arthritis / ˌnjʊrəˈpæθɪk ɑrˈθraɪtɪs / 神经病性关节炎 shénjīngbìngxìngguānjiéyán

nonunion / ˈnɑnˌjʊnjən / 骨折不愈合 gǔzhébùyùhé

old fracture / oʊld ˈfræktʃər / 陈旧性骨折 chénjiùxìnggǔzhé

open fracture / ˈoʊpən ˈfræktʃər / 开放性骨折 kāifàngxìnggǔzhé

ossifying myositis / ˈɑsəˈfaiiŋ ˌmaiəˈsaitis / 骨化性肌炎 gǔhuàxìngjīyán

osteoarthritis / ˌɑstioʊɑrˈθraɪtɪs / 骨关节炎 gǔguānjiéyán

osteoarthrosis deformaris endemica / ˌɒstɪəʊɑˈθrəʊsɪs diˈfɔməriz enˈdemɪkə / 大骨节病 dàgǔjiébìng

osteogenesis imperfecta / ˌɑstɪəˈdʒɛnəsɪs ˌɪmpəˈfɛktə / 成骨不全 chénggǔbùquán

osteoma / ˌɑstɪˈomə / 骨瘤 gǔliú

osteoporosis / ˌɑstioʊpəˈroʊsɪs / 骨质疏松症 gǔzhì shūsōngzhèng

pain in metatarsus / pein in ˌmɛtəˈtɑrsəs / 跖痛症 zhítòngzhèng

patellar chondromalacia / pəˈtɛlə ˌkɔndrəʊməˈleiʃiə / 髌骨软化症 bìngǔruǎnhuàzhèng

patellar dislocation / pəˈtɛlə ˌdɪsloʊˈkeiʃn / 髌骨脱位 bìngǔtuōwèi

patellar fracture / pəˈtɛlə ˈfræktʃər / 髌骨骨折 bìngǔgǔzhé

pathological fracture / ˌpæθəˈlɑdʒɪkl ˈfræktʃər / 病理

性骨折 bìnglǐxìnggǔzhé

pelvic fracture / ˈpelvɪk ˈfræktʃər / 骨盆骨折 gǔpén gǔzhé

periarthritis humeroscapularis / periaˈθraitis ˈhʌmərskæpjʊˈlærɪs / 肩周炎 jiānzhōuyán

perimyotenositis of extensor of radial aspect / ˈpirɪmaɪəˈtenəsaɪtis əv ɪkˈstensər əv ˈreɪdiəl ˈæspekt / 桡侧伸腕肌腱周围炎 ráocèshēnwànjījiànzhōu wéiyán

phalangeal fracture / ˌfelənˈdʒiəl ˈfræktʃər / 趾骨骨折 zhǐgǔgǔzhé

piriformis syndrome / ˌpirəˈfɔmis ˈsɪndroʊm / 梨状肌综合征 lízhuàngjīzōnghézhēng

popliteal cyst / pɔpˈlitiəl sɪst / 腘窝囊肿 guōwōnáng zhǒng

prepatellar bursitis / pripəˈtelə ˌbɜrˈsaɪtis / 髌前滑膜炎 bìnqiánhuámóyán

prolapse of lumbar intervertebral disc / ˈproʊlæps əv ˈlʌmbər ˌɪntəˈvɝˈtəbrəl dɪsk / 腰椎间盘突出症 yāozhuījiānpántūchūzhèng

pyogenic arthritis / ˌpaɪəˈdʒɛnɪk ɑrˈθraitis / 化脓性关节炎 huànóngxìngguānjiéyán

pyriformis syndrome / pɪrɪˈfɔmis ˈsɪndroʊm / 梨状肌综合征 lízhuàngjīzōnghézhēng

rheumatoid arthritis / ˈrʊmətɔɪd ɑrˈθraitis / 类风湿性关节炎 lèifēngshīxìngguānjiéyán

rotator cuff injury / ˈrotetə kʌf ˈɪndʒəri / 肩袖损伤 jiānxiùsǔnshāng

rupture / ˈrʌptʃər / 断裂伤 duànlièshāng

rupture of achilles tendon / ˈrʌptʃ ɪər əv əˈkiliz ˈtendən / 跟腱断裂 gēnjiànduànliè

rupture of coccyx / ˈrʌptʃər əv ˈkɑksɪks / 骶尾部挫伤 dǐwěibùcuòshāng

rupture of patellar tendon / ˈrʌptʃər əv pəˈtelə ˈtendən / 髌腱断裂 bìnjiànduànliè

rupture of tendon of biceps brachii / ˈrʌptʃər əv ˈtendən əv ˈbaɪseps bˈreɪtʃi / 肱二头肌腱断裂 gōng'èrtóujījiànduànliè

sacral fracture / ˈsekrəl ˈfræktʃər / 骶骨骨折 dǐgǔgǔzhé

scapular dislocation / ˈskæpjʊlə ˌdɪsloʊˈkeɪʃn / 肩关节脱位 jiānguānjiétuōwèi

sclerosing osteomyelitis / skliəˈrəusiŋ ˌɑstɪoˌmaɪəˈlaɪtɪs / 硬化性骨髓炎 yìnghuàxìnggǔsuǐyán

scoliosis / ˌskoʊliˈoʊsɪs / 脊柱侧弯 jǐzhùcèwān

sliding of long and short muscle tendon of fibula / ˈsliding əv lɔŋ ənd ʃɔrt ˈmʌsl ˈtendən əv ˈfɪbjələ / 腓骨长短肌腱滑脱 féigǔchángduǎnjījiànhuátuō

snapping hip / ˈsnæpɪŋ hɪp / 弹响髋 dànxiǎngkuān

spinal cord injury / ˈspaɪnl kɔrd injury / 脊髓损伤 jǐsuǐsǔnshāng

sprain / spreɪn / 扭伤 niǔshāng

sprain of ankle joint / spreɪn əv ˈæŋkl dʒɔɪnt / 踝关节扭伤 huáiguānjiéniǔshāng

sprain of medial and lateral ligaments of ankle joint / spreɪn əv ˈmidiəl ənd ˈlætərəl ˈlɪgəmənts əv 'æŋkl dʒɔɪnt / 踝关节内外侧副韧带损伤 huái guānjiénèiwàicèfùrèndàisǔnshāng

sprain of neck muscle / spreɪn əv nek 'mʌsl / 颈肌扭伤 jǐngjīniǔshāng

sprain of tarsometatarsal joint / spreɪn əv tɑrsoʊmetə'tɑrsl dʒɔɪnt / 跗跖关节扭伤 fūzhíguānjiéniǔshāng

sprain of wrist joint / spreɪn əv rɪst dʒɔɪnt / 腕关节扭伤 wànguānjiéniǔshāng

stenosing tenosynovitis / stɪ'noʊsɪŋ 'tenəʊˌsinə'vaitis / 狭窄性腱鞘炎 xiázhǎixìngjiànqiàoyán

sternoclavicular dislocation / ˌstənəʊklə'vikjulə ˌdɪsloʊ'keɪʃn / 胸锁关节脱位 xiōngsuǒguānjiétuōwèi

stiff neck / stɪf nek / 落枕 làozhěn

straitness of lumbar vertebrae / 'streitnis əv 'lʌmbər 'vɜrtɪbrə / 腰椎椎管狭窄症 yāozhuīzhuīguǎnxiázhǎizhèng

subacromial bursitis / ˌsʌ'bækrəmɪrl bɜr'saɪtɪs / 肩峰下滑囊炎 jiānfēngxiàhuánángyán

subluxation of radial head / sʌblʌk'seʃən əv 'reɪdiəs hed / 桡骨头半脱位 ráogǔtóubàntuōwèi

supracondylar fracture of femur / sjuprəkən'dɪla 'fræktʃər əv 'fimər / 股骨髁上骨折 gǔgǔkēshàng gǔzhé

supracondylar fracture of humerus / sjuprəkən'dɪla 'fræktʃər əv 'hjumərəs / 肱骨髁上骨折 gōnggǔkēshànggǔzhé

syndrome of aponeurotic space / 'sɪndroʊm əv ˌæpənju'rɔtik speɪs / 筋膜间隔区综合征 jīnmó jiāngéqūzōnghézhēng

syndrome of chest outlet / ˈsɪndroʊm əv tʃest ˈaʊtlet / 胸廓出口综合征 xiōngkuòchūkǒuzōnghézhēng

synovitis of ischiac tubercle / saɪnəˈvaɪtɪs əv ˈɪskɪæk ˈtu, bərkl / 坐骨结节滑囊炎 zuògǔjiéjiéhuánángyán

synovitis of olecranon / saɪnəˈvaɪtɪs əv oˈlɛkrənɑn / 尺骨鹰嘴滑囊炎 chǐgǔyīngzuǐhuánángyán

tendinitis of supraspinatus muscle / tendɪˈnaɪtəs əv sʌpraspɪˈneɪtəs ˈmʌsl / 冈上肌肌腱炎 gāngshàngjījījiànyán

thecal cyst / ˈθikl sɪst / 腱鞘囊肿 jiànqiàonángzhǒng

torticollis / ˌtɔtɪˈkɒlɪs / 斜颈 xiéjǐng

transient synovitis of hip joint / ˈtrænsiənt saɪnəˈvaɪtɪs əv hɪp dʒɔɪnt / 髋关节一过性滑膜炎 kuānguānjiéyīguòxìnghuámóyán

transverse process syndrome of third lumbar vertebra / ˈtrænzvɜrs proˈsɛs ˈsɪndroʊm əv θɜrd ˈlʌmbər ˈvɜrtɪbrə / 第三腰椎横突综合征 dìsānyāozhuī héngtūzōnghézhēng

traumatic arthritis / trəˈmætɪk ɑrˈθraɪtɪs / 创伤性关节炎 chuāngshāngxìngguānjiéyán

traumatic paraplegia / trəˈmætɪk ˌpærəˈplidʒə / 外伤性截瘫 wàishāngxìngjiétān

traumatic synovitis of knee joint / trəˈmætɪk saɪnəˈvaɪtɪs əv ni dʒɔɪnt / 膝关节创伤性滑膜炎 xīguānjié chuāngshāngxìnghuámóyán

tuberculous osteoarthropathy / tjʊˈbɜrkjələs ˌɒstiəuɑˈθrəupəθi / 骨关节结核 gǔguānjiéjiéhé

wryneck / ˈraɪnek / 斜颈 xiéjǐng

Chapter 10　Gynecology of Traditional Chinese Medicine

第十章　中医妇科学

Section 1　Menstrual Diseases

第一节　月　经　病

advanced menstruation / əd'vænst ˌmenstruˈeɪʃn / 月经先期 yuèjīngxiānqī

amenorrhea / eiˌmenəˈriə / 闭经 bìjīng

dysmenorrhea / ˌdɪsmɛnəˈriə / 痛经 tòngjīng

Fu Qingzhu Nüke / fu tʃiŋʤu nykə / 傅青主女科 fùqīngzhǔnǚkē

gynecology of traditional Chinese medicine / ˌgaɪnə ˈkɑlədʒi əv trəˈdɪʃənl ˌtʃaiˈniz ˈmedɪsn / 中医妇科学 zhōngyīfùkēxuè

intermenstrual bleeding / ɪnˈtɜrmenstruəl ˈblidɪŋ / 经间期出血 jīngjiānqīchūxiè

menarche / məˈnɑki / 初潮 chūcháo

menopathy / ˈmenəpəθɪ / 月经病 yuèjīngbìng

menostaxis / menəˈstæksɪs / 经期延长 jīngqīyáncháng

menstrual cycle / ˈmenstruəl ˈsaɪkl / 月经周期 yuèjīngzhōuqī

menstrual disorders / ˈmenstruəl dɪsˈɔrdərz / 月经不调 yuèjīngbùtiáo

menstrual period / ˈmenstruəl ˈpɪriəd / 月经期 yuèjīngqī

menstrual volume / ˈmenstruəl ˈvɑljum / 经量 jīng liàng

metrorrhagia / ˌmitrəˈredʒɪə / 崩漏 bēnglòu

mons pubis / mɔnz ˈpjubɪs / 毛际 máojì

retarded menstruation / rɪˈtɑrdɪd ˌmenstruˈeɪʃn / 月经后期 yuèjīnghòuqī

tian gui / tæn kweɪ / 天癸 tiānguǐ

uterine ostium / ˈjutərɪn ɑstɪəm / 胞门 bāomén

vagina / vəˈdʒaɪnə / 阴道 yīndào

wenjing decoction / wendʒɪŋ dɪˈkɑkʃn / 温经汤 wēnjīngtāng

Section 2 Perimenstrual and Perimenopausal Syndromes
第二节　经行前后诸证

climacteric period / ˌklaɪmækˈtɛrɪk ˈpɪriəd / 更年期 gēngniánqī

menopause / ˈmenəpɔz / 绝经 juéjīng

moody state during menstruation / ˈmudi steɪt ˈdʊrɪŋ ˌmenstruˈeɪʃn / 经行情志异常 jīngxíngqíngzhì yìcháng

Section 3 Leukorrheal Diseases
第三节　带　下　病

cold pathogen / koʊld ˈpæθədʒən / 寒邪 hánxié

congestion / kənˈdʒestʃən / 淤血 yūxuè

dampness pathogen / ˈdæmpnəs ˈpæθədʒən / 湿邪

shīxié

excessive sexual intercourse / ɪkˈsɛsɪv sɛkʃuəl ˈɪntərkɔrs / 房劳 fángláo

history of marriage / ˈhɪstri əv ˈmærɪdʒ / 婚育史 hūn yùshǐ

leukorrheal diseases / lukɒˈrel dɪˈzizɪs / 带下病 dàixià bìng

oligo-vaginal discharge / ˌɔligəu vəˈdʒaɪnl dɪsˈtʃɑrdʒ / 带下过少 dàixiàguòshǎo

Section 4　Gestational Diseases
第四节　妊　娠　病

cervical scraping smear / ˈsɜrvɪkl ˈskreɪpɪŋ smɪr / 宫颈刮片 gōngjǐngguāpiàn

cesarean section / sɪˈzɛriən ˈsekʃn / 剖宫产术 pōu gōngchǎnshù

eclampsia / ɪˈklæmpsiə / 子痫 zǐxián

Eight Extraordinary Channels / eɪt ɪkˈstrɔrdənˌeri tʃænlz / 奇经八脉 qíjīngbāmài

Eight Extraordinary Meridians / eɪt ɪkˈstrɔrdəneri məˈrɪdiəns / 奇经八脉 qíjīngbāmài

gestational diseases / dʒeˈsteiʃənəl dɪˈzizɪs / 妊娠病 rènshēnbìng

habitual abortion / həˈbɪtʃuəl əˈbɔrʃn / 滑胎 huátāi

internal treatment / ɪnˈtɜrnl ˈtritmənt / 内治法 nèizhìfǎ

labor pain / ˈlebə peɪn / 阵痛 zhèntòng

lochia / ˈlokɪə / 恶露 èlù

pregnancy pulse / ˈpregnənsi pʌls / 妊娠脉 rènshēn

mài

urine retention during pregnancy / ˈjʊrɪn rɪˈtenʃn ˈdʊrɪŋ ˈpregnənsi / 妊娠小便不通 rènshēnxiǎobiànbùtōng

Section 5　Puerperal Diseases
第五节　产　后　病

after-pains / ˈæftər peɪnz / 产后宫缩痛 chǎnhòugōngsuōtòng

encolpism / enkɒlˈpɪzəm / 阴道纳药 yīndàonàyào

external treatment / ekˈstərnəl ˈtritmənt / 外治法 wàizhìfǎ

labor / ˈlebə / 产程 chǎnchéng

lactation / lækˈteɪʃn / 哺乳期 bǔrǔqī

parturition / ˌpɑrtʃəˈrɪʃn / 分娩 fēnmiǎn

postpartum abdominal pain / ˌpostˈpɑrtəm æbˈdɑmɪnl peɪn / 产后腹痛 chǎnhòufùtòng

postpartum anemic fainting / ˌpostˈpɑrtəm ənimɪk ˈfeintiŋ / 产后血晕 chǎnhòuxuèyūn

postpartum haemorrhage / ˌpostˈpɑrtəm ˈhemərɪdʒ / 产后血崩 chǎnhòuxuèbēng

postpartum pain of body / ˌpostˈpɑrtəm peɪn əv ˈbɑdi / 产后身痛 chǎnhòushēntòng

puerperal constipation / pjuˈəpərəl ˌkɑnstɪˈpeɪʃn / 产后大便难 chǎnhòudàbiànnán

puerperal disease / pjuˈəpərəl dɪˈziz / 产后病 chǎnhòubìng

puerperal fever / pjuˈəpərəl ˈfivər / 产后发热 chǎn

hòufārè

puerperium / ˌpjuəˈpɪəriəm / 产褥期 chǎnrùqī

spontaneous sweating and night sweating after childbirth / spɑnˈteɪniəs ˈswetɪŋ ənd naɪt ˈswetɪŋ ˈæftər ˈtʃaɪld bɜrθ / 产后自汗盗汗 chǎnhòuzìhàndàohàn

vaginal douche / vəˈdʒaɪnl duʃ / 阴道冲洗 yīndào chōngxǐ

vulval steaming and douche / ˈvʌlvə ˈstimɪŋ ənd duʃ / 外阴熏洗 wàiyīnxūnxǐ

Section 6 Gynecological Miscellaneous Diseases
第六节 妇科杂病

basal body temperature / ˈbeɪsl ˈbɑdi ˈtemprətʃər / 基础体温 jīchǔtǐwēn

endometriosis / ˌɛndoˌmitriˈosɪs / 子宫内膜异位症 zǐgōngnèimóyìwèizhèng

estrogen / ˈɛstrədʒən / 雌激素 cíjīsù

external genital organs of female / ekˈstərnəl ˈdʒenɪtl ˈɔrgəns əv ˈfimeɪl / 女性外生殖器官 nǚxìngwài shēngzhíqìguān

infertility / ˌɪnfɜrˈtɪləti / 不孕症 bùyùnzhèng

internal genital organs of female / ɪnˈtɜrnl ˈdʒenɪtl ˈɔrgəns əv ˈfimeɪl / 女性内生殖器官 nǚxìngnèi shēngzhíqìguān

lutropin / lˈjutrəpɪn / 促黄体素 cùhuángtǐsù

orifice of uterus / ˈɔrɪfɪs əv ˈjutərəs / 子宫口 zǐgōng kǒu

pelvic floor / ˈpelvɪk flɔr / 骨盆底 gǔpéndǐ

pelvic mass in woman / ˈpelvɪk mæs ɪn ˈwʊmən / 妇人癥瘕 fùrénzhēngjiǎ

pelvis / ˈpelvɪs / 骨盆 gǔpén

pruritus vulvae / prʊˈraɪtəs ˈəʌlvi / 阴痒 yīnyǎng

sore of vulvae / sɔr əv ˈəʌlvi / 阴疮 yīnchuāng

sterillization / ˌsterələˈzeɪʃn / 绝育 juéyù

uterine prolapse / ˈjutəraɪn ˈproʊlæps / 阴挺 yīntǐng

Chapter 11 Pediatrics of Traditional Chinese Medicine

第十一章　中医儿科学

abnormal natural endowment / æbˈnɔrməl ˈnætʃrəl ɪnˈdaʊmənt / 禀赋异常 bǐngfùyìcháng

acute infantile convulsion / əˈkjut ˈɪnfəntaɪl kənˈvʌlʃn / 急惊风 jíjīngfēng

acute infantile convulsion due to fright / əˈkjut ˈɪnfəntaɪl kənˈvʌlʃn du tə fraɪt / 急惊风·惊恐惊风证 jíjīngfēng·jīngkǒngjīngfēngzhèng

acute infantile convulsion due to phlegm-food / əˈkjut ˈɪnfəntaɪl kənˈvʌlʃn du tə flem fud / 急惊风·痰食惊风证 jíjīngfēng·tánshíjīngfēngzhèng

acute infantile convulsion due to summer-heat / əˈkjut ˈɪnfəntaɪl kənˈvʌlʃn du tə ˈsʌmər hit / 急惊风·暑热发搐证 jíjīngfēng·shǔrèfāchùzhèng

acute infantile convulsion due to wind-heat / əˈkjut ˈɪnfəntaɪl kənˈvʌlʃn du tə wɪnd hit / 急惊风·风热发搐证 jíjīngfēng·fēngrèfāchùzhèng

acute infantile convulsion with syndrome of warm-heat and pestilent toxin / əˈkjut ˈɪnfəntaɪl kənˈvʌlʃn wɪð ˈsɪndroʊm əv wɔrm hit ənd ˈpestilənt ˈtɑksɪn / 急惊风·温热疫毒证 jíjīngfēng·wēnrèyìdúzhèng

adding food supplements / ˈædɪŋ fud ˈsʌpləmənts / 添加辅食 tiānjiāfǔshí

adolescence / ˌædəˈlesns / 青春期 qīngchūnqī

anterior fontanel / ænˈtɪriər ˌfɒntəˈnel / 前囟 qiánxìn

aphtha / ˈæfθə / 口糜 kǒumí

artificial feeding / ˌɑrtɪˈfɪʃl ˈfidɪŋ / 人工喂养 réngōng wèiyǎng

attacking stage of infantile asthma / əˈtækɪŋ steɪdʒ əv ˈɪnfəntaɪl ˈæzmə / 小儿哮喘·发作期 xiǎo'érxiào chuǎn·fāzuòqī

babyhood / ˈbeɪbihʊd / 婴儿期 yīng'érqī

birthmark / ˈbɜrθmɑrk / 胎生青记 tāishēngqīngjì

breast feeding / brest ˈfidɪŋ / 母乳喂养 mǔrǔwèi yǎng

bulging fontanel / ˈbʌldʒɪŋ ˌfɔntəˈnel / 囟门高突 xìn méngāotū

* **children's hyperkinesis syndrome with deficiency of both heart and spleen** / ˈtʃɪldrəns ˌhaɪpəkɪˈnɪsɪs ˈsɪndroʊm wɪð dɪˈfɪʃnsi əv boʊθ hɑrt ənd splin / 儿童多动综合征·心脾两虚证 értóngduōdòng zōnghézhēng·xīnpíliǎngxūzhèng

* **chronic infantile convulsion with syndrome of yang deficiency of spleen and kidney** / ˈkrɑnɪk ˈɪnfəntaɪl kənˈvʌlʃn wɪð ˈsɪndroʊm əv jæŋ dɪˈfɪʃnsi əv splin ənd ˈkɪdni / 慢惊风·脾肾阳虚证 mànjīng fēng·píshènyángxūzhèng

case of measles with favorable prognosis / keɪs əv ˈmizlz wɪð ˈfevərəbl prɑglˈnoʊsɪs / 麻疹·顺证 mázhěn·shùnzhèng

children's hyperkinesis syndrome / ˈtʃɪldrəns ˌhaɪpəkɪˈnɪsɪs ˈsɪndroʊm / 儿童多动综合征 értóng duōdòngzōnghézhēng

children's hyperkinesis syndrome with insufficiency of

heart and kidney / ˈtʃɪldrəns ˌhaɪpəkɪˈnɪsɪs ˈsɪndroʊm wɪð ˌɪnsəˈfɪʃənsi əv hɑrt ənd ˈkɪdni / 儿童多动综合征·心肾不足证 értóngduōdòng zōnghézhēng · xīnshènbùzúzhèng

children's hyperkinesis syndrome with phlegm-fire disturbing spirit / ˈtʃɪldrəns ˌhaɪpəkɪˈnɪsɪs ˈsɪndroʊm wɪð flem ˈfaɪər dɪˈstɜrbɪŋ ˈspɪrɪt / 儿童多动综合征·痰火扰神证 értóngduōdòngzōnghézhēng · tánhuǒrǎoshénzhèng

children's hyperkinesis syndrome with spleen deficiency and liver hyperactivity / ˈtʃɪldrəns ˌhaɪpəkɪˈnɪsɪs ˈsɪndroʊm wɪð splin dɪˈfɪʃnsi ənd ˈlɪvər ˌhaɪpərækˈtɪvəti / 儿童多动综合征·脾虚肝旺证 értóngduōdòngzōnghézhēng · píxūgānwàng zhèng

children's hyperkinesis syndrome with yin deficiency of liver and kidney / ˈtʃɪldrəns ˌhaɪpəkɪˈnɪsɪs ˈsɪndroʊm wɪð jɪn dɪˈfɪʃnsi əv ˈlɪvər ənd ˈkɪdni / 儿童多动综合征·肝肾阴虚证 értóngduōdòng zōnghézhēng · gānshènyīnxūzhèng

chronic infantile convulsion / ˈkrɑnɪk ˈɪnfəntaɪl kənˈvʌlʃn / 慢惊风 mànjīngfēng

chronic infantile convulsion with syndrome of deficiency of both qi and blood / ˈkrɑnɪk ˈɪnfəntaɪl kənˈvʌlʃn wɪð ˈsɪndroʊm əv dɪˈfɪʃnsi əv boʊθ tʃi ənd blʌd / 慢惊风·气血两虚证 mànjīngfēng · qìxuèliǎng xūzhèng

chronic infantile convulsion with syndrome of spleen deficiency and liver hyperactivity / ˈkrɑnɪk ˈɪnfəntaɪl kən'vʌlʃn wɪð 'sɪndroʊm əv splin dɪ'fɪʃnsi ənd 'lɪvər ˌhaɪpəræk'tɪvəti / 慢惊风 · 脾虚肝旺证 màn jīngfēng · píxūgānwàngzhèng

chronic infantile convulsion with syndrome of wind stirring due to yin deficiency / 'krɑnɪk 'ɪnfəntaɪl kən'vʌlʃn wɪð 'sɪndroʊm əv wɪnd 'stɜrɪŋ du tə jɪn dɪ'fɪʃnsi / 慢惊风 · 阴虚动风证 mànjīngfēng · yīnxūdòngfēngzhèng

closed eyes in newborn / kloʊzd aɪz ɪn 'nubɔrn / 初生目闭 chūshēngmùbì

cold asthma / koʊld 'æzmə / 寒性哮喘 hánxìng xiàochuǎn

color of venule / 'kʌlər əv 'vɛnjʊl / 纹色 wénsè

complementary feeding / ˌkɑmplɪ'mentri 'fidɪŋ / 补授法 bǔshòufǎ

contracted tongue / kən'træktɪd tʌŋ / 舌缩 shésuō

crane's joint / kreɪn's dʒɔɪnt / 鹤节 hèjié

cretinism / 'kritɪnˌɪzəm / 呆小病 dāixiǎobìng

curly tongue / 'kɜrli tʌŋ / 舌卷 shéjuǎn

* **deteriorated case of infantile diarrhea** / dɪ'tɪəriəˌreɪtɪd keɪs əv 'ɪnfəntaɪl ˌdaɪə'riə / 小儿泄泻 · 变证 xiǎo'érxièxiè · biànzhèng

* **deteriorated case of infantile edema** / dɪ'tɪəriəˌreɪtɪd keɪs əv 'ɪnfəntaɪl i'dimə / 小儿水肿 · 变证 xiǎo'érshuǐzhǒng · biànzhèng

deciduous teeth / dɪ'sɪdʒuəs tiθ / 乳牙 rǔyá

deficient type infantile common cold / dɪ'fɪʃnt taɪp 'ɪnfəntaɪl 'kɑmən koʊld / 小儿虚证感冒 xiǎo'ér xūzhènggǎnmào

deteriorated case of mumps / dɪˈtɪriəreɪtɪd keɪs əv mʌmps / 痄腮·变证 zhàsai·biànzhèng

deteriorated case of pneumonia with dyspneic cough / dɪˈtɪriəreɪtɪd keɪs əv nuˈmouniə wɪð dɪsˈpnik kɔf / 肺炎喘嗽·变证 fèiyánchuǎnsòu·biànzhèng

diphtheria / dɪfˈθɪriə / 白喉 báihóu

double tongue / ˈdʌbl tʌŋ / 重舌 chóngshé

enlarged square skull / ɪnˈlɑrdʒd skwer skʌl / 方颅 fānglú

eye gan disease / aɪ gæn dɪˈziz / 眼疳 yǎngān

* **five retardations with syndrome of deficiency of both heart and spleen** / faɪv ˌritɑrˈdeɪʃns wɪð ˈsɪndroum əv dɪˈfɪʃnsi əv bouθ hɑrt ənd splin / 五迟·心脾两虚证 wǔchí·xīnpíliǎngxūzhèng

failure of closure of fontanel / ˈfeɪljər əv ˈklouʒər əv ˌfɔntəˈnel / 囟门不合 xìnménbùhé

feeding baby / ˈfidɪŋ bebi / 婴儿喂养 yīng'érwèiyǎng

feeding with substitute / ˈfidɪŋ wɪð ˈsʌbstɪtut / 代授法 dàishòufǎ

fetal debility / ˈfitl dɪˈbɪləti / 胎怯 tāiqiè

fetal debility with syndrome of feeble kidney essence / ˈfitl dɪˈbɪləti wɪð ˈsɪndroum əv ˈfibl ˈkɪdni ˈesns / 胎怯·肾精薄弱证 tāiqiè·shènjīngbóruòzhèng

fetal debility with syndrome of qi deficiency of spleen and kidney / ˈfitl dɪˈbɪləti wɪð ˈsɪndroum əv tʃi dɪˈfɪʃnsi əv splin ənd ˈkɪdni / 胎怯·脾肾气虚证 tāiqiè·píshènqìxūzhèng

fetal jaundice / ˈfitl ˈdʒɔndɪs / 胎黄 tāihuáng

fetal jaundice with collapse syndrome / ˈfitl ˈdʒɔndɪs wɪð kəˈlæps ˈsɪndroʊm / 胎黄虚脱证 tāihuángxū tuōzhèng

fetal jaundice with syndrome of blood stasis and amassment / ˈfitl ˈdʒɔndɪs wɪð ˈsɪndroʊm əv blʌd ˈsteɪs ɪs ənd əˈmæsmənt / 胎黄·瘀积发黄证 tāi huáng·yūjīfāhuángzhèng

fetal jaundice with syndrome of stagnation and congelation of cold-damp / ˈfitl ˈdʒɔndɪs wɪð ˈsɪndroʊm əv stæɡˈneɪʃn ənd ˌkɑndʒəˈleʃən əv koʊld dæmp / 胎黄·寒湿凝滞证 tāihuáng·hánshīníngzhìzhèng

fetal jaundice with syndrome of stagnation and steaming of damp-heat / ˈfitl ˈdʒɔndɪs wɪð ˈsɪndroʊm əv stæɡˈneɪʃn ənd ˈstimɪŋ əv dæmp hit / 胎黄·湿热郁蒸证 tāihuáng·shīrèyùzhēngzhèng

fetal jaundice with syndrome of wind stirring / ˈfitl ˈdʒɔndɪs wɪð ˈsɪndroʊm əv wɪnd ˈstɜrɪŋ / 胎黄动风证 tāihuángdòngfēngzhèng

fetal stage / ˈfitl steɪdʒ / 胎儿期 tāi'érqī

fetal toxicosis / ˈfitl ˌtɔksiˈkəusis / 胎毒 tāidú

five infantile flaccidity / faɪv ˈɪnfəntaɪl flækˈsɪdɪti / 五软 wǔruǎn

five retardations / faɪv ˌritɑrˈdeɪʃns / 五迟 wǔchí

five retardations with syndrome of blockade of phlegm and static blood / faɪv ˌritɑrˈdeɪʃns wɪð ˈsɪndroʊm əv blɑˈkeɪd əv flem ənd ˈstætɪk blʌd / 五迟·痰瘀阻滞证 wǔchí·tányūzǔzhìzhèng

five retardations with syndrome of deficiency of both liver and kidney / faɪv ˌritɑrˈdeɪʃns wɪð ˈsɪndroʊm əv dɪ'fɪʃnsi əv boʊθ lɪvər ənd 'kɪdni / 五迟 · 肝肾两虚证 wǔchí · gānshènliǎngxūzhèng

five stiffness / faɪv 'stɪfnəs / 五硬 wǔyìng

flaccid tongue / 'flæsɪd tʌŋ / 舌痿 shéwěi

flaccidity of feet / flæk'sɪdɪti əv fit / 足软 zúruǎn

flaccidity of hand / flæk'sɪdɪti əv hænd / 手软 shǒuruǎn

flaccidity of mastication / flæk'sɪdɪti əv ˌmæstɪ'keɪʃn / 口软 kǒuruǎn

flaccidity of muscles / flæk'sɪdɪti əv 'mʌslz / 肌肉软 jīròuruǎn

flaccidity of neck / flæk 'sɪdɪti əv nek / 头项软 tóuxiàngruǎn

fontanel / ˌfɔntə'nel / 囟门 xìnmén

frequent protruding and wagging tongue / 'frikwənt prou'trudɪŋ ənd 'wægɪŋ tʌŋ / 弄舌 nòngshé

gan disease of five Zang-viscera / gæn dɪ'ziz əv faɪv zæŋ 'vɪsərə / 五脏疳 wǔzànggān

gan disease with edema and abdominal distention / gæn dɪ'ziz wɪð i'dimə ənd æb'dɑmɪnl dis'tenʃən / 疳肿胀 gānzhǒngzhàng

gan disease with syndrome of food stagnation / gæn dɪ'ziz wɪð 'sɪndroʊm əv fud stæg'neɪʃn / 疳积 gānjī

gan disease: infantile chronic malnutrition / gæn dɪ'ziz 'ɪnfəntaɪl 'krɑnɪk ˌmælnu'trɪʃn / 疳证 · 小儿慢性营养不良 gānzhèng · xiǎo'ér mànxìngyíngyǎng bùliáng

gingival gan disease / dʒɪnˈdʒaɪvl gæn dɪˈziz / 牙疳 yágān

harelip / ˈherlɪp / 兔缺 tùquē

head circumference / hed sərˈkʌmfərəns / 头围 tóuwéi

heart gan disease / hɑrt gæn dɪˈziz / 心疳 xīngān

heat asthma / hit ˈæzmə / 热性哮喘 rèxìngxiàochuǎn

hunchback / ˈhʌntʃbæk / 龟背 guībèi

* **indigestion with syndrome of milk and food stagnation** / ˌɪndɪˈdʒestʃən wɪð ˈsɪndroʊm əv mɪlk ənd fud stægˈneɪʃn / 积滞·乳食积滞证 jīzhì · rǔshíjīzhì zhèng

* **infantile abdominal pain with syndrome of accumulated heat in stomach and intestine** / ˈɪnfəntaɪl æbˈdɑmɪnl peɪn wɪð ˈsɪndroʊm əv əˈkjumjəˌletɪd hit ɪn ˈstʌmək ənd ɪnˈtestɪn / 小儿腹痛·胃肠积热证 xiǎo'érfùtòng · wèichángjīrèzhèng

* **infantile abdominal pain with syndrome of cold attacking abdomen** / ˈɪnfəntaɪl æbˈdɑmɪnl peɪn wɪð ˈsɪndroʊm əv koʊld əˈtækɪŋ ˈæbdəmən / 小儿腹痛·腹部中寒证 xiǎo'érfùtòng · fùbùzhōnghánzhèng

* **infantile abdominal pain with syndrome of deficient cold of spleen and stomach** / ˈɪnfəntaɪl æbˈdɑmɪnl peɪn wɪð ˈsɪndroʊm əv dɪˈfɪʃnt koʊld əv splin ənd ˈstʌmək / 小儿腹痛·脾胃虚寒证 xiǎo'érfùtòng · píwèixūhánzhèng

* **infantile abdominal pain with syndrome of milk and food stagnation** / ˈɪnfəntaɪl æbˈdɑmɪnl peɪn wɪð ˈsɪndroʊm əv mɪlk ənd fud stægˈneɪʃn / 小儿腹痛·乳食积滞证 xiǎo'érfùtòng · rǔshíjīzhìzhèng

* **infantile asthma with syndrome of external cold and internal heat** / ˈɪnfəntaɪl ˈæzmə wɪð ˈsɪndroʊm əv ɪkˈstɜrnl koʊld ənd ɪnˈtɜrnl hit / 小儿哮喘·外寒内热证 xiǎo'érxiàochuǎn · wàihánnèirè zhèng

* **infantile asthma with syndrome of qi deficiency of lung and spleen** / ˈɪnfəntaɪl ˈæzmə wɪð ˈsɪndroʊm əv tʃi dɪˈfɪʃnsi əv lʌŋ ənd splin / 小儿哮喘·肺脾气虚证 xiǎo'érxiàochuǎn · fèipíqìxūzhèng

* **infantile constipation** / ˈɪnfəntaɪl ˌkɑnstɪˈpeɪʃn / 小儿便秘 xiǎo'érbiànmì

* **infantile cough with syndrome of lung qi deficiency** / ˈɪnfəntaɪl kɔf wɪð ˈsɪndroʊm əv lʌŋ tʃi dɪˈfɪʃnsi / 小儿咳嗽·肺气虚证 xiǎo'érkésou · fèiqìxūzhèng

* **infantile cough with syndrome of phlegm-heat congesting lung** / ˈɪnfəntaɪl kɔf wɪð ˈsɪndroʊm əv flem hit kənˈdʒɛstɪŋ lʌŋ / 小儿咳嗽·痰热壅肺证 xiǎo'érkésou · tánrèyōngfèizhèng

* **infantile cough with syndrome of wind-heat invading lung** / ˈɪnfəntaɪl kɔf wɪð ˈsɪndroʊm əv wɪnd hit ɪnˈvedɪŋ lʌŋ / 小儿咳嗽·风热犯肺证 xiǎo'érkésou · fēngrèfànfèizhèng

* **infantile dementia** / ˈɪnfəntaɪl dɪˈmenʃə / 小儿痴呆 xiǎo'érchīdāi

* **infantile diarrhea** / ˈɪnfəntaɪl ˌdaɪəˈriə / 小儿泄泻 xiǎo'érxièxiè

* **infantile diarrhea with spleen deficiency syndrome** / ˈɪnfəntaɪl ˌdaɪəˈriə wɪð splin dɪˈfɪʃnsi ˈsɪndroʊm / 小儿泄泻·脾虚证 xiǎo'érxièxiè · píxūzhèng

* **infantile diarrhea with syndrome of [accumulation and binding of] damp-heat** / ˈɪnfəntaɪl ˌdaɪəˈriə wɪð ˈsɪndroʊm əv [əˌkjumjəˈleɪʃn ənd ˈbaɪndɪŋ əv] dæmp hit / 小儿泄泻·湿热蕴结证 xiǎo'ér xièxiè·shīrèyùnjiézhèng

* **infantile diarrhea with syndrome of deficiency of both qi and yin** / ˈɪnfəntaɪl ˌdaɪəˈriə wɪð ˈsɪndroʊm əv dɪˈfɪʃnsi əv boʊθ tʃi ənd jɪn / 小儿泄泻·气阴两虚证 xiǎo'érxièxiè·qìyīnliǎngxūzhèng

* **infantile diarrhea with syndrome of improper diet** / ˈɪnfəntaɪl ˌdaɪəˈriə wɪð ˈsɪndroʊm əv ɪmˈprɑpər ˈdaɪət / 小儿泄泻·伤食证 xiǎo'érxièxiè·shāngshízhèng

* **infantile diarrhea with syndrome of yang deficiency of spleen and kidney** / ˈɪnfəntaɪl ˌdaɪəˈriə wɪð ˈsɪndroʊm əv jæŋ dɪˈfɪʃnsi əv splin ənd ˈkɪdni / 小儿泄泻·脾肾阳虚证 xiǎo'érxièxiè·píshènyángxūzhèng

* **infantile diarrhea with syndrome of yin depletion and yang collapse** / ˈɪnfəntaɪl ˌdaɪəˈriə wɪð ˈsɪndroʊm əv jɪn dɪˈpliʃn ənd jæŋ kəˈlæps / 小儿泄泻·阴竭阳脱证 xiǎo'érxièxiè·yīnjiéyángtuōzhèng

* **infantile diarrhea with wind-cold syndrome** / ˈɪnfəntaɪl ˌdaɪəˈriə wɪð wɪnd koʊld ˈsɪndroʊm / 小儿泄泻·风寒证 xiǎo'érxièxiè·fēnghánzhèng

* **infantile edema with syndrome of damp retention due to spleen deficiency** / ˈɪnfəntaɪl iˈdimə wɪð ˈsɪndroʊm əv dæmp rɪˈtenʃn du tə splin dɪˈfɪʃnsi / 小儿水肿·脾虚湿困证 xiǎo'érshuǐzhǒng·píxū

shīkùnzhèng

* **infantile edema with syndrome of intermingling of wind and water** / ˈɪnfəntaɪl iˈdimə wɪð ˈsɪndroʊm əv ˌɪntəˈmɪŋglɪŋ əv wɪnd ənd wɔtər / 小儿水肿·风水相搏证 xiǎo'érshuǐzhǒng · fēngshuǐxiāngbózhèng

* **infantile edema with syndrome of internal blockade of water-poison** / ˈɪnfəntaɪl iˈdimə wɪð ˈsɪndroʊm əv ɪnˈtɜrnl blɑˈkeɪd əv ˈwɔtər ˈpɔɪzn / 小儿水肿·水毒内闭证 xiǎo'érshuǐzhǒng · shuǐdúnèibìzhèng

* **infantile edema with syndrome of internal invasion of damp-heat** / ˈɪnfəntaɪl iˈdimə wɪð ˈsɪndroʊm əv ɪnˈtɜrnl ɪnˈveɪʒn əv dæmp hit / 小儿水肿·湿热内侵证 xiǎo'érshuǐzhǒng · shīrènèiqīnzhèng

* **infantile edema with syndrome of pathogen invading heart and liver** / ˈɪnfəntaɪl iˈdimə wɪð ˈsɪndroʊm əv ˈpæθədʒən ɪnˈvedɪŋ hɑrt ənd ˈlɪvər / 小儿水肿·邪陷心肝证 xiǎo'érshuǐzhǒng · xiéxiànxīngānzhèng

* **infantile edema with syndrome of qi deficiency of lung and spleen** / ˈɪnfəntaɪl iˈdimə wɪð ˈsɪndroʊm əv tʃi dɪˈfɪʃnsi əv lʌŋ ənd splin / 小儿水肿·肺脾气虚证 xiǎo'érshuǐzhǒng · fèipíqìxūzhèng

* **infantile edema with syndrome of water qi invading heart** / ˈɪnfəntaɪl iˈdimə wɪð ˈsɪndroʊm əv ˈwɔtər tʃi ɪnˈvedɪŋ hɑrt / 小儿水肿·水气凌心证 xiǎo'érshuǐzhǒng · shuǐqìlíngxīnzhèng

* **infantile edema with syndrome of yang deficiency of spleen and kidney** / ˈɪnfəntaɪl iˈdimə wɪð

'sɪndroʊm əv jæŋ dɪ'fɪʃnsi əv splin ənd 'kɪdni / 小儿水肿 · 脾肾阳虚证 xiǎo'érshuǐzhǒng · pí shènyángxūzhèng

* **infantile edema** / 'ɪnfəntaɪl i'dimə / 小儿水肿 xiǎo'érshuǐzhǒng

* **infantile enuresis** / 'ɪnfəntaɪl ˌenjʊ'rɪsɪs / 小儿遗尿 xiǎo'éryíniào

* **infantile enuresis with syndrome of damp-heat in liver channel** / 'ɪnfəntaɪl enjʊ'rɪsɪs wɪð 'sɪndroʊm əv dæmp hit ɪn 'lɪvər 'tʃænl / 小儿遗尿 · 肝经湿热证 xiǎo'éryíniào · gānjīngshīrèzhèng

* **infantile enuresis with syndrome of incoordination between heart and kidney** / 'ɪnfəntaɪl ˌenjʊ'rɪsɪs wɪð 'sɪndroʊm əv ˌɪnkoˌɔrdn'eʃən bɪ'twin hɑrt ənd 'kɪdni / 小儿遗尿 · 心肾不交证 xiǎo'éryíniào · xīnshènbùjiāozhèng

* **infantile enuresis with syndrome of qi deficiency of lung and spleen** / 'ɪnfəntaɪl enjʊ'rɪsɪs wɪð 'sɪndroʊm əv tʃi dɪ'fɪʃnsi əv lʌŋ ənd splin / 小儿遗尿 · 肺脾气虚证 xiǎo'éryíniào · fèipíqìxūzhèng

* **infantile enuresis with syndrome of unconsolidated kidney qi** / 'ɪnfəntaɪl ˌenjʊ'rɪsɪs wɪð 'sɪndroʊm əv ˌʌnkən'sɑlɪˌdetɪd 'kɪdni tʃi / 小儿遗尿 · 肾气不固证 xiǎo'éryíniào · shènqìbùgùzhèng

* **infantile epilepsy with syndrome of damp retention due to spleen deficiency** / 'ɪnfəntaɪl 'epɪlepsi wɪð 'sɪndroʊm əv dæmp rɪ'tenʃn du tə splin dɪ'fɪʃnsi / 小儿癫 · 脾虚湿困证 xiǎo'érdiān · píxūshīkùn zhèng

* **infantile epilepsy with syndrome of deficiency of both heart and spleen** / ˈɪnfəntaɪl ˈepɪlepsi wɪð ˈsɪndroʊm əv dɪˈfɪʃnsi əv boʊθ hɑrt ənd splin / 小儿癫·心脾两虚证 xiǎo'érdiān · xīnpíliǎng xūzhèng

* **infantile frequent urination** / ˈɪnfəntaɪl ˈfrikwənt ˌjʊrɪˈneɪʃn / 小儿尿频 xiǎo'érniàopín

* **infantile frequent urination with internal heat due to yin deficiency** / ˈɪnfəntaɪl ˈfrikwənt ˌjʊrɪˈneɪʃn wɪð ɪnˈtɜrnl hit du tə jɪn dɪˈfɪʃnsi / 小儿尿频·阴虚内热证 xiǎo'érniàopín · yīnxūnèirèzhèng

* **infantile frequent urination with syndrome of qi deficiency of spleen and kidney** / ˈɪnfəntaɪl ˈfrikwənt ˌjʊrɪˈneɪʃn wɪð ˈsɪndroʊm əv tʃi dɪˈfɪʃnsi əv splin ənd ˈkɪdni / 小儿尿频·脾肾气虚证 xiǎo'érniàopín · píshènqìxūzhèng

* **infantile oral ulcer with syndrome of accumulated heat in heart and spleen** / ˈɪnfəntaɪl ˈɔrəl ˈʌlsər wɪð ˈsɪndroʊm əv əˈkjʊmjəˌletɪd hit ɪn hɑrt ənd splin / 小儿口疮·心脾积热证 xiǎo'érkǒuchuāng · xīnpíjīrèzhèng

* **infantile oral ulcer with syndrome of flaring up of heart fire** / ˈɪnfəntaɪl ˈɔrəl ˈʌlsər wɪð ˈsɪndroʊm əv ˈflɛrɪŋ ʌp əv hɑrt ˈfaɪər / 小儿口疮·心火上炎证 xiǎo'érkǒuchuāng · xīnhuǒshàngyánzhèng

* **infantile palpitation with syndrome of blockade due to heart blood stasis** / ˈɪnfəntaɪl ˌpælpɪˈteɪʃn wɪð ˈsɪndroʊm əv blɑˈkeɪd du tə hɑrt blʌd ˈsteɪsɪs / 小儿心悸·心血瘀阻证 xiǎo'érxīnjì · xīnxuèyūzǔzhèng

* **infantile palpitation with syndrome of deficiency of both heart and spleen** / ˈɪnfəntaɪl ˌpælpɪˈteɪʃn wɪð ˈsɪndroʊm əv dɪˈfɪʃnsi əv boʊθ hɑrt ənd splin / 小儿心悸·心脾两虚证 xiǎo'érxīnjì · xīnpíliǎng xūzhèng

* **infantile palpitation with syndrome of exuberant fire due to yin deficiency** / ˈɪnfəntaɪl ˌpælpɪˈteɪʃn wɪð ˈsɪndroʊm əv ɪgˈzubərənt ˈfaɪər du tə jɪn dɪˈfɪʃnsi / 小儿心悸·阴虚火旺证 xiǎo'érxīnjì · yīnxūhuǒwàng zhèng

* **infantile palpitation with syndrome of heart deficiency and timidity** / ˈɪnfəntaɪl ˌpælpɪˈteɪʃn wɪð ˈsɪndroʊm əv hɑrt dɪˈfɪʃnsi ənd tɪˈmɪdəti / 小儿心悸·心虚胆怯证 xiǎo'érxīnjì · xīnxūdǎnqièzhèng

* **infantile palpitation with syndrome of heart yang deficiency** / ˈɪnfəntaɪl ˌpælpɪˈteɪʃn wɪð ˈsɪndroʊm əv hɑrt jæŋ dɪˈfɪʃnsi / 小儿心悸·心阳虚证 xiǎo'érxīnjì · xīnyángxūzhèng

* **infantile palpitation with syndrome of water qi invading heart** / ˈɪnfəntaɪl ˌpælpɪˈteɪʃn wɪð ˈsɪndroʊm əv ˈwɔtər tʃi ɪnˈvedɪŋ hɑrt / 小儿心悸·水气凌心证 xiǎo'érxīnjì · shuǐqìlíngxīnzhèng

* **infantile palpitations** / ˈɪnfəntaɪl ˌpælpɪˈteɪʃnz / 小儿心悸 xiǎo'érxīnjì

* **infantile paralysis with syndrome of pathogen diffusing into channel-collaterals** / ˈɪnfəntaɪl pəˈræləsɪs wɪð ˈsɪndroʊm əv ˈpæθədʒən dɪˈfjuzɪŋ ˈɪntə ˈtʃænl kəˈlætərəlz / 小儿麻痹症·邪注经络证 xiǎo'érmá bìzhèng · xiézhùjīngluòzhèng

* **infantile purpura with syndrome of yang deficiency of spleen and kidney** / ˈɪnfəntaɪl ˈpɜrpjʊrə wɪð ˈsɪndroʊm əv jæŋ dɪˈfɪʃnsi əv splin ənd ˈkɪdni / 小儿紫癜·脾肾阳虚证 xiǎo'érzǐdiàn · píshèn yángxūzhèng

* **infantile strangury with syndrome of damp-heat in bladder** / ˈɪnfəntaɪl ˈstræŋgjəri wɪð ˈsɪndroʊm əv dæmp hit ɪn ˈblædər / 小儿淋证·膀胱湿热证 xiǎo'érlínzhèng · pángguāngshīrèzhèng

* **infantile summer-heat warm disease with syndrome of disharmony between nutrient and defense phases** / ˈɪnfəntaɪ ˈsʌmər hit wɔrm dɪˈziz wɪð ˈsɪndroʊm əv dɪsˈharməni bɪˈtwin ˈnutriənt ənd dɪˈfɛns ˈfesiz / 小儿暑温·营卫不和证 xiǎo'érshǔwēn · yíng wèibùhézhèng

* **infantile summer-heat warm disease with syndrome of internal heat due to yin deficiency** / ˈɪnfəntaɪ ˈsʌmər hit wɔrm dɪˈziz wɪð ˈsɪndroʊm əv ɪnˈtɜrnl hit du tə jɪn dɪˈfɪʃnsi / 小儿暑温·阴虚内热证 xiǎo'ér shǔwēn · yīnxūnèirèzhèng

* **infantile tonsillitis** / ˈɪnfəntaɪl ˌtɑnsəˈlaɪtɪs / 小儿乳蛾 xiǎo'érrǔ'é

* **infantile tonsillitis with blazing heat-toxin** / ˈɪnfəntaɪl ˌtɑnsəˈlaɪtɪs wɪð bleɪzɪŋ hit ˈtɑksɪn / 小儿乳蛾·热毒炽盛证 xiǎo'érrǔ'é · rèdúchìshèngzhèng

* **infantile tonsillitis with syndrome of intermingling of wind-heat** / ˈɪnfəntaɪl ˌtɑnsəˈlaɪtɪs wɪð ˈsɪndroʊm əv ˌɪntəˈmɪŋglɪŋ əv wɪnd hit / 小儿乳蛾·风热搏结证 xiǎo'érrǔ'é · fēngrèbójiézhèng

* **infantile tonsillitis with syndrome of yin deficiency of lung and stomach** / ˈɪnfəntaɪl tɑnsəˈlaɪtɪs wɪð ˈsɪndroʊm əv jɪn dɪˈfɪʃnsi əv lʌŋ ənd ˈstʌmək / 小儿乳蛾·肺胃阴虚证 xiǎo'érrǔ'é · fèiwèiyīn xūzhèng

* **infantile urinary turbidity** / ˈɪnfəntaɪl ˈjʊrɪneri tɜrˈbɪdəti / 小儿尿浊 xiǎo'érniàozhuó

* **infantile vomiting with syndrome of deficient cold of spleen and stomach** / ˈɪnfəntaɪl ˈvɑmɪtɪŋ wɪð ˈsɪndroʊm əv dɪˈfɪʃnt koʊld əv splin ənd ˈstʌmək / 小儿呕吐·脾胃虚寒证 xiǎo'érǒutù · píwèixūhán zhèng

* **infantile vomiting with syndrome of milk and food stagnation** / ˈɪnfəntaɪl ˈvɑmɪtɪŋ wɪð ˈsɪndroʊm əv mɪlk ənd fud stægˈneɪʃn / 小儿呕吐·乳食积滞证 xiǎo'érǒutù · rǔshíjīzhìzhèng

indigestion / ˌɪndɪˈdʒestʃən / 积滞 jīzhì

indigestion with syndrome of malnutrition due to spleen deficiency / ˌɪndɪˈdʒestʃən wɪð ˈsɪndroʊm əv ˌmælnuˈtrɪʃn du tə splin dɪˈfɪʃnsi / 积滞·脾虚夹积证 jīzhì · píxūjiájīzhèng

inextensible fist / ˌɪnɪkˈstɛnsəbl fɪst / 手拳不展 shǒu quánbùzhǎn

inextensible toes / ˌɪnɪkˈstɛnsəbl toʊs / 脚拳不展 jiǎo quánbùzhǎn

infancy / ˈɪnfənsi / 幼儿期 yòuérqī

infantile abdominal pain / ˈɪnfəntaɪl æbˈdɑmɪnl peɪn / 小儿腹痛 xiǎo'érfùtòng

infantile abdominal pain with syndrome of qi stagnation

and blood stasis / ˈɪnfəntaɪl æbˈdɑmɪnl peɪn wɪð ˈsɪndroʊm əv tʃi stæɡˈneɪʃn ənd blʌd ˈsteɪsɪs / 小儿腹痛·气滞血瘀证 xiǎo'érfùtòng · qìzhìxuè yūzhèng

infantile ancylostomiasis / ˈɪnfəntaɪl ˌænsɪˌlɑstəˈmaɪəsɪs / 小儿钩虫病 xiǎo'érgōuchóngbìng

infantile anorexia / ˈɪnfəntaɪl ˌænəˈrɛksiə / 小儿厌食 xiǎo'éryànshí

infantile anorexia with syndrome of qi deficiency of spleen and stomach / ˈɪnfəntaɪl ˌænəˈrɛksiə wɪð ˈsɪndroʊm əv tʃi dɪˈfɪʃnsi əv splin ənd ˈstʌmək / 小儿厌食·脾胃气虚证 xiǎo'éryànshí · píwèiqì xūzhèng

infantile anorexia with syndrome of yin deficiency of spleen and stomach / ˈɪnfəntaɪl ˌænəˈrɛksiə wɪð ˈsɪndroʊm əv jɪn dɪˈfɪʃnsi əv splin ənd ˈstʌmək / 小儿厌食·脾胃阴虚证 xiǎo'éryànshí · píwèiyīn xūzhèng

infantile ascariasis / ˈɪnfəntaɪl ˌæskəˈraɪəsɪs / 小儿蛔虫病 xiǎo'érhuíchóngbìng

infantile ascariasis with syndrome of accumulation of worms in intestine / ˈɪnfəntaɪl ˌæskəˈraɪəsɪs wɪð ˈsɪndroʊm əv əˌkjumjəˈleɪʃn əv wərmz ɪn ɪnˈtestɪn / 小儿蛔虫病·虫积肠道证 xiǎo'érhuíchóngbìng · chóngjīchángdàozhèng

infantile ascariasis with syndrome of qi deficiency of spleen and stomach / ˈɪnfəntaɪl ˌæskəˈraɪəsɪs wɪð ˈsɪndroʊm əv tʃi dɪˈfɪʃnsi əv splin ənd ˈstʌmək / 小儿蛔虫病·脾胃气虚证 xiǎo'érhuíchóngbìng ·

píwèiqìxūzhèng

infantile asthma / ˈɪnfəntaɪl ˈæzmə / 小儿哮喘 xiǎoʼérxiàochuǎn

infantile asthma with syndrome of failure to receive Qi due to kidney deficiency / ˈɪnfəntaɪl ˈæzmə wɪð ˈsɪndroʊm əv ˈfeɪljər tə rɪˈsiv tʃi du tə ˈkɪdni dɪˈfɪʃnsi / 小儿哮喘·肾虚不纳证 xiǎoʼérxiàochuǎn · shèn xūbúnàzhèng

infantile asthma with syndrome of intermingling of deficiency and excess / ˈɪnfəntaɪl ˈæzmə wɪð ˈsɪndroʊm əv ˌɪntəˈmɪŋglɪŋ əv dɪˈfɪʃnsi ənd ɪkˈses / 小儿哮喘·虚实夹杂证 xiǎoʼérxiàochuǎn · xūshíjiāzázhèng

infantile asthma with syndrome of spleen qi deficiency / ˈɪnfəntaɪl ˈæzmə wɪð ˈsɪndroʊm əv splin tʃi dɪˈfɪʃnsi / 小儿哮喘·脾气虚证 xiǎoʼérxiàochuǎn · píqìxūzhèng

infantile blood syncope / ˈɪnfəntaɪl blʌd ˈsɪŋkəpi / 小儿厥证·血厥 xiǎoʼérjuézhèng · xuèjué

infantile body of pure yang / ˈɪnfəntaɪl ˈbɑdi əv pjʊr jæŋ / 纯阳之体 chúnyángzhītǐ

infantile cold syncope / ˈɪnfəntaɪl koʊld ˈsɪŋkəpi / 小儿厥证·寒厥 xiǎoʼérjuézhèng · hánjué

infantile collapse / ˈɪnfəntaɪl kəˈlæps / 小儿脱证 xiǎoʼértuōzhèng

infantile collapse with syndrome of collapse of both yin and yang / ˈɪnfəntaɪl kəˈlæps wɪð ˈsɪndroʊm əv kəˈlæps əv boʊθ jɪn ənd jæŋ / 小儿脱证·阴阳两脱证 xiǎoʼértuōzhèng · yīnyángliǎngtuōzhèng

infantile collapse with syndrome of fluid depletion and yin deficiency / ˈɪnfəntaɪl kəˈlæps wɪð ˈsɪndroʊm əv ˈfluɪd dɪˈpliʃn ənd jɪn dɪˈfɪʃnsi / 小儿脱证·阴虚液脱证 xiǎo'értuōzhèng · yīnxūyètuōzhèng

infantile collapse with syndrome of sudden collapse of yangqi / ˈɪnfəntaɪl kəˈlæps wɪð ˈsɪndroʊm əv ˈsʌdn kəˈlæps əv jæŋ tʃi / 小儿脱证·阳气暴脱证 xiǎo'értuōzhèng · yángqìbàotuōzhèng

infantile common cold / ˈɪnfəntaɪl ˈkɑmən koʊld / 小儿感冒 xiǎo'érgǎnmào

infantile common cold complicated with dyspepsia / ˈɪnfəntaɪl ˈkɑmən koʊld ˈkɑmplɪkeɪtɪd wɪð dɪsˈpepʃə / 小儿感冒·夹滞 xiǎo'érgǎnmào · jiázhì

infantile common cold complicated with fright / ˈɪnfəntaɪl ˈkɑmən koʊld ˈkɑmplɪkeɪtɪd wɪð fraɪt / 小儿感冒·夹惊 xiǎo'érgǎnmào · jiájīng

infantile common cold complicated with phlegm / ˈɪnfəntaɪl ˈkɑmən koʊld ˈkɑmplɪkeɪtɪd wɪð flem / 小儿感冒·夹痰 xiǎo'érgǎnmào · jiátán

infantile common cold with syndrome of summer-heat damp invading superficies / ˈɪnfəntaɪl ˈkɑmən koʊld wɪð ˈsɪndroʊm əv ˈsʌmər hit dæmp ɪnˈvedɪŋ ˌsupəˈfɪʃɪˌiz / 小儿感冒·暑湿袭表证 xiǎo'érgǎnmào · shǔshīxíbiǎozhèng

infantile common cold with syndrome of wind-cold tightening superficies / ˈɪnfəntaɪl ˈkɑmən koʊld wɪð ˈsɪndroʊm əv wɪnd koʊld ˈtaɪtnɪŋ ˌsupəˈfɪʃɪiz / 小儿感冒 · 风寒束表证 xiǎo'érgǎnmào ·

fēnghánshùbiǎozhèng

infantile common cold with syndrome of wind-heat invading superficies / ˈɪnfəntaɪl ˈkɑmən koʊld wɪð ˈsɪndroʊm əv wɪnd hit ɪnˈvedɪŋ ˌsupəˈfɪʃɪˌiz / 小儿感冒·风热袭表证 xiǎo'érgǎnmào · fēngrèxí biǎozhèng

infantile convulsion / ˈɪnfəntaɪl kənˈvʌlʃn / 惊风 jīng fēng

infantile cough / ˈɪnfəntaɪl kɔf / 小儿咳嗽 xiǎo'ér késou

infantile cough with syndrome of lung yin deficiency / ˈɪnfəntaɪl kɔf wɪð ˈsɪndroʊm əv lʌŋ jɪn dɪˈfɪʃnsi / 小儿咳嗽·肺阴虚证 xiǎo'érkésou · fèiyīn xūzhèng

infantile cough with syndrome of phlegm-damp amassing in lung / ˈɪnfəntaɪl kɔf wɪð ˈsɪndroʊm əv flem dæmp əˈmæsɪŋ ɪn lʌŋ / 小儿咳嗽·痰湿蕴肺证 xiǎo'érkésou · tánshīyùnfèizhèng

infantile cough with syndrome of wind-cold invading lung / ˈɪnfəntaɪl kɔf wɪð ˈsɪndroʊm əv wɪnd koʊld ɪnˈvedɪŋ lʌŋ / 小儿咳嗽·风寒袭肺证 xiǎo'érkésou · fēnghánxífèizhèng

infantile crapulent syncope / ˈɪnfəntaɪl ˈkræpjulənt ˈsɪŋkəpi / 小儿厥证·食厥 xiǎo'érjuézhèng · shíjué

infantile cysticercosis / ˈɪnfəntaɪl ˌsɪstɪsəˈkosɪs / 小儿囊虫病 xiǎo'érnángchóngbìng

infantile disease due to fetal injury / ˈɪnfəntaɪl dɪˈziz du tə ˈfitl ˈɪndʒəri / 胎产损伤 tāichǎnsǔnshāng

infantile dysentery / ˈɪnfəntaɪl ˈdɪsənteri / 小儿痢疾

xiǎo'érlìji

infantile eczema / ˈɪnfəntaɪl ɪgˈzimə / 奶癣 nǎixuǎn

infantile eczema with syndrome of blood deficiency and wind-dryness / ˈɪnfəntaɪl ɪgˈzimə wɪð ˈsɪndroʊm əv blʌd dɪˈfɪʃnsi ənd wɪnd ˈdraɪnəs / 奶癣·血虚风燥证 nǎixuǎn·xuèxūfēngzàozhèng

infantile eczema with syndrome of inundated damp-heat / ˈɪnfəntaɪl ɪgˈzimə wɪð ˈsɪndroʊm əv ˈɪnəndetɪd dæmp-hit / 奶癣·湿热浸淫证 nǎixuǎn·shīrèjìnyínzhèng

infantile eczema with syndrome of lingering wind-heat / ˈɪnfəntaɪl ɪgˈzimə wɪð ˈsɪndroʊm əv ˈlɪŋgərɪŋ wɪnd hit / 奶癣·风热留恋证 nǎixuǎn·fēngrèliúliànzhèng

infantile endogenous cough / ˈɪnfəntaɪl enˈdɑdʒənəs kɔf / 小儿内伤咳嗽 xiǎo'érnèishāngkésou

infantile epilepsy with syndrome of deficiency of both liver and kidney / ˈɪnfəntaɪl ˈepɪlepsi wɪð ˈsɪndroʊm əv dɪˈfɪʃnsi əv boʊθ ˈlɪvər ənd ˈkɪdni / 小儿癫·肝肾两虚证 xiǎo'érdiān·gānshènliǎngxūzhèng

infantile epilepsy with syndrome of qi deficiency of spleen and kidney / ˈɪnfəntaɪl ˈepɪlepsi wɪð ˈsɪndroʊm əv tʃi dɪˈfɪʃnsi əv splin ənd ˈkɪdni / 小儿癫·脾肾气虚证 xiǎo'érdiān·píshènqìxūzhèng

infantile epilepsy / ˈɪnfəntaɪl ˈepɪlepsi / 小儿癫 xiǎo'érdiān

infantile exogenous cough / ˈɪnfəntaɪl ekˈsɑdʒənəs kɔf / 小儿外感咳嗽 xiǎo'érwàigǎnkésou

infantile fasciolopsiasis / ˈɪnfəntaɪl fəsiəlɔpˈsaiəsis /

小儿姜片虫病 xiǎo'érjiāngpiànchóngbìng

infantile feeding / ˈɪnfəntaɪl ˈfidɪŋ / 幼儿喂养 yòu'ér wèiyǎng

infantile filariasis / ˈɪnfəntaɪl fɪˌleərɪˈeɪsɪs / 小儿丝虫病 xiǎo'érsīchóngbìng

infantile flaccidity / ˈɪnfəntaɪl flækˈsɪdɪti / 小儿痿病 xiǎo'érwěibìng

infantile frightened epilepsy / ˈɪnfəntaɪl ˈfraɪtnd ˈepɪlepsi / 小儿惊 xiǎo'érjīng

infantile fulminant dysentery / ˈɪnfəntaɪl ˈfʌlminənt ˈdɪsənteri / 小儿疫毒痢 xiǎo'éryìdúlì

infantile fulminant dysentery with syndrome of internal blockade of pestilent toxin / ˈɪnfəntaɪl ˈfʌlminənt ˈdɪsənteri wɪð ˈsɪndroʊm əv ɪnˈtɜrnl blɑˈkeɪd əv ˈpestilənt ˈtɑksɪn / 小儿疫毒痢 · 疫毒内闭证 xiǎo'éryìdúlì · yìdúnèibìzhèng

infantile fulminant dysentery with syndrome of internal blockade and external collapse / ˈɪnfəntaɪl ˈfʌlminənt ˈdɪsənteri wɪð ˈsɪndroʊm əv ɪnˈtɜrnl blɑˈkeɪd ənd ɪkˈstɜrnl kəˈlæps / 小儿疫毒痢 · 内闭外脱证 xiǎo'éryìdúlì · nèibìwàituōzhèng

infantile heat syncope / ˈɪnfəntaɪl hit ˈsɪŋkəpi / 小儿厥证 · 热厥 xiǎo'érjuézhèng · rèjué

infantile oral ulcer / ˈɪnfəntaɪl ˈɔrəl ˈʌlsər / 小儿口疮 xiǎo'érkǒuchuāng

infantile oral ulcer with syndrome of deficiency of both qi and blood / ˈɪnfəntaɪl ˈɔrəl ˈʌlsər wɪð ˈsɪndroʊm əv dɪˈfiʃnsi əv boʊθ tʃi ənd blʌd / 小儿口疮 · 气血两虚证 xiǎo'érkǒuchuāng · qìxuè liǎngxūzhèng

infantile oral ulcer with upward floating of deficient fire / ˈɪnfəntaɪl ˈɔrəl ˈʌlsər wɪð ˈʌpwərd ˈfloʊtɪŋ əv dɪˈfɪʃnt ˈfaɪər / 小儿口疮 · 虚火上浮证 xiǎo'ér kǒuchuāng · xūhuǒshàngfúzhèng

infantile oxyuriasis / ˌɪnfəntaɪl ˌɒksɪjʊəˈraɪəsɪs / 小儿蛲虫病 xiǎo'érnáochóngbìng

infantile paralysis / ˈɪnfəntaɪl pəˈræləsɪs / 小儿麻痹症 xiǎo'érmábìzhèng

infantile paralysis with syndrome of deficiency of both liver and kidney / ˈɪnfəntaɪl pəˈræləsɪs wɪð ˈsɪndroʊm əv dɪˈfɪʃnsi əv boʊθ ˈlɪvər ənd ˈkɪdni / 小儿麻痹症 · 肝肾两虚证 xiǎo'érmábìzhèng · gānshènliǎngxūzhèng

infantile paralysis with syndrome of pathogen stagnated in lung and stomach / ˈɪnfəntaɪl pəˈræləsɪs wɪð ˈsɪndroʊm əv ˈpæθədʒən ˈstæɡneɪtɪd ɪn lʌŋ ənd ˈstʌmək / 小儿麻痹症 · 邪郁肺胃证 xiǎo'érmábìzhèng · xiéyùfèiwèizhèng

infantile paralysis with syndrome of qi deficiency and blood stasis / ˈɪnfəntaɪl pəˈræləsɪs wɪð ˈsɪndroʊm əv tʃi dɪˈfɪʃnsi ənd blʌd ˈsteɪsɪs / 小儿麻痹症 · 气虚血瘀证 xiǎo'érmábìzhèng · qìxūxuèyūzhèng

infantile phlegm epilepsy / ˈɪnfəntaɪl flem ˈepɪlepsi / 小儿痰 xiǎo'értán

infantile phlegm syncope / ˈɪnfəntaɪl flem ˈsɪŋkəpi / 小儿厥证 · 痰厥 xiǎo'érjuézhèng · tánjué

infantile proctoptosis / ˈɪnfəntaɪl prɒktɒp ˈtəʊsɪs / 小儿脱肛 xiǎo'értuōgāng

infantile purpura / ˈɪnfəntaɪl ˈpɜrpjʊrə / 小儿紫癜 xiǎo'érzǐdiàn

infantile purpura with syndrome of blood-heat injuring collaterals / ˈɪnfəntaɪl ˈpɜrpjʊrə wɪð ˈsɪndroʊm əv blʌd hit ˈɪndʒərɪŋ kəˈlætərəlz / 小儿紫癜·血热伤络证 xiǎo'érzǐdiàn · xuèrèshāngluòzhèng

infantile purpura with syndrome of exuberant fire due to yin deficiency / ˈɪnfəntaɪl ˈpɜrpjʊrə wɪð ˈsɪndroʊm əv ɪgˈzubərənt ˈfaɪər du tə jɪn dɪˈfɪʃnsi / 小儿紫癜·阴虚火旺证 xiǎo'érzǐdiàn · yīnxūhuǒwàngzhèng

infantile purpura with syndrome of failure of qi to keep blood / ˈɪnfəntaɪl ˈpɜrpjʊrə wɪð ˈsɪndroʊm əv ˈfeɪljər əv tʃi tə kip blʌd / 小儿紫癜·气不摄血证 xiǎo'érzǐdiàn · qìbùshèxuèzhèng

infantile purpura with syndrome of qi stagnation and blood stasis / ˈɪnfəntaɪl ˈpɜrpjʊrə wɪð ˈsɪndroʊm əv tʃi stægˈneɪʃn ənd blʌd ˈsteɪsɪs / 小儿紫癜·气滞血瘀证 xiǎo'érzǐdiàn · qìzhìxuèyūzhèng

infantile purpura with syndrome of wind-heat disturbing collaterals / ˈɪnfəntaɪl ˈpɜrpjʊrə wɪð ˈsɪndroʊm əv wɪnd hit dɪˈstɜrbɪŋ kəˈlætərəlz / 小儿紫癜·风热扰络证 xiǎo'érzǐdiàn · fēngrèrǎoluòzhèng

infantile qi syncope / ˈɪnfəntaɪl tʃi ˈsɪŋkəpi / 小儿厥证·气厥 xiǎo'érjuézhèng · qìjué

infantile scarlet fever / ˈɪnfəntaɪl ˈskarlət ˈfivər / 小儿烂喉丹痧 xiǎo'érlànhóudānshā

infantile scarlet fever with syndrome of blazing heat in both qi and nutrient phases / ˈɪnfəntaɪl ˈskarlət ˈfivər wɪð ˈsɪndroʊm əv bleɪzɪŋ hit ɪn boʊθ tʃi

ənd ˈnutriənt ˈfesiz / 小儿烂喉丹痧·气营两燔证
xiǎo'érlànhóudānshā · qìyíngliǎngfánzhèng

infantile scarlet fever with syndrome of pathogen invading lung-defense phase / ˈɪnfəntaɪl ˈskarlət ˈfivər wɪð ˈsɪndroʊm əv pæθədʒən ɪnˈveɪdɪŋ lʌŋ dɪˈfens feɪz / 小儿烂喉丹痧·邪侵肺卫证
xiǎo'érlànhóudānshā · xiéqīnfèiwèizhèng

infantile scarlet fever with syndrome of yin injury after pathogen subsidence / ˈɪnfəntaɪl ˈskarlət ˈfivər wɪð ˈsɪndroʊm əv jɪn ˈɪndʒəri ˈaftər ˈpæθədʒən səbˈsaɪdns / 小儿烂喉丹痧·邪退阴伤证
xiétuìyīnshāngzhèng

infantile schistosomiasis / ˈɪnfəntaɪl ˌskɪstəsoˈmaɪəsɪs / 小儿血吸虫病 xiǎo'érxuèxīchóngbìng

infantile strangury / ˈɪnfəntaɪl ˈstræŋgjəri / 小儿淋证
xiǎo'érlínzhèng

infantile strangury with syndrome of qi deficiency of spleen and kidney / ˈɪnfəntaɪl ˈstræŋgjəri wɪð ˈsɪndroʊm əv tʃi dɪˈfɪʃnsi əv splin ənd ˈkɪdni / 小儿淋证·脾肾气虚证 xiǎo'érlínzhèng · píshèn qìxūzhèng

infantile summer-heat warm disease / ˈɪnfəntaɪl ˈsʌmər hit wɔrm dɪˈziz / 小儿暑温 xiǎo'érshǔwēn

infantile summer-heat warm disease with syndrome of blazing heat in both qi and nutrient phases / ˈɪnfəntaɪl ˈsʌmər hit wɔrm dɪˈziz wɪð ˈsɪndroʊm əv ˈbleɪzɪŋ hit ɪn boʊθ tʃi ənd ˈnutriənt ˈfesiz / 小儿暑温·气营两燔证 xiǎo'érshǔwēn · qìyíng liǎngfánzhèng

infantile summer-heat warm disease with syndrome of heat invading nutrient and blood phases / ˈɪnfəntaɪl ˈsʌmər hit wɔrm dɪˈziz wɪð ˈsɪndroʊm əv hit ɪnˈvedɪŋ ˈnutriənt ənd blʌd ˈfesiz / 小儿暑温·热入营血证 xiǎo'érshǔwēn·rèrùyíngxuèzhèng

infantile summer-heat warm disease with syndrome of internal blockade and external collapse / ˈɪnfəntaɪl ˈsʌmər hit wɔrm dɪˈziz wɪð ˈsɪndroʊm əv ɪnˈtɜrnl blaˈkeɪd ənd ɪkˈstɜrnl kəˈlæps / 小儿暑温·内闭外脱证 xiǎo'érshǔwēn·nèibìwàituōzhèng

infantile summer-heat warm disease with syndrome of internal disturbance of phlegm-fire / ˈɪnfəntaɪl ˈsʌmər hit wɔrm dɪˈziz wɪð ˈsɪndroʊm əv ɪnˈtɜrnl dɪ ˈstɜrbəns əv flem ˈfaɪər / 小儿暑温·痰火内扰证 xiǎo'érshǔwēn·tánhuǒnèirǎozhèng

infantile summer-heat warm disease with syndrome of internal stirring of liver wind / ˈɪnfəntaɪl ˈsʌmər hit wɔrm dɪˈziz wɪð ˈsɪndroʊm əv ɪnˈtɜrnl ˈstɜrɪŋ əv ˈlɪvər wɪnd / 小儿暑温·肝风内动证 xiǎo'érshǔwēn·gānfēngnèidòngzhèng

infantile summer-heat warm disease with syndrome of involving both defense and qi phases / ˈɪnfəntaɪl ˈsʌmər hit wɔrm dɪˈziz wɪð ˈsɪndroʊm əv ɪnˈvalvɪŋ boʊθ dɪˈfɛns ənd tʃi ˈfesiz / 小儿暑温·卫气同病证 xiǎo'érshǔwēn·wèiqìtóngbìngzhèng

infantile summer-heat warm disease with syndrome of phlegm clouding clear orifices / ˈɪnfəntaɪl ˈsʌmər hit wɔrm dɪˈziz wɪð ˈsɪndroʊm əv flem ˈklaudɪŋ klɪr 'ɔrəfɪsɪz / 小儿暑温·痰蒙清窍证 xiǎo'érshǔwēn · tánméngqīngqiàozhèng

infantile summer-heat warm disease with syndrome of qi deficiency and blood stasis / 'ɪnfəntaɪl 'sʌmər hit wɔrm dɪ'ziz wɪð 'sɪndroʊm əv tʃi dɪ'fɪʃnsi ənd blʌd 'steɪsɪs / 小儿暑温·气虚血瘀证 xiǎo'érshǔwēn · qìxūxuèyūzhèng

infantile summer-heat warm disease with syndrome of wind pathogen stagnating in collaterals / 'ɪnfəntaɪl 'sʌmər hit wɔrm dɪ'ziz wɪð 'sɪndroʊm əv wɪnd 'pæθədʒən 'stægneɪtɪŋ ɪn kə'lætərəlz / 小儿暑温·风邪留络证 xiǎo'érshǔwēn · fēngxiéliúluòzhèng

infantile syncope / 'ɪnfəntaɪl 'sɪŋkəpi / 小儿厥证 xiǎo'érjuézhèng

infantile taeniasis / 'ɪnfəntaɪl ti'naɪəsɪs / 小儿绦虫病 xiǎo'értāochóngbìng

infantile venule of index finger / 'ɪnfəntaɪl 'vɛnjʊl əv 'ɪndeks 'fɪŋgər / 小儿指纹 xiǎo'érzhǐwén

infantile vomiting / 'ɪnfəntaɪl 'vɑmɪtɪŋ / 小儿呕吐 xiǎo'érǒutù

infantile vomiting with syndrome of exogenous pathogen invading stomach / 'ɪnfəntaɪl 'vɑmɪtɪŋ wɪð 'sɪndroʊm əv ek'sɑdʒənəs 'pæθədʒən ɪn'vedɪŋ 'stʌmək / 小儿呕吐·外邪犯胃证 xiǎo'érǒutù · wàixiéfànwèizhèng

infantile vomiting with syndrome of liver qi invading stomach / 'ɪnfəntaɪl 'vɑmɪtɪŋ wɪð 'sɪndroʊm əv 'lɪvər tʃi ɪn'vedɪŋ 'stʌmək / 小儿呕吐·肝气犯胃

证 xiǎo'érǒutù · gānqìfànwèizhèng

infantile vomiting with syndrome of stomach heat and qi counter-flowing / ˈɪnfəntaɪl ˈvɑmɪtɪŋ wɪð ˈsɪndroʊm əv ˈstʌmək hit ənd tʃi ˈkaʊntər ˈfloɪŋ / 小儿呕吐 · 胃热气逆证 xiǎo'érǒutù · wèirèqìnìzhèng

infantile wind epilepsy / ˈɪnfəntaɪl wɪnd ˈepɪlepsi / 小儿风 xiǎo'érfēng

infantile yang edema / ˈɪnfəntaɪl jæŋ ɪˈdimə / 小儿阳水 xiǎo'éryángshuǐ

infantile yin edema / ˈɪnfəntaɪl jɪn ɪˈdimə / 小儿阴水 xiǎo'éryīnshuǐ

insufficiency of natural endowment / ˌɪnsəˈfɪʃənsi əv ˈnætʃrəl ɪnˈdaʊmənt / 禀赋不足 bǐngfùbùzú

keen visceral qi / kin ˈvɪsərəl tʃi / 脏气清灵 zàngqì qīnglíng

kidney gan disease / ˈkɪdni gæn dɪˈziz / 肾疳 shèngān

lack of neonatal meconium / læk əv ˌnioʊˈneɪtl məˈkonɪəm / 初生大便不通 chūshēngdàbiànbù tōng

liver gan disease / ˈlɪvər gæn dɪˈziz / 肝疳 gāngān

lung gan disease / lʌŋ gæn dɪˈziz / 肺疳 fèigān

measles / ˈmizlz / 麻疹 mázhěn

measles with syndrome of exuberant heat in lung and stomach / ˈmizlz wɪð ˈsɪndroʊm əv ɪgˈzubərənt hit ɪn lʌŋ ənd ˈstʌmək / 麻疹 · 肺胃热盛证 má zhěn · fèiwèirèshèngzhèng

measles with syndrome of lung blocked by pathogenic toxin / mizlz wɪð ˈsɪndrəʊm əv lʌŋ blakt baɪ

ˌpæθəˈdʒenɪk ˈtɒksɪn / 麻疹·邪毒闭肺证 má zhěn·xiédúbìfèizhèng

measles with syndrome of pathogen invading lung defense phase / ˈmizlz wɪð ˈsɪndroʊm əv ˈpæθədʒən ɪnˈveɪdɪŋ lʌŋ dɪˈfɛns feɪz / 麻疹·邪犯肺卫证 mázhěn·xiéfànfèiwèizhèng

measles with syndrome of pathogenic toxin attacking throat / mizlz wɪð ˈsɪndrəʊm əv ˌpæθəˈdʒenɪkɪŋ ˈtɒksɪn əˈtækɪŋ θrəʊt / 麻疹·邪毒攻喉证 mázhěn·xiédúgōnghóuzhèng

measles with syndrome of toxin invading heart and liver / mizlz wɪð ˈsɪndrəʊm əv ˈtɒksɪn ɪnˈveɪdɪŋ hart ənd ˈlɪvər / 麻疹·毒陷心肝证 mázhěn·dúxiànxīngānzhèng

measles with syndrome of yin injury after pathogen subsidence / ˈmizlz wɪð ˈsɪndroʊm əv jɪn ˈɪndʒəri ˈaftər ˈpæθədʒən səbˈsaɪdns / 麻疹·邪退阴伤证 mázhěn·xiétuìyīnshāngzhèng

metopism / ˈmetəˌpɪzəm / 解颅 jiělú

metopism with syndrome of congestion and stagnation of heat-toxin / ˈmetəˌpɪzəm wɪð ˈsɪndroʊm əv kənˈdʒestʃən ənd stægˈneɪʃn əv hit ˈtɒksɪn / 解颅·热毒壅滞证 jiělú·rèdúyōngzhìzhèng

metopism with syndrome of kidney qi deficiency / ˈmetəˌpɪzəm wɪð ˈsɪndroʊm əv ˈkɪdni tʃi dɪˈfɪʃnsi / 解颅·肾气虚证 jiělú·shènqìxūzhèng

metopism with syndrome of spleen deficiency and liver hyperactivity / ˈmetəˌpɪzəm wɪð ˈsɪndroʊm əv splin dɪˈfɪʃnsi ənd ˈlɪvər ˌhaɪpərækˈtɪvəti / 解

颅 · 脾虚肝旺证 jiělú · píxūgānwàngzhèng

metopism with syndrome of water overflowing due to spleen deficiency / ˈmetəˌpɪzəm wɪð ˈsɪndroʊm əv ˈwɔtər ˌəʊvəˈfloʊɪŋ du tə splin dɪˈfɪʃnsi / 解颅 · 脾虚水泛证 jiělú · píxūshuǐfànzhèng

mild gan disease / maɪld gæn dɪˈziz / 疳气 gānqì

mixed feeding / mɪkst ˈfidɪŋ / 混合喂养 hùnhéwèiyǎng

mumps / mʌmps / 痄腮 zhàsai

mumps with accumulation and binding of warm-toxin syndrome / mʌmps wɪð əˌkjumjəˈleɪʃn ənd ˈbaɪndɪŋ əv wɔrm ˈtaksɪn ˈsɪndroʊm / 痄腮 · 温毒蕴结证 zhàsai · wēndúyùnjiézhèng

mumps with syndrome of pathogen invading heart and liver / mʌmps wɪð ˈsɪndroʊm əv pæˈθədʒən ɪnˈveɪdɪŋ hart ənd ˈlɪvər / 痄腮 · 邪陷心肝证 zhà sai · xiéxiànxīngānzhèng

mumps with syndrome of warm-toxin invading superficies / mʌmps wɪð ˈsɪndroʊm əv wɔrm ˈtaksɪn ɪnˈvedɪŋ ˌsʊpəˈfɪʃɪiz / 痄腮 · 温毒袭表证 zhàsai · wēndúxíbiǎozhèng

mumps with toxin attacking testes / mʌmps wɪð ˈtɑksɪn əˈtækɪŋ ˈtestiz / 痄腮 · 毒窜睾腹证 zhà sai · dúcuàngāofùzhèng

* **neonatal pneumonia with syndrome of wind-heat invading lung** / ˌnioʊˈneɪtl nuˈmoʊniə wɪð ˈsɪndroʊm əv wɪnd hit ɪnˈvedɪŋ lʌŋ / 新生儿肺炎 · 风热犯肺证 xīnshēng'érfèiyán · fēngrèfànfèizhèng

* **nocturnal crying with syndrome of accumulated heat in Heart Channel** / nɑkˈtɜrnl kraɪɪŋ wɪð ˈsɪndroʊm əv əˈkjʊmjəˌleɪtɪd hit ɪn hɑrt ˈtʃænl / 夜啼·心经积热证 yètí · xīnjīngjīrèzhèng

* **nocturnal crying with syndrome of spleen deficiency and cold attack** / nɑkˈtɜrnl kraɪɪŋ wɪð ˈsɪndroʊm əv splin dɪˈfɪʃnsi ənd koʊld əˈtæk / 夜啼·脾虚中寒证 yètí · píxūzhōnghánzhèng

neonatal adiposis / ˌnioʊˈneɪtl ˌædiˈpəʊsis / 胎肥 tāiféi

neonatal anal blockade / ˌnioʊˈneɪtl ˈeɪnl blɑˈkeɪd / 初生肛门内合 chūshēnggāngménnèihé

neonatal anuria / ˌnioʊˈneɪtl əˈnjʊəriə / 初生小便不通 chūshēngxiǎobiànbùtōng

neonatal cold / ˌnioʊˈneɪtl koʊld / 胎寒 tāihán

neonatal fetal mass / ˌnioʊˈneɪtl ˈfitl mæs / 胎瘤 tāiliú

neonatal fever / ˌnioʊˈneɪtl ˈfivər / 胎热 tāirè

neonatal lockjaw / ˌnioʊˈneɪtl ˈlɑkdʒɔ / 初生口噤 chūshēngkǒujìn

neonatal mammary nodule / ˌnioʊˈneɪtl ˈmæməri ˈnɑdʒul / 初生乳核 chūshēngrǔhé

neonatal pneumonia / ˌnioʊˈneɪtl nuˈmoʊniə / 新生儿肺炎 xīnshēng'érfèiyán

neonatal pneumonia with syndrome of lung heat and blood stasis / ˌnioʊˈneɪtl nuˈmoʊniə wɪð ˈsɪndroʊm əv lʌŋ hit ənd blʌd ˈsteɪsɪs / 新生儿肺炎·肺热血瘀证 xīnshēng'érfèiyán · fèirèxuèyūzhèng

neonatal pneumonia with syndrome of wind-cold invading lung / ˌnioʊˈneɪtl nuˈmoʊniə wɪð ˈsɪndroʊm əv wɪnd koʊld ɪnˈvedɪŋ lʌŋ / 新生儿肺炎·风寒袭肺证 xīnshēng'érfèiyán · fēnghánxífèizhèng

neonatal stage / ˌniouˈneɪtl steɪdʒ / 新生儿期 xīn shēng'érqī

neonatal vaginal bleeding / ˌniouˈneɪtl vəˈdʒaɪnl ˈblidɪŋ / 初生女婴阴道出血 chūshēngnǚyīngyīndàochūxuè

newborn asphyxia / ˈnubɔrn æsˈfɪksɪə / 初生不啼 chū shēngbùtí

nocturnal crying / nɑkˈtɜrnl kraɪɪŋ / 夜啼 yètí

nocturnal crying with syndrome of fright injuring spirit / nɑkˈtɜrnl kraɪɪŋ wɪð ˈsɪndroum əv fraɪt ˈɪndʒərɪŋ ˈspɪrɪt / 夜啼·惊恐伤神证 yètí · jīngkǒngshāng shénzhèng

noma / ˈnəumə / 走马疳 zǒumǎgān

oral gan disease / ˈɔrəl gæn dɪˈziz / 口疳 kǒugān

over growth of skull / ˈouvər grouθ əv skʌl / 头围增长过速 tóuwéizēngzhǎngguòsù

＊ **pneumonia with dyspneic cough with syndrome of phlegm-heat congesting lung** / nuˈmouniə wɪð dɪsˈpnik kɔf wɪð ˈsɪndroum əv flem hit kənˈdʒɛstɪŋ lʌŋ / 肺炎喘嗽·痰热壅肺证 fèiyán chuǎnsòu · tánrèyōngfèizhèng

＊ **pneumonia with dyspneic cough with syndrome of qi deficiency of lung and spleen** / nuˈmouniə wɪð dɪsˈpnik kɔf wɪð ˈsɪndroum əv tʃi dɪˈfɪʃənsi əv lʌŋ ənd splin / 肺炎喘嗽·肺脾气虚证 fèiyán chuǎnsòu · fèipíqìxūzhèng

＊ **pneumonia with dyspneic cough with syndrome of wind-heat invading lung** / nuˈmouniə wɪð dɪsˈpnik kɔf wɪð ˈsɪndroum əv wɪnd hit ɪnˈvedɪŋ lʌŋ / 肺炎喘嗽·风热犯肺证 fèiyánchuǎnsòu · fēngrè fànfèizhèng

* **pneumonia with dyspneic cough with syndrome of yin deficiency and lung heat** / nuˈmoʊniə wɪð dɪsˈpnik kɔf wɪð ˈsɪndroʊm əv jɪn dɪˈfɪʃənsi ənd lʌŋ hit / 肺炎喘嗽·阴虚肺热证 fèiyánchuǎnsòu · yīnxūfèirèzhèng

parasitic abdominal mass / ˌpærəˈsɪtɪk æbˈdɑmɪnl mæs / 虫瘕 chóngjiǎ

paroxia / pəˈrɒksɪr / 嗜异 shìyì

pigeon breast / ˈpɪdʒɪn brest / 鸡胸 jīxiōng

pneumonia with dyspneic cough / nuˈmoʊniə wɪð dɪsˈpnik kɔf / 肺炎喘嗽 fèiyánchuǎnsòu

pneumonia with dyspneic cough with syndrome of heart yang exhaustion / nuˈmoʊniə wɪð dɪsˈpnik kɔf wɪð ˈsɪndroʊm əv hɑrt jæŋ ɪgˈzɔstʃən / 肺炎喘嗽·心阳虚衰证 fèiyánchuǎnsòu · xīnyángxūshuāizhèng

pneumonia with dyspneic cough with syndrome of pathogen invading Jueyin / nuˈmoʊniə wɪð dɪsˈpnik kɔf wɪð ˈsɪndroʊm əv ˈpæθədʒən ɪnˈvedɪŋ dʒuəjɪn / 肺炎喘嗽·邪陷厥阴证 fèiyánchuǎnsòu · xiéxiànjuéyīnzhèng

pneumonia with dyspneic cough with syndrome of wind-cold invading lung / nuˈmoʊniə wɪð dɪsˈpnik kɔf wɪð ˈsɪndroʊm əv wɪnd koʊld ɪnˈvedɪŋ lʌŋ / 肺炎喘嗽·风寒袭肺证 fèiyánchuǎnsòu · fēnghánxífèizhèng

posterior fontanel / pɑˈstɪriər ˌfɒntəˈnel / 后囟 hòuxìn

premature closure of fontanel / ˌprɪməˈtʃʊr ˈkloʊʒər əv ˌfɒntəˈnel / 囟门早闭 xìnménzǎobì

preschool stage / ˈpriskul steɪdʒ / 学龄前期 xuélíng qiánqī

protracted tongue / prəˈtræktɪd tʌŋ / 舌纵 shézòng

protruding tongue / prouˈtrudɪŋ tʌŋ / 吐舌 tǔshé

puberty / ˈpjubərti / 青春期 qīngchūnqī

quiescent stage of infantile epilepsy / kwiˈesnt steɪdʒ əv ˈɪnfəntaɪl ˈepɪlepsi / 小儿癫·休止期 xiǎo'érdiān· xiūzhǐqī

* **regular case of infantile diarrhea** / ˈregjələr keɪs əv ˈɪnfəntaɪl ˌdaɪəˈriə / 小儿泄泻·常证 xiǎo'érxiè xiè·chángzhèng

* **regular case of infantile edema** / ˈregjələr keɪs əv ˈɪnfəntaɪl iˈdimə / 小儿水肿·常证 xiǎo'érshuǐ zhǒng·chángzhèng

* **rickets with syndrome of qi deficiency of lung and spleen** / ˈrɪkɪts wɪð ˈsɪndroum əv tʃi dɪˈfɪʃnsi əv lʌŋ ənd splin / 佝偻病·肺脾气虚证 gōulóubìng· fèipíqìxūzhèng

* **thrush with syndrome of accumulated heat in heart and spleen** / θrʌʃ wɪð ˈsɪndroum əv əˈkjumjəˌletɪd hit ɪn hart ənd splin / 鹅口疮·心脾积热证 é'kǒu chuāng·xīnpíjīrèzhèng

red buttock / red ˈbʌtək / 臀红 túnhóng

regular case of mumps / ˈregjələr keɪs əv mʌmps / 痄腮·常证 zhàsai·chángzhèng

regular case of pneumonia with dyspneic cough / ˈregjələr keɪs əv nuˈmouniə wɪð dɪsˈpnik kɔf / 肺炎喘嗽·常证 fèiyánchuǎnsòu·chángzhèng

remitting stage of infantile asthma / rɪˈmɪtɪŋ steɪdʒ əv 'ɪnfəntaɪl 'æzmə / 小儿哮喘 · 缓解期 xiǎo'érxiào chuǎn · huǎnjiěqī

retardation in hair growth / ˌritɑr'deɪʃn ɪn her groʊθ / 发迟 fàchí

retardation in speaking / ˌritɑr'deɪʃn ɪn 'spikɪŋ / 语迟 yǔchí

retardation in standing / ˌritɑr'deɪʃn ɪn 'stændɪŋ / 立迟 lìchí

retardation in tooth eruption / ˌritɑr'deɪʃn ɪn tuθ ɪ'rʌpʃn / 齿迟 chǐchí

retardation in walking / ˌritɑr'deɪʃn ɪn 'wɔkɪŋ / 行迟 xíngchí

retraction of testes in newborn / rɪ'trækʃn əv 'testiz ɪn 'nubɔrn / 初生肾缩 chūshēngshènsuō

rickets / 'rɪkɪts / 佝偻病 gōulóubìng

rickets with syndrome of qi deficiency of spleen and kidney / 'rɪkɪts wɪð 'sɪndroʊm əv tʃi dɪ'fɪʃnsi əv splin ənd 'kɪdni / 佝偻病 · 脾肾气虚证 gōulóubìng · píshènqìxūzhèng

rickets with syndrome of spleen deficiency and liver hyperactivity / 'rɪkɪts wɪð 'sɪndroʊm əv splin dɪ'fɪʃnsi ənd 'lɪvər ˌhaɪpəræk'tɪvəti / 佝偻病 · 脾虚肝旺证 gōulóubìng · píxūgānwàngzhèng

rickets with syndrome of yin deficiency of liver and kidney / 'rɪkɪts wɪð 'sɪndroʊm əv jɪn dɪ'fɪʃnsi əv lɪvər ənd 'kɪdni / 佝偻病 · 肝肾阴虚证 gōulóubìng · gānshènyīnxūzhèng

rigid swollen tongue / 'rɪdʒɪd 'swoʊlən tʌŋ / 木舌 mùshé

roseola infantum / roʊzi'oʊlə ɪn'fæntəm / 奶麻 nǎimá

roseola infantum with syndrome of pathogen diffusing into muscles and skin / rouziˈoulə inˈfæntəm wɪð ˈsɪndroʊm əv pæθədʒən dɪˈfjuzɪŋ ˌɪntə ˈmʌslz ənd skɪn / 奶麻 · 邪透肌肤证 nǎimá · xiétòujīfūzhèng

roseola infantum with syndrome of pathogen stagnated in lung and stomach / rouziˈoulə inˈfæntəm wɪð ˈsɪndroʊm əv pæθədʒən ˈstæɡneɪtɪd ɪn lʌŋ ənd ˈstʌmək / 奶麻 · 邪郁肺胃证 nǎimá · xiéyùfèiwèizhèng

rubella / ruˈbelə / 风疹 fēngzhěn

rubella with syndrome of blazing heat in both qi and nutrient phases / ruˈbelə wɪð ˈsɪndroʊm əv bleɪzɪŋ hit ɪn boʊθ tʃi ənd ˈnutriənt ˈfesiz / 风疹 · 气营两燔证 fēngzhěn · qìyíngliǎngfánzhèng

rubella with syndrome of internal exuberance of pathogenic toxin / ruˈbelə wɪð ˈsɪndroʊm əv ɪnˈtɜrnl ɪɡˈzubərəns əv ˌpæθəˈdʒenɪk ˈtaksɪn / 风疹 · 邪毒内盛证 fēngzhěn · xiédúnèishèngzhèng

rubella with syndrome of pathogen invading lung-defense phase / ruˈbelə wɪð ˈsɪndroʊm əv pæθədʒən ɪnˈveɪdɪŋ lʌŋ dɪˈfɛns feɪz / 风疹 · 邪犯肺卫证 fēngzhěn · xiéfànfèiwèizhèng

school stage / skul steɪdʒ / 学龄期 xuélíngqī

scleredema neonatorum / sklɪrɪˈdimə niɒnæˈtɔrʌm / 新生儿硬肿病 xīnshēng'éryìngzhǒngbìng

scleredema neonatorum of cold congelation and blood stasis / sklɪrɪˈdimə niɒnæˈtɔrʌm əv koʊld ˌkɑndʒəˈleʃən ənd blʌd ˈsteɪsɪs / 新生儿硬肿病 · 寒凝血瘀

证 xīnshēng'éryìngzhǒngbìng · hánníngxuè
yūzhèng

scleredema neonatorum of yang qi exhaustion
/ sklɪrɪ'dimə nɪɒnæ'tɔrʌm əv jæŋ tʃi ɪg'zɔstʃən /
新生儿硬肿病 · 阳气虚衰证 xīnshēng'éryìng
zhǒngbìng · yángqìxūshuāizhèng

seizure stage of infantile epilepsy / 'siʒər steɪdʒ əv
'ɪnfəntaɪl 'epɪlepsi / 小儿癫 · 发作期 xiǎo'ér
diān · fāzuòqī

severe gan disease / sɪ'vɪr gæn dɪ'ziz / 干疳 gāngān

sexual prematurity / 'sekʃuəl primə'tjʊrəti / 性早熟
xìngzǎoshú

**sexual prematurity with syndrome of exuberant fire due
to yin deficiency** / 'sekʃuəl primə'tjʊrəti wɪð
'sɪndroʊm əv ɪg'zubərənt 'faɪər du tə jɪn dɪ'fɪʃnsi /
性早熟 · 阴虚火旺证 xìngzǎoshú · yīnxūhuǒ
wàngzhèng

**sexual prematurity with syndrome of liver depression
transforming into fire** / 'sekʃuəl primə'tjʊrəti wɪð
'sɪndroʊm əv 'lɪvər dɪ'preʃn træns'fɔmɪŋ 'ɪntə
'faɪər / 性早熟 · 肝郁化火证 xìngzǎoshú · gān
yùhuàhuǒzhèng

skin erosion in newborn / skɪn ɪ'rəʊʒn ɪn 'nubɔrn / 初
生无皮 chūshēngwúpí

smallpox / 'smɔlpɑks / 天花 tiānhuā

spinal pinching / 'spaɪnl pɪntʃɪŋ / 捏脊 niējǐ

spinal pushing / 'spaɪnl pʊʃɪŋ / 推脊 tuījǐ

spleen gan disease / splin gæn dɪ'ziz / 脾疳 pígān

static blood epilepsy / 'stætɪk blʌd 'epɪlepsi / 小儿瘀

血 xiǎo'éryūxuè

steaming changes in infant / ˈstimɪŋ tʃendʒz ɪn ˈɪnfənt /
变蒸 biànzhēng

stiff flesh / stɪf fleʃ / 肉硬 ròuyìng

stiff foot / stɪf fʊt / 足硬 zúyìng

stiff hand / stɪf hænd / 手硬 shǒuyìng

stiff loin / stɪf lɔɪn / 腰硬 yāoyìng

stiff neck / stɪf nek / 颈硬 jǐngyìng

sudden frightening in infant / ˈsʌdn ˈfraɪtnɪŋ ɪn ˈɪnfənt /
客忤 kèwǔ

summer fever / ˈsʌmər ˈfivər / 夏季热 xiàjìrè

summer fever with summer heat injuring lung and stomach / ˈsʌmər ˈfivər wɪð ˈsʌmər hit inˈʃuəɪɪŋ lʌŋ ənd ˈstʌmək / 夏季热·暑伤肺胃证 xiàjìrè·shǔshāngfèiwèizhèng

summer fever with syndrome of upper excess and lower deficiency / ˈsʌmər ˈfivər wɪð ˈsɪndroʊm əv ˈʌpər ɪkˈses ənd ˈloʊər dɪˈfɪʃnsi / 夏季热·上盛下虚证 xiàjìrè·shàngshèngxiàxūzhèng

summer non-acclimatization in infant / ˈsʌmər nɑn əˌklaɪmətəˈzeɪʃn ɪn ˈɪnfənt / 小儿疰夏 xiǎo'érzhùxià

summer non-acclimatization in infant with syndrome of dampness retaining in spleen and stomach / ˈsʌmər nɑn əˌklaɪmətəˈzeɪʃn ɪn ˈɪnfənt wɪð ˈsɪndroʊm əv ˈdæmpnəs rɪˈteɪnɪŋ ɪn splin ənd ˈstʌmək / 小儿疰夏·湿困脾胃证 xiǎo'érzhùxià·shīkùnpíwèizhèng

summer non-acclimatization in infant with syndrome of qi deficiency of spleen and stomach / ˈsʌmər nɑn əˌklaɪmətəˈzeɪʃɪn ɪn ˈɪnfənt wɪð ˈsɪndroʊm əv tʃi dɪˈfɪʃnsi əv splin ənd ˈstʌmək / 小儿疰夏·脾胃气虚证 xiǎo'érzhùxià · píwèiqìxūzhèng

sunken fontanel / ˈsʌŋkən ˌfɑntəˈnel / 囟门下陷 xìn ménxiàxiàn

swollen gums / ˈswoʊlən gʌmz / 重龈 chóngyín

swollen upper palate / ˈswoʊlən ʌpər ˈpælət / 重腭 chóng'è

tender yang / ˈtendər jæŋ / 稚阳 zhìyáng

tender yin / ˈtendər jɪn / 稚阴 zhìyīn

tense fontanel / tens ˌfɔntəˈnel / 囟门紧张 xìnménjǐn zhāng

tetanus neonatorum / ˈtetnəs niɒnæˈtɔrʌm / 脐风 qífēng

tetanus neonatorum with channel-collateral blockage syndrome / ˈtetnəs niɒnæˈtɔrʌm wɪð ˈtʃænl kəˈlætərəl ˈblɑkɪdʒ ˈsɪndroʊm / 脐风·经络闭阻证 qífēng · jīngluòbìzǔzhèng

tetanus neonatorum with syndrome of pathogenic toxin attacking Zang-viscera / ˈtetnəs niɒnæˈtɔrʌm wɪð ˈsɪndroʊm əv ˌpæθəˈdʒenɪk ˈtɑksɪn əˈtækɪŋ zæŋ-ˈvɪsərə / 脐风·邪毒中脏证 qífēng · xiédúzhòng zàngzhèng

thrush / θrʌʃ / 鹅口疮 ékǒuchuāng

thrush with syndrome of heat-toxin attacking throat / θrʌʃ wɪð ˈsɪndroʊm əv hit ˈtɑksɪn əˈtækɪŋ θroʊt / 鹅口疮·热毒攻喉证 ékǒuchuāng · rè dúgōnghóuzhèng

thrush with upward floating of deficient fire / θrʌʃ wɪð ˈʌpwərd ˈfloʊtɪŋ əv dɪˈfɪʃnt ˈfaɪər / 鹅口疮·虚火

上浮证 ékǒuchuāng · xūhuǒshàngfúzhèng

trembling tongue / ˈtrɛmblɪŋ tʌŋ / 舌颤 shéchàn

umbilical bleeding / ʌmˈbɪlɪkl ˈblidɪŋ / 脐血 qíxuè

umbilical dampness / ʌmˈbɪlɪkl ˈdæmpnəs / 脐湿 qíshī

umbilical hernia / ʌmˈbɪlɪkl ˈhɜrniə / 脐突 qítū

umbilical sore / ʌmˈbɪlɪkl sɔr / 脐疮 qíchuāng

umbilical swelling / ʌmˈbɪlɪkl ˈswelɪŋ / 脐肿 qízhǒng

unable to suck in newborn / ʌnˈeɪbl tə sʌk ɪn ˈnubɔrn /
初生不乳 chūshēngbùrǔ

unfavorable case of measles / ʌnˈfevrəbl keɪs əv ˈmizlz /
麻疹 · 逆证 mázhěn · nìzhèng

vaccination / ˌvæksəˈneʃən / 预防接种 yùfángjiēzhòng

varicella / ˌværəˈsɛlə / 水痘 shuǐdòu

varicella with syndrome of blazing heat-toxin
/ ˌværəˈsɛlə wɪð ˈsɪndroʊm əv bleɪzɪŋ hit ˈtaksɪn /
水痘 · 热毒炽盛证 shuǐdòu · rèdúchìshèngzhèng

varicella with syndrome of pathogen stagnated in lung-defense phase / ˌværəˈsɛlə wɪð ˈsɪndroʊm əv
pæθədʒən ˈstæɡneɪtɪd ɪn lʌŋ dɪˈfɛns feɪz / 水痘 ·
邪郁肺卫证 shuǐdòu · xiéyùfèiwèizhèng

venule going through all passes to reach nail / ˈvɛnjʊl
ˈɡoʊɪŋ θru ɔl ˈpasiz tə ritʃ neɪl / 透关射甲 tòu
guānshèjiǎ

vomiting ascaris / ˈvɑmɪtɪŋ ˈæskəris / 吐蛔 tǔhuí

vulnerable to manifestation of deficiency and excess
/ ˈvʌlnərəbl tə ˌmænɪfeˈsteɪʃn əv dɪˈfɪʃnsi ənd
ɪkˈses / 易虚易实 yìxūyìshí

vulnerable to manifestation of heat and cold / ˈvʌlnərəbl
tə ˌmænɪfeˈsteɪʃn əv hit ənd koʊld / 易寒易热 yìhányìrè

* **whooping cough with syndrome of qi deficiency of lung and spleen** / ˈhupiŋ kɔf wɪð ˈsɪndroʊm əv tʃi dɪˈfɪʃnsi əv lʌŋ ənd splin / 顿咳·肺脾气虚证 dùn ké·fèipíqìxūzhèng

wandering erysipelas / ˈwɑndərɪŋ ˌeriˈsipiləs / 赤游丹 chìyóudān

wandering erysipelas with syndrome of toxin invading heart and liver / ˈwɑndərɪŋ ˌeriˈsipiləs wɪð ˈsɪndroʊm əv ˈtɑksɪn ɪnˈvedɪŋ hɑrt ənd ˈlɪvər / 赤游丹·毒传心肝证 chìyóudān·dúchuánxīngānzhèng

wandering erysipelas with syndrome of toxin invading muscle and skin / ˈwɑndərɪŋ ˌeriˈsipiləs wɪð ˈsɪndroʊm əv ˈtɑksɪn ɪnˈvedɪŋ ˈmʌsl ənd skɪn / 赤游丹·毒在肌肤证 chìyóudān·dúzàijīfūzhèng

whooping cough / ˈhupiŋ kɔf / 顿咳 dùnké

whooping cough with syndrome of lung yin deficiency / ˈhupiŋ kɔf wɪð ˈsɪndroʊm əv lʌŋ jɪn dɪˈfɪʃnsi / 顿咳·肺阴虚证 dùnké·fèiyīnxūzhèng

whooping cough with syndrome of pathogen invading lung-defense phase / ˈhupiŋ kɔf wɪð ˈsɪndroʊm əv pæθədʒən ɪnˈveidɪŋ lʌŋ dɪˈfɛns feɪz / 顿咳·邪犯肺卫证 dùnké·xiéfànfèiwèizhèng

whooping cough with syndrome of phlegm-fire blocking lung / ˈhupiŋ kɔf wɪð ˈsɪndroʊm əv flem ˈfaɪər ˈblakɪŋ lʌŋ / 顿咳·痰火阻肺证 dùnké·tánhuǒzǔfèizhèng

widened fontanel / ˈwaɪdnd ˌfɔntəˈnel / 囟门宽大 xìnménkuāndà

wry tongue / raɪ tʌŋ / 舌歪 shéwāi

Chapter 12   The Five Sense Organs of Traditional Chinese Medicine

第十二章　中医五官科学

Section 1　Eye Diseases

第一节　眼　病

conjunctival follicle / ˌkɒndʒʌŋkˈtaɪvə ˈfɑlɪkl / 粟疮 sùchuāng

conjunctival lithiasis / ˌkɒndʒʌŋkˈtaɪvə lɪˈθaɪəsɪs / 睑内结石 jiǎnnèijiéshí

ectropion / ɛkˈtropɪən / 胞睑外翻 bāojiǎnwàifān

erysipelas of eyelid / ɛrɪˈsɪpələs əv ˈaɪlɪd / 眼丹 yǎndān

eyelid disease / ˈaɪlɪd dɪˈziz / 胞睑病 bāojiǎnbìng

frequent nictitation / ˈfrikwənt ˌnɪktɪˈteɪʃən / 目劄 mùzhá

hordeolum / hɔrˈdiələm / 针眼 zhēnyǎn

phlegmatic nodule in eyelid / fleɡˈmætɪk ˈnɑdʒul ɪn ˈaɪlɪd / 胞生痰核 bāoshēngtánhé

ptosis of eyelid / ˈtosɪs əv ˈaɪlɪd / 上胞下垂 shàngbāoxiàchuí

puffiness of eyelid / ˈpʌfinəs əv ˈaɪlɪd / 胞虚如球 bāoxūrúqiú

red ulcerated eyelid / red ˈʌlsəreɪtɪd ˈaɪlɪd / 睑弦赤烂 jiǎnxiánchìlàn

severe inflammatory edema of eyelid / sɪˈvɪr ɪnˈflæmə

tɔri iˈdimə əv ˈaɪlɪd / 胞肿如桃 bāozhǒngrútáo

sticking of cornea and eyelid / stɪkɪŋ əv ˈkɔrni ənd ˈaɪlɪd / 胞肉粘轮 bāoròuzhānlún

trachoma / trəˈkomə / 沙眼 shāyǎn

trichiasis and entropion / trɪˈkaɪəsɪs ənd ɛnˈtropɪˌɑn / 倒睫拳毛 dǎojiéquánmáo

twitching of eyelid / ˈtwɪtʃɪŋ əv ˈaɪlɪd / 胞轮振跳 bāolúnzhèntiào

vesiculated dermatitis of eyelid / vɪˈsɪkjʊˌleɪtɪd ˌdɜrməˈtaɪtɪs əv ˈaɪlɪd / 风赤疮痍 fēngchìchuāngyí

acute dacryocystitis / əˈkjut ˌdækriausisˈtaitis / 漏睛疮 lòujīngchuāng

canthus disease / ˈkænθəs dɪˈziz / 眦病 zìbìng

cold tear / koʊld ˈtir / 冷泪 lěnglèi

cold tear induced by wind / koʊld ˈtir ɪnˈdjʊst baɪ wɪnd / 迎风冷泪 yíngfēnglěnglèi

constant cold tear / ˈkɑnstənt koʊld ˈtir / 无时冷泪 wúshílěnglèi

constant epiphora / ˈkɑnstənt ɪˈpɪfərə / 无时冷泪 wúshílěnglèi

dacryocystitis / ˌdækriausisˈtaitis / 漏睛 lòujīng

pterygium / təˈrɪdʒɪəm / 胬肉攀睛 nǔròupānjīng

red vessels invading white eye / red ˈvɛslz ɪnˈvedɪŋ waɪt aɪ / 赤脉传睛 chìmàichuánjīng

blue sclera / blu ˈsklɪrə / 白睛青蓝 báijīngqīnglán

constant eye itching / ˈkɑnstənt aɪ ˈɪtʃɪŋ / 时复目痒 shífùmùyǎng

disease of white eye / dɪˈziz əv waɪt aɪ / 白睛病 bái

jīngbìng

dry astringent eye / draɪ əˈstrɪndʒənt aɪ / 白涩症 bái sèzhèng

epidemic red eye / ˌepɪˈdemɪk red aɪ / 天行赤眼 tiān xíngchìyǎn

epidemic red eye with acute nebula / ˌepɪˈdemɪk red aɪ wɪð əˈkjut ˈnebjələ / 天行赤眼暴翳 tiānxíngchì yǎnbàoyì

fire malnutrition of eye / ˈfaɪər ˌmælnuˈtrɪʃn əv aɪ / 火疳 huǒgān

golden malnutrition of eye / ˈɡoʊldən ˌmælnuˈtrɪʃn əv aɪ / 金疳 jīngān

hemorrhagic white eye / ˈhemərædʒɪk waɪt aɪ / 白睛溢血 báijīngyìxuè

sudden wind and invading fever / ˈsʌdn wɪnd ənd ɪnˈvedɪŋ ˈfivər / 暴风客热 bàofēngkèrè

coagulated fatty nebula / koʊˈæɡjuleɪtid ˈfæti ˈnebjələ / 凝脂翳 níngzhīyì

cornea disease / ˈkɔrniə dɪˈziz / 黑睛病 hēijīngbìng

crab eye / kræb aɪ / 蟹睛 xièjīng

keratohelcosis / kerætoʊˈhelkəʊsɪs / 花翳白陷 huāyì báixiàn

malnutrition of eye / ˌmælnuˈtrɪʃn əv aɪ / 疳积上目 gānjīshàngmù

mixed nebula / mɪkst ˈnebjələ / 混睛障 hùnjīng zhàng

old nebula / oʊld ˈnebjələ / 宿翳 xiǔyì

petal nebula / ˈpetl ˈnebjələ / 花翳白陷 huāyìbáixiàn

prolapse of red membrane / ˈproʊlæps əv red ˈmembreɪn / 赤膜下垂 chìmóxiàchuí

red wind wheel / red wɪnd wil / 风轮赤豆 fēnglún chìdòu

starred nebula / stɑd ˈnebjələ / 聚星障 jùxīngzhàng

upward rushing of yellow fluid / ˈʌpwərd ˈrʌʃɪŋ əv ˈjeloʊ ˈfluɪd / 黄液上冲 huángyèshàngchōng

vascular nebula / ˈvæskjələr ˈnebjələ / 血翳包睛 xuèyìbāojīng

white membrane invading eye / waɪt ˈmembreɪn ɪnˈvedɪŋ aɪ / 白膜侵睛 báimóqīnjīng

blue blindness / blu ˈblaɪndnəs / 青盲 qīngmáng

blue wind glaucoma / blu wɪnd glaʊˈkoʊmə / 青风内障 qīngfēngnèizhàng

blurred vision / blɜrd ˈvɪʒn / 视瞻昏渺 shìzhānhūnmiǎo

congenital cataract / kənˈdʒenɪtl ˈkætərækt / 胎患内障 tāihuànnèizhàng

dry defective pupil / draɪ dɪˈfektɪv ˈpjupl / 瞳神干缺 tóngshéngànquē

fog moving into eye / fɑg ˈmuvɪŋ ˈɪntə aɪ / 云雾移睛 yúnwùyíjīng

green wind glaucoma / grin wɪnd glaʊˈkoʊmə / 绿风内障 lǜfēngnèizhàng

hyphema and vitreous hemorrhage / haiˈfimə ənd ˈvɪtriə ˈhɛmərɪdʒ / 血灌瞳神 xuèguàntóngshén

papillary seclusion / pəˈpɪləri sɪˈkluʒn / 瞳神紧小 tóngshénjǐnxiǎo

pupil disease / ˈpjupl dɪˈziz / 瞳神病 tóngshénbìng

senile cataract / ˈsinaɪl ˈkætərækt / 圆翳内障 yuányì nèizhàng

sparrow eye / ˈspæroʊ aɪ / 高风雀目 gāofēngquèmù

straight things seen as crooked / streɪt θɪŋz sin əz ˈkrʊkɪd / 视直如曲 shìzhírúqǔ

sudden visual loss / ˈsʌdn ˈvɪʒuəl lɔs / 暴盲 bàománg

contusion of palpebra / kənˈtuʒn əv ˈpælpəbrə / 振胞瘀痛 zhènbāoyūtòng

eye injured by acid and alkali / aɪ ˈɪndʒərd baɪ ˈæsɪd ənd ˈælkəlaɪ / 酸碱伤目 suānjiǎnshāngmù

eye injured by overheat / aɪ ˈɪndʒərd baɪ ˌoʊvərˈhit / 热烫伤目 rètàngshāngmù

foreign body in eye / ˈfɔrən ˈbɑdi ɪn aɪ / 异物入目 yìwùrùmù

ocular contusion / ˈɑkjələr kənˈtuʒn / 撞击伤目 zhuàngjīshāngmù

traumatic cataract / trəˈmætɪk ˈkætərækt / 惊震内障 jīngzhènnèizhàng

traumatic injury of lens / trəˈmætɪk ˈɪndʒəri əv lenz / 物损真睛 wùsǔnzhēnjīng

Section 2   Ear Diseases
第二节　耳　病

acute retroauricular lymphadenitis / əˈkjut retroʊjuˈrɪkjʊlə lɪmˌfædɪˈnaɪtɪs / 耳根毒 ěrgēndú

blocked ear / blɑkt ɪr / 耳闭 ěrbì

catarrhal otitis media / kəˈtɑrəl oʊˈtaɪtɪs ˈmidiə / 耳胀

ěrzhàng

ceruminal ear / sɪˈrumɪnəl ɪr / 耵耳 dīng'ěr

chronic deafness / ˈkrɑnɪk ˈdefnəs / 久聋 jiǔlóng

deafness / ˈdefnəs / 耳闭 ěrbì

deafness-mutism / ˈdefnəs ˈmjutɪzəm / 聋哑 lóngyǎ

ear disease / ɪr dɪˈziz / 耳病 ěrbìng

ear furuncle / ɪr ˈfjʊərʌŋk(ə)l / 耳疖 ěrjiē

ear polyp / ɪr ˈpɑlɪp / 耳蕈 ěrxùn

exogenous cold pathogenic disease with yellowish ear / ekˈsɑdʒənəs koʊld ˌpæθəˈdʒenɪk dɪˈziz wɪð ˈjeloʊɪʃ ɪr / 黄耳伤寒 huáng'ěrshānghán

facial hemiparalysis due to purulent ear / ˈfeɪʃl hemɪpɑˈrələsɪs du tə ˈpjʊrələnt ɪr / 脓耳口眼歪斜 nóng'ěrkǒuyǎnwāixié

foreign body in ear / ˈfɔrən ˈbɑdi ɪn ɪr / 异物入耳 yìwùrù'ěr

high fever otitis media / haɪ ˈfivər oʊˈtaɪtɪs ˈmidiə / 黄耳伤寒 huáng'ěrshānghán

Meniere's syndrome / meinˈjɛərz ˈsɪndroʊm / 耳眩晕 ěrxuànyūn

otitis media / oʊˈtaɪtɪs ˈmidiə / 耵耳 dīng'ěr

phlegm cover auricle / flem ˈkʌvər ˈɔrɪkl / 耳壳痰包 ěrkétánbāo

phlegmatic nodule of auricle / flegˈmætɪk ˈnɑdʒul əv ˈɔrɪkl / 耳壳痰包 ěrkétánbāo

purulent ear lead to wry mouth and eye / ˈpjʊrələnt ɪr lid tə raɪ maʊθ ənd ɪr / 脓耳口眼歪斜 nóng'ěrkǒuyǎnwāixié

sore of external auditory meatus / sɔr əv ɪkˈstɜrnl ˈɔdətɔri mɪˈeɪtəs / 耳疮 ěrchuāng

sore severing auricle / sɔr ˈsɛvərɪŋ ˈɔrɪkl / 断耳疮 duàn'ěrchuāng

sudden hearing loss / ˈsʌdn ˈhɪrɪŋ lɔs / 暴聋 bàolóng

suppurative otitis media / ˈsʌpjʊəretɪv oʊˈtaɪtɪs ˈmidiə / 脓耳 nóng'ěr

swollen ear / ˈswoʊlən ɪr / 耳胀 ěrzhàng

Section 3 Nasal Diseases
第三节 鼻 病

acute and chronic sinusitis / əˈkjut ənd ˈkrɑnɪk ˌsaɪnəˈsaɪtɪs / 鼻渊 bíyuān

allergic rhinitis / əˈlɜrdʒɪk raɪˈnaɪtɪs / 鼻鼽 bíqiú

atrophic rhinitis / əˈtrɑfɪk raɪˈnaɪtɪs / 鼻槁 bígǎo

carcinoma of nasopharynx / ˌkɑrsɪˈnoʊmə əv ˌnezoˈfærɪŋks / 颃颡岩 hángsǎngyán

hematoma of nose / ˌhɛməˈtomə əv noʊz / 鼻血瘤 bíxuèliú

injury of nose / ˈɪndʒəri əv noʊz / 鼻损伤 bísǔnshāng

lingering nasal-sore / ˈlɪŋgərɪŋ ˈneɪzl sɔr / 鼻疳 bígān

nasal blockade / ˈneɪzl blɑˈkeɪd / 鼻窒 bízhì

nasal diseases / ˈneɪzl dɪˈziz / 鼻病 bíbìng

nasal furunculosis / ˈneɪzl fjʊˌrʌnkjəˈlosɪs / 鼻疔 bídīng

nasal malnutrition / ˈneɪzl ˌmælnuˈtrɪʃn / 鼻疳 bígān

nasal polyp / ˈneɪzl ˈpɑlɪp / 鼻息肉 bíxīròu

phlegmatic mass in nasal sinus / flegˈmætɪk mæs ɪn

'neɪzl 'saɪnəs / 鼻窦痰包 bídòutánbāo

withered nose / 'wɪðərd noʊz / 鼻槁 bígǎo

Section 4　Throat Diseases

第四节　咽　喉　病

* acute nippled moth / ə'kjut nɪpəld mɔθ / 急乳蛾 jírǔ'é

* acute tonsillitis / ə'kjut ˌtɑnsə'laɪtɪs / 急乳蛾 jírǔ'é

abscess of throat pass / 'æbses əv θroʊt pæs / 喉关痈 hóuguānyōng

abscess of upper palate / 'æbses əv 'ʌpər 'pælət / 上腭痈 shàng'èyōng

acute hoarseness / ə'kjut 'hɔrsnəs / 急喉喑 jíhóuyīn

acute laryngeal infection / ə'kjut lə'rɪndʒɪəl ɪn'fekʃn / 急喉风 jíhóufēng

acute pharyngitis / ə'kjut ˌfærɪn'dʒaɪtɪs / 急喉痹 jíhóubì

acute throat obstruction / ə'kjut θroʊt əb'strʌkʃn / 急喉痹 jíhóubì

* chronic nippled moth / 'krɑnɪk nɪpəld mɔθ / 慢乳蛾 mànrǔ'é

* chronic tonsillitis / 'krɑnɪk ˌtɑnsə'laɪtɪs / 慢乳蛾 mànrǔ'é

carcinoma of larynx / ˌkɑrsɪ'noʊmə əv 'lærɪŋks / 喉菌 hóujūn

carcinoma of pharynx / ˌkɑrsɪ'noʊmə əv 'færɪŋks / 咽菌 yānjūn

chronic hoarseness / 'krɑnɪk 'hɔrsnəs / 慢喉喑 mànhóuyīn

chronic pharyngitis / 'krɑnɪk ˌfærɪn'dʒaɪtɪs / 慢喉痹

mànhóubì

chronic throat obstruction / ˈkrɑnɪk θroʊt əbˈstrʌkʃn / 慢喉痹 mànhóubì

globus hysterics / gˈləʊbʌs hɪˈsterɪks / 梅核气 méihéqì

hoarseness / ˈhɔrsnəs / 喉喑 hóuyīn

laryngeal foreign body / ləˈrɪndʒɪəl ˈfɔrən ˈbɑdi / 异物梗喉 yìwùgěnghóu

laryngeal polypus / ləˈrɪndʒɪəl ˈpɑlɪpəs / 喉息肉 hóuxīròu

lingering dysphonia / ˈlɪŋgərɪŋ dɪsˈfəʊnɪə / 久喑 jiǔyīn

membranous pharyngitis / ˈmembrənəs ˌfærɪnˈdʒaɪtɪs / 喉癣 hóuxuǎn

* **nippled moth** / nɪpəld mɔθ / 乳蛾 rǔ'é

peritonsillar abscess / ˌperiˈtɔnsɪlə ˈæbses / 喉关痈 hóuguānyōng

pharyngitis / ˌfærɪnˈdʒaɪtɪs / 喉痹 hóubì

postpartum dysphonia / ˌpostˈpɑrtəm dɪsˈfəʊnɪə / 产后喑 chǎnhòuyīn

retropharyngeal abscess / retrəʊfəˈrɪndʒɪəl ˈæbses / 里喉痈 lǐhóuyōng

stony moth / ˈstoʊni mɔθ / 石蛾 shí'é

stony tonsillitis / ˈstoʊni ˌtɑnsəˈlaɪtɪs / 石蛾 shí'é

submandibular abscess / ˌsʌbmænˈdibjulə ˈæbses / 颌下痈 héxiàyōng

sudden loss of voice / ˈsʌdn lɔs əv vɔɪs / 暴喑 bàoyīn

* **tonsillitis** / ˌtɑnsəˈlaɪtɪs / 乳蛾 rǔ'é

throat abscess / θroʊt ˈæbses / 喉痈 hóuyōng

throat coughing / θroʊt ˈkɔfɪŋ / 喉咳 hóuké

throat disease / θroʊt dɪˈziz / 咽喉病 yānhóubìng

throat obstruction / θroʊt əbˈstrʌkʃn / 喉痹 hóubì

throat tinea / θroʊt ˈtɪnɪə / 喉癣 hóuxuǎn

tumor of throat / ˈtjʊmə əv θroʊt / 喉瘤 hóuliú

Section 5　Diseases of Mouth and Teeth

第五节　口　齿　病

ankyloglossia / ˌæŋkələuˈglɔsiə / 结连舌 jiéliánshé

carcinoma of cheek / ˌkɑrsɪˈnoʊmə əv tʃik / 腮岩 sāiyán

carcinoma of gum / ˌkɑrsɪˈnoʊmə əv gʌm / 牙岩 yáyán

dental caries / ˈdentl ˈkeriz / 龋齿 qǔchǐ

disease of mouth and teeth / dɪˈziz əv maʊθ ənd tiθ / 口齿病 kǒuchǐbìng

double tongue / ˈdʌbl tʌŋ / 重舌 chóngshé

exfoliative inflammation of lips / eksˈfəʊlɪətɪv ˌɪnflə ˈmeɪʃn əv lɪps / 唇风 chúnfēng

gingival abscess / dʒɪnˈdʒaɪvl ˈæbses / 牙痈 yáyōng

gingival atrophy / dʒɪnˈdʒaɪvl ˈætrəfi / 牙宣 yáxuān

gingival malnutrition / dʒɪnˈdʒaɪvl ˌmælnuˈtrɪʃn / 牙疳 yágān

gum abscess / gʌm ˈæbses / 牙咬痈 yáyǎoyōng

hematoma of uvula / ˌhɛmэˈtomə əv ˈjuvjələ / 飞扬喉 fēiyánghóu

jaw wind / dʒɔ wɪnd / 齿槽风 chǐcáofēng

labial wind / ˈleɪbiəl wɪnd / 唇风 chúnfēng

lip cancer / lɪp ˈkænsər / 唇菌 chúnjūn

noma / ˈnəʊmə / 走马牙疳 zǒumǎyágān

oral aphthae / ˈɔrəl ˈæfθi / 口疮（病）kǒuchuāng
（bìng）

phlegmatic mass in mouth and tongue / flegˈmætɪk
mæs ɪn maʊθ ənd tʌŋ / 口舌痰包 kǒushétánbāo

salivary stone / ˈsæləveri stoʊn / 涎石 xiánshí

sialolith / saiˈæləliθ / 涎石 xiánshí

sublingual swollen tongue / sʌbˈlɪŋgwəl ˈswoʊlən tʌŋ /
重舌 chóngshé

tie up tongue / taɪ ʌp tʌŋ / 结连舌 jiéliánshé

tongue carcinoma / tʌŋ ˌkɑrsɪˈnoʊmə / 舌菌 shéjūn

ulcerative gingivitis / ˈʌlsərətɪv ˌdʒɪndʒɪˈvaɪtɪs / 牙疳
yágān

Appendix

附　录

1. International Classification of Diseases 11th Edition(ICD – 11)(Tradilional Medicine Chapter)

一、国际疾病分类第十一次修订本
（ICD – 11）（传统医药章节）

L1 – SA0 Traditional medicine disorders 传统医学疾病（TM1）

　L2 – SA0 Organ system disorders 脏腑系统疾病(TM1)

　L3 – SA0 Liver system disorders 肝系病类(TM1)

　　SA00 Hypochondrium pain disorder 胁痛(TM1)

　　SA01 Jaundice disorder 黄疸(TM1)

　　SA02 Liver distension disorder 肝著(TM1)

　　SA03 Tympanites disorder 鼓胀(TM1)

　　SA04 Liver abscess disorder 肝痈(TM1)

　　SA05 Gallbladder distension disorder 胆胀(TM1)

　　SA0Y Other specified liver system disorders 其他特指的肝系病类(TM1)

　　SA0Z Liver system disorders, unspecified 未特指的肝系病类(TM1)

　L3 – SA1 Heart system disorders 心系病类(TM1)

　　L4 –SA1 Palpitation disorders 心悸(TM1)

　　SA10 Inducible palpitation disorder 惊悸(TM1)

　　SA11 Spontaneous palpitation disorder 怔忡(TM1)

　　SA1Y Other specified palpitation disorders 其他特指的心悸(TM1)

　　SA1Z Palpitation disorders, unspecified 未特指的心悸(TM1)

L4-SA2 Chest impediment disorders 胸痹(TM1)

SA20 True heart pain disorder 真心痛(TM1)

SA2Y Other specified chest impediment disorders 其他
特指的胸痹(TM1)

SA2Z Chest impediment disorders, unspecified 未特指
的胸痹(TM1)

SA4Y Other specified heart system disorders 其他特指
的心系病类(TM1)

SA4Z Heart system disorders, unspecified 未特指的心
系病类(TM1)

L3-SA5 Spleen system disorders 脾系病类(TM1)

SA50 Dysphagia disorder 噎膈(TM1)

SA51 Stomach ache disorder 胃脘痛(TM1)

SA52 Epigastric distension disorder 胃胀(TM1)

SA53 Epigastric upset disorder 嘈杂(TM1)

SA54 Food retention disorder 食积(TM1)

SA55 Diarrhea disorder 泄泻(TM1)

SA56 Dysentery disorder 痢疾(TM1)

SA57 Constipation disorder 便秘(TM1)

SA58 Abdominal pain disorder 腹痛(TM1)

SA59 Intestinal abscess disorder 肠痈(TM1)

SA5Y Other specified spleen system disorders 其他特
指的脾系病类(TM1)

SA5Z Spleen system disorders, unspecified 未特指的
脾系病类(TM1)

L3-SA6 Lung system disorders 肺系病类(TM1)

SA60 Common cold disorder 感冒(TM1)

L4-SA7 Cough disorders 咳嗽(TM1)

SA70 Cough with dyspnea disorder 咳逆(TM1)

SA7Y Other specified cough disorders 其他特指的咳嗽
(TM1)

SA7Z Cough disorders, unspecified 未特指的咳嗽（TM1）

SA80 Dyspnea disorder 喘证（TM1）

SA81 Wheezing disorder 哮病（TM1）

SA82 Lung distension disorder 肺胀（TM1）

SA83 Pleural fluid retention disorder 悬饮（TM1）

SA84 Lung heat disorder 肺热病（TM1）

SA85 Lung withering disorder 肺痿（TM1）

SA86 Chest bind disorder 结胸（TM1）

SA8Y Other specified lung system disorders 其他特指的肺系病类（TM1）

SA8Z Lung system disorders, unspecified 未特指的肺系病类（TM1）

L3–SA9 Kidney system disorders 肾系病类（TM1）

L4–SA9 Strangury disorders 淋证（TM1）

SA90 Stony stranguria disorder 石淋（TM1）

SA91 Heat stranguria disorder 热淋（TM1）

SA9Y Other specified strangury disorders 其他特指的淋证（TM1）

SA9Z Strangury disorders, unspecified 未特指的淋证（TM1）

SB00 Kidney stagnation disorder 肾著（TM1）

SB01 Flooding urine disorder 尿崩（TM1）

SB02 Enuresis disorder 遗尿（TM1）

SB03 Turbid urine disorder 尿浊（TM1）

SB04 Dribbling urinary block disorder 癃闭（TM1）

SB05 Block and repulsion disorder 关格（TM1）

SB06 Edema disorders 水肿（TM1）

SB06. 0 Kidney edema disorders 肾水（TM1）

SB06. 1 Wind edema disorders 风水（TM1）

SB06. Y Other specified edena disorders 其他特指的水

肿(TM1)

SB06. Z Edema disorders, unspecified 未特指的水肿
(TM1)

SB07 Lower abdominal colic disorder 疝气(TM1)

SB08 Premature ejaculation disorder 早泄(TM1)

SB09 Involuntary ejaculation disorder 遗精(TM1)

SB0A Persistent erection disorder 阳强(TM1)

SB0B Impotence disorder 阳痿(TM1)

SB0C Male Infertility disorder 不育(TM1)

SB0Y Other specified kidney system disorders 其他特
指的肾系病类(TM1)

SB0Z Kidney system disorders, unspecified 未特指的
肾系病类(TM1)

SB2Y Other specified organ system disorders 其他特指
的脏腑系统疾病(TM1)

SB2Z Organ system disorders, unspecified 未特指的脏
腑系统疾病(TM1)

L2-SB3 Other body system disorders 其他身体系统疾病
(TM1)

L3-SB3 Skin and mucosa system disorders 皮肤黏膜系统
病类(TM1)

SB30 Dampness sore disorder 湿疮(TM1)

SB31 Impetigo disorder 黄水疮(TM1)

L4-SB4 Furuncle disorders 疔疮(TM1)

SB40 Septicemic furunculosis disorder 疔疮走黄
(TM1)

SB4Y Other specified furuncle disorders 其他特指的疔
疮(TM1)

SB4Z Furuncle disorders, unspecified 未特指的疔疮
(TM1)

SB50 Bed sore disorder 褥疮(TM1)

L4 – SB6 Abscess disorders 痈证(TM1)

SB60 Deep multiple abscess disorder 流注(TM1)

SB61 Anal abscess disorder 肛痈(TM1)

SB6Y Other specified abscess disorders 其他特指的痈证(TM1)

SB6Z Abscess disorders, unspecified 未特指的痈证(TM1)

SB70 Headed carbuncle disorder 疽证(TM1)

SB71 Foot dampness itch disorder 脚湿气(TM1)

SB72 Tinea circinate disorder 圆癣(TM1)

SB73 Dry skin disorder 蛇皮癣(TM1)

SB74 Gangrene disorder 脱疽(TM1)

SB75 Wart disorder 疣(TM1)

SB76 Hand dampness itch disorder 鹅掌风(TM1)

SB77 Erysipelas disorder 丹毒(TM1)

SB78 Cellulitis disorder 发证(TM1)

SB79 Thrush disorder 鹅口疮(TM1)

SB7A Herpes zoster disorder 蛇串疮(TM1)

SB7B Interior haemorroid disorder 内痔(TM1)

SB7C Fissured anus disorder 肛裂(TM1)

SB7Y Other specified skin and mucosa system disorders 其他特指的皮肤黏膜系统病类(TM1)

SB7Z Skin and mucosa system disorders, unspecified 未特指的皮肤黏膜系统病类(TM1)

L3–SB8 Female reproductive system disorders (including childbirth) 女性生殖系统(包括分娩)病类(TM1)

L4–SB8 Menstruation associated disorders 月经病类(TM1)

L5–SB8 Menstruation cycle disorders 月经周期病(TM1)

SB80 Advanced menstruation disorder 月经先期(TM1)

SB81 Delayed menstruation disorder 月经后期(TM1)

SB82 Irregular menstruation disorders 月经先后无定期 (TM1)

SB8Y Other specified menstruation cycle disorders 其他特指的月经周期病(TM1)

SB8Z Menstruation cycle disorders, unspecified 未特指的月经周期病(TM1)

SB90 Menorrhagia disorder 月经过多(TM1)

SB91 Decreased menstruation disorder 月经过少 (TM1)

SB92 Prolonged menstruation disorder 经期延长(TM1)

SB93 Metrorrhagia disorder 崩漏(TM1)

SB94 Amenorrhea disorder 闭经(TM1)

SB95 Menopausal disorder 绝经前后诸症(TM1)

SB96 Dysmenorrhea disorder 痛经(TM1)

SB9Y Other specified menstruation associated disorders 其他特指的月经病类(TM1)

SB9Z Menstruation associated disorders, unspecified 未特指的月经病类(TM1)

L4 – SC0 Pregnancy associated disorders 妊娠病类 (TM1)

SC00 Morning sickness disorder 恶阻(TM1)

SC01 Unstable fetus disorder 胎动不安(TM1)

SC02 Bladder pressure disorder 转胞(TM1)

SC03 Eclampsia disorder 子痫(TM1)

SC04 Floating sensation pregnancy disorder 子悬 (TM1)

SC0Y Other specified pregnancy associated disorders 其他特指的妊娠病类(TM1)

SC0Z Pregnancy associated disorders, unspecified 未特指的妊娠病类(TM1)

L4 – SC1 Puerperium associated disorders 产后病类 (TM1)

SC10 Puerperal abdominal pain disorder 儿枕痛 (TM1)

SC11 Puerperal wind disorder 产后风(TM1)

SC12 Hypogalactia disorder 缺乳(TM1)

SC13 Postpartum lochiorrhea disorder 恶露不绝(TM1)

SC1Y Other specified puerperium associated disorders 其他特指的产后病类(TM1)

SC1Z Puerperium associated disorders, unspecified 未特指的产后病类(TM1)

L4–SC2 Other female reproductive system associated disorders 其他女性生殖系统病类(TM1)

SC20 Leukorrhea disorder 带下病(TM1)

SC21 Vaginal flatus disorder 阴吹(TM1)

SC22 Infertility disorder 不孕(TM1)

SC23 Uterine mass disorder 石瘕(TM1)

SC24 Breast lump disorder 乳癖(TM1)

SC2Y Other specified other female reproductive system associated disorders 其他特指的其他女性生殖系统病类(TM1)

SC2Z Other female reproductive system associated disorders, unspecified 未特指的其他女性生殖系统病类(TM1)

SC4Y Other specified female reproductive system disorders(including childbirth)其他特指的女性生殖系统(包括分娩)病类(TM1)

SC4Z Female reproductive system disorders (including childbirth), unspecified 未特指的女性生殖系统(包括分娩)病类(TM1)

L3–SC5 Bone, joint and muscle system disorders 骨、关

节和肌肉系统病类（TM1）

L4-SC5 Joint impediment disorders 痹病（TM1）

SC50 Cold impediment disorder 寒痹（TM1）

SC51 Wind impediment disorder 风痹（TM1）

SC52 Dampness impediment disorder 著痹（TM1）

SC5Y Other specified joint impediment disorders 其他特指的痹病（TM1）

SC5Z Joint impediment disorders, unspecified 未特指的痹病（TM1）

SC60 Muscle spasm disorder 转筋（TM1）

SC61 Lumbago disorder 腰痛（TM1）

SC62 Numbness disorder 麻木（TM1）

SC63 Wilting disorder 痿证（TM1）

SC6Y Other specified bone, joint and muscle system disorders 其他特指的骨、关节和肌肉系统病类（TM1）

SC6Z Bone, joint and muscle system disorders, unspecified 未特指的骨、关节和肌肉系统病类（TM1）

L3-SC7 Eye, ear, nose and throat system disorders 眼、耳、鼻和喉系统病类（TM1）

SC70 Night blindness disorder 高风内障［雀目］（TM1）

SC71 Wind glaucoma disorder 五风内障（TM1）

SC72 Inflammatory eyelid disorder 胞肿如桃（TM1）

SC73 Non-inflammatory eyelid disorder 胞虚如球（TM1）

SC74 Corneal opacity disorder 混睛障（TM1）

SC75 Tinnitus disorder 耳鸣（TM1）

L4-SC8 Deafness disorders 耳聋（TM1）

SC80 Sudden deafness disorder 暴聋（TM1）

SC81 Gradual deafness disorder 渐聋（TM1）

SC8Y Other specified deafness disorders 其他特指的耳聋(TM1)

SC8Z Deafness disorders, unspecified 未特指的耳聋(TM1)

SC90 Allergic rhinitis disorder 鼻鼽(TM1)

SC91 Nasal sinusitis disorder 鼻渊(TM1)

SC92 Hoarseness disorder 喉暗(TM1)

SC93 Tonsillitis disorder 乳蛾(TM1)

SC9Y Other specified eye, ear, nose and throat system disorders 其他特指的眼、耳、鼻和喉系统病类(TM1)

SC9Z Eye, ear, nose and throat system disorders, unspecified 未特指的眼、耳、鼻和喉系统病类(TM1)

L3–SD0 Brain system disorders 脑系病类(TM1)

SD00 Facial paralysis disorder 口僻(TM1)

L4–SD1 Headache disorders 头痛(TM1)

SD10 Migraine disorder 偏头风(TM1)

SD11 Head wind disorder 头风(TM1)

SD1Y Other specified headache disorders 其他特指的头痛(TM1)

SD1Z Headache disorders, unspecified 未特指的头痛(TM1)

SD20 Convulsion disorder 痉痉(TM1)

SD21 Cerebral tinnitus disorder 脑鸣(TM1)

SD22 Vertigo disorder 眩晕(TM1)

SD23 Forgetfulness disorder 健忘(TM1)

SD24 Frequent protrusion of tongue disorder 弄舌(TM1)

L4–SD3 Wind stroke disorders 中风(TM1)

SD30 Prodrome of wind stroke disorder 中风先兆证

（TM1）

SD31 Sequela of wind stroke disorder 中风后遗证（TM1）

SD3Y Other specified wind stroke disorders 其他特指的中风（TM1）

SD3Z Wind stroke disorders, unspecified 未特指的中风（TM1）

SD40 Syncope disorder 厥症（TM1）

SD4Y Other specified brain system disorders 其他特指的脑系病类（TM1）

SD4Z Brain system disorders, unspecified 未特指的脑系病类（TM1）

SD6Y Other specified other body system disorders 其他特指的其他身体系统疾病（TM1）

SD6Z Other body system disorders, unspecified 未特指的其他身体系统疾病（TM1）

L2-SD7 qi, blood and fluid disorders 气血津液病（TM1）

SD70 qi goiter disorder 气瘿（TM1）

SD71 Wasting thirst disorder 消渴（TM1）

SD72 Consumptive disorder 虚劳（TM1）

SD7Y Other specified qi, blood and fluid disorders 其他特指的气血津液病（TM1）

SD7Z qi, blood and fluid disorders, unspecified 未特指的气血津液病（TM1）

L2-SD8 Mental and emotional disorders 精神情志病类（TM1）

SD80 Lily disorder 百合病（TM1）

SD81 Manic disorder 躁病（TM1）

SD82 Depression disorder 郁证（TM1）

SD83 Uneasiness disorder 脏躁（TM1）

SD84 Insomnia disorder 不寐（TM1）

SD85 Somnolence disorder 多寐(TM1)

SD86 Dementia disorder 痴呆(TM1)

SD87 Repressed fire disorder 火病(TM1)

SD8Y Other specified mental and emotional disorders 其他特指的精神情志病类(TM1)

SD8Z Mental and emotional disorders, unspecified 未特指的精神情志病类(TM1)

L2-SD9 External contraction disorders 外感病(TM1)

SD90 Seasonal cold disorder 时行感冒(TM1)

SD91 Fatigue consumption disorder 劳瘵(TM1)

SD92 Severe vomiting and diarrhoea disorder 霍乱(TM1)

SD93 Alternating fever and chills disorder 疟疾(TM1)

SD94 Parasitic disorder 蛊病(TM1)

SD95 Flowing phlegm disorder 流痰(TM1)

L3-SE0 Warmth disorders 温病(TM1)

SE00 Summer-heat disorder 暑温(TM1)

SE01 Spring warmth disorder 春温(TM1)

SE02 Dampness and warmth disorder 湿温(TM1)

SE0Y Other specified warmth disorders 其他特指的温病(TM1)

SE0Z Warmth disorders, unspecified 未特指的温病(TM1)

SE2Y Other specified external contraction disorders 其他特指的外感病(TM1)

SE2Z External contraction disorders, unspecified 未特指的外感病(TM1)

L2-SE3 Childhood and adolescence associated disorders 儿童期与青少年期病类(TM1)

SE30 Developmental delay disorder 迟证(TM1)

SE31 Growth fever disorder 变蒸热(TM1)

SE32 Growth pain disorder 生长痛（TM1）

SE33 Acute convulsion disorder 急惊风（TM1）

SE34 Recurrent convulsion disorder 慢惊风（TM1）

SE35 Fright seizure disorder 客忤（TM1）

SE36 Night crying disorder 夜啼（TM1）

SE37 Infantile malnutrition disorder 疳病（TM1）

SE38 Dribbling disorder 滞遗（TM1）

SE39 Diaper dermatitis disorder 臀红（TM1）

SE3A Infant stiffness disorder 硬证（TM1）

SE3B Infant limpness disorder 软证（TM1）

SE3Y Other specified childhood and adolescence associated disorders 其他特指的儿童期与青少年期病类（TM1）

SE3Z Childhood and adolescence associated disorders, unspecified 未特指的儿童期与青少年期病类（TM1）

SE5Y Other specified traditional medicine disorders 其他特指的传统医学疾病（TM1）

SE5Z Traditional medicine disorders, unspecified 未特指的传统医学疾病（TM1）

L1–SE7 Traditional medicine patterns 传统医学证候（TM1）

L2–SE7 Principle–based patterns 八纲证（TM1）

SE70 Yang pattern 阳证（TM1）

SE71 Yin pattern 阴证（TM1）

SE72 Heat pattern 热证（TM1）

SE73 Cold pattern 寒证（TM1）

SE74 Excess pattern 实证（TM1）

SE75 Deficiency pattern 虚证（TM1）

SE76 Exterior pattern 表证（TM1）

SE77 Interior pattern 里证（TM1）

SE78 Moderate （Heat/Cold） pattern 寒热中间证

(TM1)

SE79 Medium (Excess/Deficiency) pattern 虚实中间证(TM1)

SE7A Tangled cold and heat pattern 寒热错杂证(TM1)

SE7Y Other specified principle-based patterns 其他特指的八纲证(TM1)

SE7Z Principle-based patterns, unspecified 未特指的八纲证(TM1)

L2-SE8 Environmental factor patterns 外感证(TM1)

SE80 Wind factor pattern 风淫证(TM1)

SE81 Cold factor pattern 寒淫证(TM1)

SE82 Dampness factor pattern 湿淫证(TM1)

SE83 Dryness factor pattern 燥淫证(TM1)

SE84 Fire-heat factor pattern 火热淫证(TM1)

SE85 Summer-heat factor pattern 暑淫证(TM1)

SE86 Pestilent factor pattern 疫疠证(TM1)

SE8Y Other specified environmental factor patterns 其他特指的外感证(TM1)

SE8Z Environmental factor patterns, unspecified 未特指的外感证(TM1)

L2-SE9 Body constituents patterns 气血津液证(TM1)

L3-SE9 qi patterns 气证(TM1)

SE90 qi deficiency pattern 气虚证(TM1)

SE91 qi stagnation pattern 气滞证(TM1)

SE92 qi uprising pattern 气逆证(TM1)

SE93 qi sinking pattern 气陷证(TM1)

SE94 qi collapse pattern 气脱证(TM1)

SE9Y Other specified qi patterns 其他特指的气证(TM1)

SE9Z qi patterns, unspecified 未特指的气证(TM1)

L3-SF0 Blood patterns 血证(TM1)

SF00 Blood deficiency pattern 血虚证(TM1)

SF01 Blood stasis pattern 血瘀证(TM1)

SF02 Blood heat pattern 血热证(TM1)

SF03 Blood cold pattern 血寒证(TM1)

SF04 Blood dryness pattern 血燥证(TM1)

SF0Y Other specified blood patterns 其他特指的血证(TM1)

SF0Z Blood patterns, unspecified 未特指的血证(TM1)

L3-SF1 Fluid patterns 津液证(TM1)

SF10 Fluid deficiency pattern 津液亏虚证(TM1)

SF11 Fluid disturbance pattern 水毒证(TM1)

SF12 Dry-phlegm pattern 燥痰证(TM1)

SF13 Damp phlegm pattern 湿痰证(TM1)

SF14 Phlegm-fire harassing the heart system pattern 痰火扰心证(TM1)

SF15 Wind-phlegm pattern 风痰证(TM1)

SF1Y Other specified fluid patterns 其他特指的津液证(TM1)

SF1Z Fluid patterns, unspecified 未特指的津液证(TM1)

L3-SF2 Essence patterns 精证(TM1)

SF20 Essence deficiency pattern 精虚证(TM1)

SF2Y Other specified essence patterns 其他特指的精证(TM1)

SF2Z Essence patterns, unspecified 未特指的精证(TM1)

SF4Y Other specified body constituents patterns 其他特指的气血津液证(TM1)

SF4Z Body constituents patterns, unspecified 未特指的

气血津液证(TM1)

L2-SF5 Organ system patterns 脏腑证(TM1)

L3-SF5 Liver system patterns 肝系证类(TM1)

SF50 Liver yin deficiency pattern 肝阴虚证(TM1)

SF51 Liver yang deficiency pattern 肝阳虚证(TM1)

SF52 Liver yang ascendant hyperactivity pattern 肝阳上亢证(TM1)

SF53 Liver qi deficiency pattern 肝气虚证(TM1)

SF54 Liver blood deficiency pattern 肝血虚证(TM1)

SF55 Liver depression and blood stasis pattern 肝郁血瘀证(TM1)

SF56 Liver wind stirring the interior pattern 肝风内动证(TM1)

SF57 Liver qi stagnation pattern 肝气化火证(TM1)

SF58 Liver fire flaming upward pattern 肝火上炎证(TM1)

SF59 Liver heat stirring wind pattern 肝热动风证(TM1)

SF5A Liver-gallbladder dampness-heat pattern 肝胆湿热证(TM1)

SF5B Liver meridian dampness-heat pattern 肝经湿热证(TM1)

SF5C Liver meridian cold stagnation pattern 寒滞肝脉证(TM1)

SF5D Gallbladder qi deficiency pattern 胆气虚证(TM1)

SF5E Gallbladder depression with phlegm harassment pattern 胆郁痰扰证(TM1)

SF5F Gallbladder heat pattern 胆热证(TM1)

SF5G Gallbladder cold pattern 胆寒证(TM1)

SF5H Liver and kidney yin deficiency pattern 肝肾阴虚

证(TM1)

SF5J Disharmony of liver and spleen systems pattern 肝脾不和证(TM1)

SF5K Disharmony of liver and stomach systems pattern 肝胃不和证(TM1)

SF5L Liver fire invading the stomach system pattern 肝火犯胃证(TM1)

SF5M Liver fire invading the lung system pattern 肝火犯肺证(TM1)

SF5Y Other specified liver system patterns 其他特指的肝系证类(TM1)

SF5Z Liver system patterns, unspecified 未特指的肝系证类(TM1)

L3-SF6 Heart system patterns 心系证类(TM1)

SF60 Heart qi deficiency pattern 心气虚证(TM1)

SF61 Heart blood deficiency pattern 心血虚证(TM1)

SF62 Dual deficiency of heart qi and blood pattern 心气血两虚证(TM1)

SF63 Heart meridian obstruction pattern 心脉痹阻证(TM1)

SF64 Heart yin deficiency pattern 心阴虚证(TM1)

SF65 Deficiency of heart qi and yin pattern 心气阴两虚证(TM1)

SF66 Heart yang deficiency pattern 心阳虚证(TM1)

SF67 Heart yang collapse pattern 心阳暴脱证(TM1)

SF68 Heart fire flaming upward pattern 心火上炎证(TM1)

SF69 Fire harassing heart spirit pattern 热扰心神证(TM1)

SF6A Water qi intimidating the heart system pattern 水气凌心证(TM1)

SF6B Heart spirit restlessness pattern 心神不宁证 (TM1)

SF6C Anxiety damaging the spirit pattern 忧伤神气证 (TM1)

SF6D Small intestine qi stagnation pattern 小肠气滞证 (TM1)

SF6E Small intestine excess heat pattern 小肠实热证 (TM1)

SF6F Small intestine deficiency cold pattern 小肠虚寒证(TM1)

SF6G Heart and liver blood deficiency pattern 心肝血虚证(TM1)

SF6H Heart and gallbladder qi deficiency pattern 心胆气虚证(TM1)

SF6J Heart and spleen systems deficiency pattern 心脾两虚证(TM1)

SF6K Heart and lung qi deficiency pattern 心肺气虚证 (TM1)

SF6L Heart and kidney systems disharmony pattern 心肾不交证(TM1)

SF6M Heart and kidney yang deficiency pattern 心肾阳虚证(TM1)

SF6Y Other specified heart system patterns 其他特指的心系证类(TM1)

SF6Z Heart system patterns, unspecified 未特指的心系证类(TM1)

L3-SF7 Spleen system patterns 脾系证类(TM1)

SF70 Spleenqi deficiency pattern 脾气虚证(TM1)

SF71 Spleenqi sinking pattern 脾气下陷证(TM1)

SF72 Spleen deficiency with qi stagnation pattern 脾虚气滞证(TM1)

SF73 Spleen deficiency with food retention pattern 脾虚食积证(TM1)

SF74 Spleen failing to control the blood pattern 脾不统血证(TM1)

SF75 Spleen deficiency and blood depletion pattern 脾虚血亏证(TM1)

SF76 Spleen yin deficiency pattern 脾阴虚证(TM1)

SF77 Spleen yang deficiency pattern 脾阳虚证(TM1)

SF78 Dampness-heat encumbering the spleen system pattern 湿热蕴脾证(TM1)

SF79 Spleen deficiency with dampness accumulation pattern 脾虚湿困证(TM1)

SF7A Spleen deficiency with water flooding pattern 脾虚水泛证(TM1)

SF7B Cold-dampness encumbering the spleen system pattern 寒湿困脾证(TM1)

SF7C Stomach qi deficiency pattern 胃气虚证(TM1)

SF7D Stomach qi uprising pattern 胃气上逆证(TM1)

SF7E Stomach yin deficiency pattern 胃阴虚证(TM1)

SF7F Stomach heat pattern 胃热证(TM1)

SF7G Dampness in the intestines pattern 湿阻肠道证(TM1)

SF7H Cold invading the stomach system pattern 寒邪犯胃证(TM1)

SF7J Intestine cold stagnation pattern 寒滞肠道证(TM1)

SF7K Anxiety damaging the spleen system pattern 思伤脾气证(TM1)

SF7L Lung and spleen deficiency pattern 肺脾两虚证(TM1)

SF7M Spleen and kidney yang deficiency pattern 脾肾

阳虚证(TM1)

SF7Y Other specified spleen system patterns 其他特指的脾系证类(TM1)

SF7Z Spleen system patterns, unspecified 未特指的脾系证类(TM1)

L3–SF8 Lung system patterns 肺病证类(TM1)

SF80 Lung qi deficiency pattern 肺气虚证(TM1)

SF81 Lung yin deficiency pattern 肺阴虚证(TM1)

SF82 Lung and kidney yin deficiency pattern 肺肾阴虚证(TM1)

SF83 Lung qi and yin deficiency pattern 肺气阴两虚证(TM1)

SF84 Lung yang deficiency pattern 肺阳虚证(TM1)

SF85 Cold phlegm obstructing the lung pattern 寒痰阻肺证(TM1)

SF86 Turbid phlegm accumulation in the lung pattern 痰浊阻肺证(TM1)

SF87 Exterior cold with lung heat pattern 表寒肺热证(TM1)

SF88 Intense congestion of lung heat pattern 肺热炽盛证(TM1)

SF89 Phlegm heat obstructing the lung pattern 痰热壅肺证(TM1)

SF8A Wind–heat invading the lung pattern 风热犯肺证(TM1)

SF8B Lung heat transmitting into the intestine pattern 肺热移肠证(TM1)

SF8C Wind–cold fettering the lung pattern 风寒束肺证(TM1)

SF8D Dryness invading the lung pattern 燥邪犯肺证(TM1)

SF8E Lung dryness with intestinal obstruction pattern 肺燥肠闭证(TM1)

SF8F Large intestine excess heat pattern 大肠实热证(TM1)

SF8G Large intestine dampness heat pattern 大肠湿热证(TM1)

SF8H Large intestine fluid deficiency pattern 大肠津亏证(TM1)

SF8J Large intestine deficiency cold pattern 大肠虚寒证(TM1)

SF8Y Other specified lung system patterns 其他特指的肺系证类(TM1)

SF8Z Lung system patterns, unspecified 未特指的肺系证类(TM1)

L3-SF9 Kidney system patterns 肾病证类(TM1)

SF90 Kidney qi deficiency pattern 肾气虚证(TM1)

SF91 Kidney failing to receive qi pattern 肾不纳气证(TM1)

SF92 Kidney qi deficiency with water retention pattern 肾气虚水泛证(TM1)

SF93 Kidney yin deficiency pattern 肾阴虚证(TM1)

SF94 Kidney yin and yang deficiency pattern 肾阴阳两虚证(TM1)

SF95 Kidney deficiency with marrow depletion pattern 肾虚髓亏证(TM1)

SF96 Kidney essence deficiency pattern 肾精亏虚证(TM1)

SF97 Kidney yang deficiency pattern 肾阳虚证(TM1)

SF98 Fear damaging the kidney system pattern 惊恐伤肾证(TM1)

SF99 Blood and heat accumulation in the uterus pattern

胞宫血热证(TM1)

SF9A Phlegm obstructing the uterus pattern 痰凝胞宫证(TM1)

SF9B Dampness–heat in the uterus pattern 胞宫湿热证(TM1)

SF9C Cold stagnation in the uterus pattern 寒凝胞宫证(TM1)

SF9D Uterine deficiency cold pattern 胞宫虚寒证(TM1)

SF9E Blood accumulation in the bladder pattern 膀胱蓄血证(TM1)

SF9F Bladder heat accumulation pattern 膀胱蕴热证(TM1)

SF9G Bladder dampness – heat pattern 膀胱湿热证(TM1)

SF9H Bladder water accumulation pattern 膀胱蓄水证(TM1)

SF9J Bladder deficiency cold pattern 膀胱虚寒证(TM1)

SF9Y Other specified kidney system patterns 其他特指的肾系证类(TM1)

SF9Z Kidney system patterns, unspecified 未特指的肾系证类(TM1)

SG1Y Other specified organ system patterns 其他特指的脏腑证类(TM1)

SG1Z Organ system patterns, unspecified 未特指的脏腑证类(TM1)

L2–SG2 Meridian and collateral patterns 经络证(TM1)

L3–SG2 Main meridian patterns 十二正经证(TM1)

SG20 Lung meridian pattern 手太阴肺经是动病证(TM1)

SG21 Large intestine meridian pattern 手阳明大肠经是动病证(TM1)

SG22 Stomach meridian pattern 足阳明胃经是动病证(TM1)

SG23 Spleen meridian pattern 足太阴脾经是动病证(TM1)

SG24 Heart meridian pattern 手少阴心经是动病证(TM1)

SG25 Small intestine meridian pattern 手太阳小肠经是动病证(TM1)

SG26 Bladder meridian pattern 足太阳膀胱经是动病证(TM1)

SG27 Kidney meridian pattern 足少阴肾经是动病证(TM1)

SG28 Pericardium meridian pattern 手厥阴心包经是动病证(TM1)

SG29 Triple energizer meridian pattern 手少阳三焦经是动病证(TM1)

SG2A Gallbladder meridian pattern 足少阳胆经是动病证(TM1)

SG2B Liver meridian pattern 足厥阴肝经是动病证(TM1)

SG2Y Other specified main meridian patterns 其他特指的十二正经证(TM1)

SG2Z Main meridian patterns, unspecified 未特指的十二正经证(TM1)

L3-SG3 Extra meridian patterns 奇经八脉证(TM1)

SG30 Governor vessel pattern 督脉病证(TM1)

SG31 Conception vessel pattern 任脉病证(TM1)

SG32 Yin heel vessel pattern 阴跷脉病证(TM1)

SG33 Yang heel vessel pattern 阳跷脉病证(TM1)

SG34 Yin link vessel pattern 阴维脉病证(TM1)

SG35 Yang link vessel pattern 阳维脉病证(TM1)

SG36 Thoroughfare vessel pattern 冲脉病证(TM1)

SG37 Belt vessel pattern 带脉病证(TM1)

SG3Y Other specified extra meridian patterns 其他特指的奇经八脉证(TM1)

SG3Z Extra meridian patterns, unspecified 未特指的奇经八脉证(TM1)

SG5Y Other specified meridian and collateral patterns 其他特指的经络证(TM1)

SG5Z Meridian and collateral patterns, unspecified 未特指的经络证(TM1)

L2-SG6 Six stage patterns 六经证(TM1)

SG60 Early yang stage pattern 太阳病证(TM1)

SG61 Middle yang stage pattern 阳明病证(TM1)

SG62 Late yang stage pattern 少阳病证(TM1)

SG63 Early yin stage pattern 太阴病证(TM1)

SG64 Middle yin stage pattern, middle yin stage pattern 少阴病证(TM1)

SG65 Late yin stage patterns 厥阴病证(TM1)

SG6Y Other specified six stage patterns 其他特指的六经证(TM1)

SG6Z Six stage patterns, unspecified 未特指的六经证(TM1)

L2-SG7 Triple energizer stage patterns 三焦证(TM1)

SG70 Upper energizer stage patterns 上焦证(TM1)

SG71 Middle energizer stage patterns 中焦证(TM1)

SG72 Lower energizer stage patterns 下焦证(TM1)

SG7Y Other specified triple energizer stage patterns 其他特指的三焦证(TM1)

SG7Z Triple energizer stage patterns, unspecified 未特

指的三焦证(TM1)

L2-SG8 Four phase patterns 卫气营血证(TM1)

L3-SG8 Defense phase patterns 卫分证(TM1)

SG80 Dampness obstructing the defense yang pattern 湿遏卫阳证(TM1)

SG81 Heat attacking the lung defense pattern 温邪侵袭肺卫证(TM1)

SG8Y Other specified defense phase patterns 其他特指的卫分证(TM1)

SG8Z Defense phase patterns, unspecified 未特指的卫分证(TM1)

L3-SG9 qi phase patterns 气分证(TM1)

SG90 Heat entering the qi phase pattern 热入气分证(TM1)

SG91 qi phase dampness and heat pattern 气分湿热证(TM1)

SG92 Dampness obstructing the qi phase pattern 湿阻气分证(TM1)

SG9Y Other specified qi phase patterns 其他特指的气分证(TM1)

SG9Z qi phase patterns, unspecified 未特指的气分证(TM1)

L3-SH0 Nutrient phase patterns 营分证(TM1)

SH00 Nutrient qi and defense qi disharmony pattern 营卫不和证(TM1)

SH01 Heat in the nutrient phase pattern 热入营分证(TM1)

SH02 Heat entering the nutrient and blood phase pattern 热入营血证(TM1)

SH0Y Other specified nutrient phase patterns 其他特指的营分证(TM1)

SH0Z Nutrient phase patterns, unspecified 未特指的营分证(TM1)

L3-SH1 Blood phase patterns 血分证(TM1)

SH10 Blood phase pattern 血分证(TM1)

SH11 Heat entering the blood phase pattern 热入血分证(TM1)

SH1Y Other specified blood phase patterns 其他特指的血分证(TM1)

SH1Z Blood phase patterns, unspecified 未特指的血分证(TM1)

SH3Y Other specified four phase patterns 其他特指的卫气营血证(TM1)

SH3Z Four phase patterns, unspecified 未特指的卫气营血证(TM1)

L2-SH4 Four constitution medicine patterns 四象医学病证(TM1)

L3-SH4 Large yang type patterns 太阳人病证(TM1)

SH40 Large yang type exterior origin lower back pattern 太阳人外感腰脊病证(TM1)

SH41 Large yang type interior origin small intestine pattern 太阳人内触小肠病证(TM1)

SH42 Large yang type exterior interior combined pattern 太阳人表里兼病证(TM1)

SH4Y Other specified large yang type patterns 其他特指的太阳人病证(TM1)

SH4Z Large yang type patterns, unspecified 未特指的太阳人病证(TM1)

L3-SH5 Small yang type patterns 少阳人病证(TM1)

SH50 Small yang type lesser yang wind damage pattern 少阳人少阳伤风证(TM1)

SH51 Small yang type yin depletion pattern 少阳人亡

阴证（TM1）

SH52 Small yang type chest heat congested pattern 少阳人胸膈热证（TM1）

SH53 Small yang type yin deficit pattern 少阳人阴虚证（TM1）

SH54 Small yang type exterior interior combined pattern 少阳人表里兼病证（TM1）

SH5Y Other specified small yang type patterns 其他特指的少阳人病证（TM1）

SH5Z Small yang type patterns, unspecified 未特指的少阳人病证（TM1）

L3–SH6 Large yin type patterns 太阴人病证（TM1）

SH60 Large yin type supraspinal exterior pattern 太阴人背顀表病证（TM1）

SH61 Large yin type esophagus cold pattern 太阴人胃脘寒证（TM1）

SH62 Large yin type liver heat pattern 太阴人肝热证（TM1）

SH63 Large yin type dryness heat pattern 太阴人燥热证（TM1）

SH64 Large yin type exterior interior combined pattern 太阴人表里兼病证（TM1）

SH6Y Other specified large yin type patterns 其他特指的太阴人病证（TM1）

SH6Z Large yin type patterns, unspecified 未特指的太阴人病证（TM1）

L3–SH7 Small yin type patterns 少阴人病证（TM1）

SH70 Small yin type congestive hyperpsychotic pattern 少阴人郁狂证（TM1）

SH71 Small yin type yang depletion pattern 少阴人亡阳证（TM1）

SH72 Small yin type greater yin pattern 少阴人太阴证
（TM1）

SH73 Small yin type lesser yin pattern 少阴人少阴证
（TM1）

SH74 Small yin type exterior interior combined pattern
少阴人表里兼病证（TM1）

SH7Y Other specified small yin type patterns 其他特指
的少阴人病证（TM1）

SH7Z Small yin type patterns, unspecified 未特指的少
阴人病证（TM1）

SH9Y Other specified four constitution medicine patterns 其他特指的四象医学病证（TM1）

SH9Z Four constitution medicine patterns, unspecified
未特指的四象医学病证（TM1）

SJ1Y Other specified traditional medicine patterns 其他
特指的传统医学证候（TM1）

SJ1Z Traditional medicine patterns, unspecified 未特指
的传统医学证候（TM1）

SJ3Y Other specified supplementary Chapter Traditional
Medicine Conditions – Module I 其他特指的传统
医学补充章节

SJ3Z Supplementary Chapter Traditional Medicine Con-
ditions-Module I, unspecified 未特指的传统医学
补充章节

2. Index

二、索　引

A

C

D

E

G

H

K

L

M

Q

R

T

U

V

X